THE FAMILY GUIDE TO
FOOD
AND
HEALTH

THE FAMILY GUIDE TO

FOOD

AND

HEALTH

ELISABETH MORSE (EDITOR)
JOHN RIVERS
ANNE HEUGHAN

BARRIE & JENKINS
— LONDON —

First published in Great Britain by
Barrie & Jenkins Ltd.
289 Westbourne Grove, London W11 2QA

British Library Cataloguing in Publication
Data
Rivers, John
    The family guide to food and health.
    1. Health food
    I. Title   II. Heughan, Anne   III. Morse,
    Elisabeth
    641.3'02

    ISBN 0-7126-2030-2 (cased)
            0-7126-1814-7 (paperback)

Typesetting by SX Composing Limited,
Rayleigh, Essex
Printed and bound by Butler & Tanner,
Frome, Somerset.

CONTENTS

PART I

FOOD AND THE BODY

Elisabeth Morse

INTRODUCTION

A little girl may be made of sugar and spice but her 10-stone (65-kg) father is likely to be made of 8½ gallons (40 litres) of water, 24lb (11kg) of protein, 2¼lb (1kg) of carbohydrate, 9lb (4kg) of minerals and 20lb (9kg) of fat. The minerals in his body include about 10oz (280g) salt, 2½lb (1.1kg) calcium, 1lb (450g) phosphate, 1oz (28g) magnesium, ¾ teaspoon of iron and ½ teaspoon of zinc, as well as minute traces of a great many other minerals and elements, including iodine, fluoride, copper, cobalt, chromium, manganese, selenium, tin, aluminium, arsenic, mercury and many more besides.

The most essential of all these components is water. Without water people cannot survive for more than a few days, whereas they can live for several weeks or longer without food, depending on the size of their fat stores and their general state of health. The human body has a number of reserves built into it. In theory it should be possible to lose 7 pints (4 litres) of water and 4½lb (2kg) of protein from lean muscle tissue, 17½lb (8kg) of fat, 3lb (1.5kg) of minerals and 7oz (200g) of carbohydrate without coming to any harm.

All these components – or nutrients – are held in and make up millions of cells: blood cells, fat cells, muscle cells and bone marrow cells. Each cell both contains and is surrounded by water. The cell walls are not solid, however; they are porous membranes through which tiny particle-sized nutrients can pass in and out. These nutrients are not allowed to go just anywhere; they are strictly regimented and are moved about by a vast quantity of genetically coded electrical impulses and chemical reactions, which are going on all the time. This continual activity is known as the body metabolism.

In order for this metabolism to take place, energy is needed. The energy, the water and the basic materials that the body needs to keep itself alive, growing and in good condition all come from the great variety of food and drink that we consume. The contents of the stomach are rather like a vast scrap-yard, which the digestive system has to break down, sort out, recycle and store. The body is remarkably efficient at this and wastes little. Indeed, one of the reasons for man's evolutionary success has been the ability of the human body to make use of, and survive on, an enormous range of foods. However, staying alive is not always the same as thriving, and, as we will see in this book, what we eat and drink can have a profound impact on our health.

CHAPTER 1

WHAT IS FOOD?

*F*ood – which comes from animals and plants – is made up of the same proteins, fats and other nutrients of which all living tissues, including those of the human body, consist. Food is needed both for energy and nutrients. Some nutrients, such as fat, carbohydrates and alcohol, mainly provide energy; others, such as fibre, water, vitamins and minerals, provide virtually no energy but are essential in other ways. Protein provides energy but is also necessary for the structure of body cells.

Food may also contain a number of miscellaneous substances, such as plant fibre, colours and flavours as well as toxic chemicals, which may be necessary for a particular plant but which can be harmful to man unless they are treated in some way. For example, beans contain substances called haemagglutinins, which can damage red blood cells unless they have been destroyed by heat during cooking. Other toxins may do little harm if small quantities are eaten, but could be highly poisonous if taken in large amounts. Thus an acid called oxalate in rhubarb stalks can be tolerated, but not in the amounts found in rhubarb leaves, which are therefore poisonous. (Oxalic acid is useful for removing ink stains and iron mould but can be a severe irritant in the human body where it can cause certain forms of bladder stones.)

The chemicals that colour and flavour plants may be present naturally (e.g., the orange carotenoids in carrots and the essential oils that give fruits their flavours), or they may be added during the preparation and manufacture of foods. The quantities added artificially are not known to be harmful – otherwise they would not be allowed by law – but a few can cause sensitivity reactions in some people, particularly children, in the same way as strawberries arouse allergies in a few unfortunate people (see page 91).

—ENERGY—

Energy is a word with more than one meaning. To the nutritionist, energy relates very precisely to the body's ability to function, whether running upstairs or keeping its metabolism operating. The body obtains the energy it needs through a series of chemical processes which convert the stored energy in food into metabolic, mechanical and heat energy. Food is thus a fuel, and if the energy obtained from it is not used immediately, it is stored in fuel depots in the body called fat tissue.

All metabolic processes involve energy. Some store it, others release it. When food or fat from the fat stores in the body is combined with oxygen from the lungs,

> *Eating has the same effect on the body as topping up the fuel tank of a car. Eating more will not help energy to be released more quickly simply because there is more fuel.*

energy in the form of heat is released and carbon dioxide and water are formed. When energy has to be manufactured quickly the lungs breathe more rapidly in order to get the extra oxygen required to speed up the breakdown of the energy reserves. Eating has the same effect on the body as topping up the fuel tank of a car. Eating more will not help energy to be released more quickly simply because there is more fuel.

The amount of energy that can be obtained from food and the amount of energy that is needed to perform a task are measured in units called either calories or joules. A calorie is a unit measuring the amount of heat energy that would be given off if a food were burnt. One ounce of fat would give off more heat than one ounce of sugar. A joule is a unit that measures the amount of mechanical work or energy that would be needed for all the activities that the body performs. Since all forms of energy are interchangeable, it does not matter whether energy is measured as units of heat or of mechanical work. For practical purposes, calories are as different from joules as Fahrenheit is from Centigrade. Many of the foods that carry a declaration of their energy content use both calories and joules on the labels. Because calories and joules are tiny measurements, the energy content of food is usually measured in thousands of these units – i.e., kilocalories and kiloJoules (1 kilocalorie equals 4.184kJ). When people talk about calories nowadays they are almost always referring to kilocalories.

The popular meaning of "energy" is, however, much broader than the strict scientific meaning, and this sometimes causes confusion. Energy in its broader sense means vigour and effort as well as fuel. In this sense energy is something that most of us would like more of, whereas calories may be thought of as undesirable substances that somehow cause the body to gain weight. But for nutritional purposes, energy means a fuel and calories are simply the units by which this fuel is measured.

At best, the body can use a quarter of the energy contained in food in order to keep alive and active. The rest is given off as heat. Heat escapes during the chemical processes that extract the energy from food, and ten to twelve people sitting in a room together can give off as much heat as a small electric fire. The digestion of food gives off far more heat to warm the body than is gained from, say, eating a hot dish rather than a cold one. For example, a bowl of hot soup providing 140 kilocalories would give off approximately 105 kilocalories as body heat. The extra kilocalories or heat that might be obtained from the temperature of the soup would be minuscule – only about 6 kilocalories. On the other hand, hot food is psychologically more welcoming than cold food in cold weather!

> *Heat escapes during the chemical processes that extract the energy from food, and ten to twelve people sitting in a room together can give off as much heat as a small electric fire.*

About two-thirds of the energy people need is used simply to keep the body alive. Ninety per cent of this energy is used up in maintaining the metabolic pumps that keep a balance between the minerals in the water inside the cells and those outside. The remaining 10 per cent is used for breathing and for the beating of the heart. The amount of energy needed to keep an adult alive is approximately 1 kilocalorie for each minute of

‘ *The amount of energy needed to keep an adult alive is approximately 1 kilocalorie for each minute of the day.* ’

the day. This is called the basal or resting metabolism. The rate at which it operates depends on age, the amount of muscle tissue and the balance of hormones. Babies who are growing fast have a basal metabolic rate that is proportionately twice that of an adult, while as adults get older their basal metabolic rate gradually slows down. Women on average have a slightly lower metabolic rate than men for a number of reasons, but mainly because, again on average, they are smaller.

The remaining one-third of the calories eaten each day is used up performing tasks like washing, dressing and the general business of everyday life. The way in which energy might be used up by a young female office worker is set out in the table below:

ENERGY CONSUMPTION OF YOUNG FEMALE OFFICE WORKER

Activity	Rate Energy Used per Minute		Time Spent	Amount of Energy Used Daily	
	kcal	*kJ*		*kcal*	*mj*
Asleep	1	4.2	8 hr	480	2.0
Sitting at work	1.3	6	6 hr	468	1.9
Standing and walking at work	1.7-3	7-13	2 hr	240	1.0
Travelling by bus	1.6	7	2 hr	192	0.8
Walking and running to catch a bus	5	21	15 min	75	0.3
Washing and dressing	3.5	15	15 min	50	0.2
Domestic chores	2.5	13	2 hr	300	1.3
Watching TV	1.3	6	3 hr	234	1.0
Exercise class	5	21	30 min	150	0.6
TOTAL			24 hr	2189	9.1

EXERCISE

From the above table it can be seen that a total of three-quarters of an hour's moderately strenuous activity – i.e., running to catch a bus and one exercise session – uses up less energy than two hours' worth of household chores. Although this can help to explain why seemingly idle people are not necessarily overweight, it is a mistake to look at exercise simply from the point of view of the calories used up. People who choose to exercise very often make other changes to their lifestyle as well, whether deliberately or inadvertently. For example, half an hour's gardening to unwind after work instead of slumping in a chair with a beer will not only use up a few more calories but will also save additional calories from the beer that is not drunk. Exercise can improve the appetite, too, and eating better at mealtimes may help to reduce the attractions of nibbling biscuits and sweets between meals. Exercise can also make people feel fitter, which in turn may motivate them to improve their health in other ways – including their diet. Thus exercise can help to trigger a positive approach to the whole subject of health. On the other hand, someone who takes exercise without enjoying it may end up compensating with extra drinks and bars of chocolate so that they end up taking in more calories than they are using up!

FOOD ENERGY

The energy in food and drink comes from the proteins, fats, carbohydrates and alcohol they contain. Each of these nutrients supplies different amounts of energy:

    1g of fat provides 9kcal (37kJ)
    1g of alcohol provides 7kcal (29kJ)
    1g of protein provides 4kcal (17kJ)
    1g of carbohydrate provides 3.75kcal (16kJ)

Minerals and vitamins provide no energy at all, and fibre almost none.

However, looking at the energy value of individual nutrients is not very useful when it comes to identifying which foods provide the bulk of the calories in the diet. Most foods are mixtures of nutrients, and foods are eaten in very variable amounts. For example, bread provides useful quantities of protein as well as of carbohydrate, and if it is spread thickly with butter and honey it will also supply a lot of fat and sugar. Thus bread on its own is a moderate source of calories but, used as a vehicle for other high energy items, it becomes a rich source of calories. Similarly a lettuce, being made up of little more than water and fibre, is low in calories, but once it is covered with an oily dressing the calorie content may increase tenfold or more. Thus bread is not necessarily "bad" and lettuce not necessarily "good" for slimmers when put in context with everything else that is eaten or drunk.

—PROTEIN—

Proteins are found in all cells, either as part of the structure, giving the cell its shape, or as components of all the regulatory factors like enzymes and hormones that make possible the whole complicated chemistry of life. Besides being made up of elements such as carbon, hydrogen and oxygen, proteins are also composed of nitrogen and sometimes sulphur. Proteins are continually being worn out and they therefore have to be replaced by other proteins entering the stomach from food.

Proteins consist of long chains of individual units called amino acids. Each protein may be made up of hundreds, even thousands, of these units strung together. The sequence in which these chains are ordered determines their particular characteristics, so producing composite substances with names like insulin, albumin, pepsin, casein and collagen. If amino acids are thought of as words, the chains can be thought of as sentences made up from these words. During digestion the protein "sentences" from foods such as eggs, bread and milk are broken down into their constituent "words", which are absorbed and then arranged in the protein "sentences" needed by human hair, muscle and nails, etc.

There are about twenty principal amino acids within the plant and animal kingdoms. The human body can convert some amino acids into the kinds it needs, but there are eight (nine in the case of infants) that the human body cannot put together. These are called essential amino acids.

Essential amino acids: isoleucine, leucine, lysine, methionine, phenylalanine, threonine, tryptophan, valine, and, for babies and children, histidine.

Non-essential amino acids: alanine, arginine, aspartic acid, cysteine, glutamic acid, glycine, hydroxyproline, ornithine, proline, serine and tyrosine.

PROTEIN QUALITY

Protein and quality are two words that have gone together for a long time. Indeed, the protein content of a food has, in the past, been used as a rough guide to its nutritional value. Of course, proteins are important, as every cell in the body is partly composed of protein and there have to be either adequate stores or supplies of protein for cells to go through the continuous process of growing and replacing themselves. However, fears for the quality of our diet in the West, at least as far as protein is concerned, are unfounded.

The rise and fall in the status of protein is an interesting story and may have parallels with our understanding of other nutrients today. In the early part of the century it was discovered that animal and vegetable proteins differed in their ability to promote growth and repair of human cells. It was found that foods containing only animal proteins were more efficient in promoting the growth of laboratory animals than those containing vegetable protein. From this developed the notion of first- and second-class proteins. Since first-class proteins corresponded with foods such as milk, eggs and meat, which were popular, and second-class proteins with the duller staples such as bread and flour, it is perhaps not surprising that the belief that the diet would be improved with extra milk and meat, etc., met with such widespread approval by both scientists and the public. This enthusiasm, in turn, shaped much of the mounting international effort in the 1950s and 1960s to improve the world food situation.

However, subsequent research has undermined the distinction between first- and second-class proteins. Not only have virtually all diets around the world been shown to provide about 10-15 per cent of total calorie requirements as protein, which exceeds the minimum protein requirement of 5-9.5 per cent, but the protein quality has been found to be much the same, whatever the proportion of animal to vegetable protein. Closer analysis has shown that not only are some vegetable proteins such as potatoes, rice and soya very good quality proteins, but also that mixtures of plant proteins can complement each other to produce high-quality proteins. Cereals are short of the amino acid lysine, and pulses are short of the sulphur-containing amino acids methionine and cysteine, whereas animal proteins are usually rich in both. How-

> *Subsequent research has undermined the distinction between first- and second-class proteins. Not only have virtually all diets around the world been shown to provide about 10-15 per cent of total calorie requirements as protein, which exceeds the minimum protein requirement of 5-9.5 per cent, but the protein quality has been found to be much the same, whatever the proportion of animal to vegetable protein.*

> *Unless calorie requirements are satisfied, protein – whatever its quality – will not be used to promote cell growth but instead will be burnt up to supply essential energy (which is rather like using pound notes to fuel a fire).*

ever, when cereals and pulses are eaten together they compensate for each other's shortcomings, and a combination like rice and lentils or beans and toast is as good protein as meat.

Lastly, but perhaps most importantly, it has never been realized that unless calorie requirements are satisfied, protein – whatever its quality – will not be used to promote cell growth but instead will be burnt up to supply essential energy (which is rather like using pound notes to fuel a fire).

The tragedy of this disproportionate emphasis on protein was that millions of pounds and many years were wasted trying to make new forms of protein foods for people who did not have enough to eat. In general, starving people don't need such special foods, simply larger amounts of the foods normally available to them.

Today the emphasis is on the advantages of vegetable foods rather than those rich in animal protein such as meat, cheese and milk. Cereals and vegetables are thought to have an advantage because they tend to contain less fat compared with dairy foods and meat. Protein is now almost taken for granted by nutritionists in much the same way as fibre was during World War II. Of course, the danger of taking anything for granted is that it can easily become neglected.

RECOMMENDED INTAKES

Protein usually makes up 10-15 per cent of the calories consumed and 10 per cent is the amount usually recommended. This works out at just over 2oz (60g) a day for the average adult. Those who use up larger or smaller quantities of energy need to make corresponding adjustments to their protein intakes. The exception to this is anyone eating a very low energy diet (such as someone who is ill or trying to lose weight) who will need to eat a relatively larger proportion of protein.

2oz (60g) of protein is found in:
16 fishfingers
19 slices wholemeal bread
3 portions of beef, chicken or fish
3 pints (1.6 litres) cow's milk (skimmed or unskimmed)
6¼lbs (2.8kg) potatoes

TOO MUCH PROTEIN?

Although most people eat roughly 2oz (60g) of protein a day, it is possible to eat much more. However, larger quantities of protein are wasteful because the kidneys simply break down the surplus and pass it out as urea in the urine. The maximum amount of protein that the kidneys can break down in a day is 10-14oz (300-400g). Although such high intakes of protein are extremely difficult to achieve from a diet of ordinary foods, synthetic diet mixes – such as those to help weight loss – can make large protein intakes possible, so risking harm to those taking them. There is a theory that intakes only two or three times the average could, if taken over long periods of time, injure the kidneys.

—FATS—

Fats are made from fatty acids consisting of carbon, hydrogen and oxygen. They form a concentrated source of energy from food, and surplus energy is stored as fat in the body. Fats are also structural components of cell walls.

There are three kinds of fat in the body: triglycerides, phospholipids and sterols. Triglycerides make up most of the fat that is stored in adipose tissue – i.e., the fat that can be felt and seen in food. All surplus calories, whether from fat, carbohydrate, protein or alcohol, can be converted into triglycerides. Although triglycerides are a storage fat, they still play an active role in the continuous metabolism of the body, which needs a steady supply of calories. When it receives a glut of calories – as at mealtimes – the surplus has to be put aside and small quantities withdrawn in the amounts needed. The adipose tissue is therefore like a bank with money – or calories – being deposited and withdrawn at intervals throughout the day.

Phospholipids are the principal structural fats, which, like proteins, help to maintain the shape of the cell walls. One well-known phospholipid is lecithin whose property of stabilizing cell structures also makes it a useful additive in certain manufactured foods such as salad creams, in which it helps to keep emulsions of oil and vinegar constant. The body is able to make all the phospholipids, including lecithin, that it needs.

Among the third group, the sterols, which are also found in cell membranes, the best known is cholesterol. All animals, but not plants, make cholesterol, so some cholesterol is obtained from food and some is made in the body. Cholesterol has three roles: like the phospholipids, it is a structural component of all cell walls; second, it is needed for the formation of certain hormones and vitamin D; and third, it is the basic material from which bile is made in the liver. Although the liver is the principal site for the manufacture of cholesterol, cholesterol is also made in many other cells in the body.

When large amounts of cholesterol are in the blood, the risk of coronary heart disease is known to increase (see pages 77-8). Although a little cholesterol is already obtained ready-made from food, most cholesterol is manufactured in the body. The amount of cholesterol that is made in the body depends on the kinds of fatty acids obtained from the fats in the diet. Fats containing saturated fatty acids particularly stimulate the production of cholesterol.

FATTY ACIDS

All fats are made up from smaller particles called fatty acids. There are over forty different kinds of fatty acids in our diet. These fatty acids resemble chains of units bonded together, and the chains can be short, medium or long. If the chains are made up of single bonds between the units, they form straight lines and are described as "saturated". All the dietary short- and medium-chain fatty acids, and a few of the long-chain fatty

The amount of cholesterol that is made in the body depends on the kinds of fatty acids obtained from the fats in the diet. Fats containing saturated fatty acids particularly stimulate the production of cholesterol.

acids, are saturated. However, most of the long-chain fatty acids have one or more double bonds. Instead of being neat, straight lines, these double bonds create kinks in the chain causing the fatty acid to fold, and the more kinks or double bonds, the more complicated the folds. These folded shapes are needed for the structure of the cell walls and chains like these are described as "unsaturated". If they have only one double bond they are termed monounsaturated, and if there are two or more double bonds they are called polyunsaturated.

KEYWORDS

Saturated fatty acids are found mainly, but not entirely, in animal products. Saturates increase the levels of cholesterol in the blood. Saturated fatty acids are "saturated" with hydrogen atoms, which means there is a single bond between each link in the chain.
Unsaturated fatty acids are found in most fatty foods but particularly rich sources are found in certain vegetable oils and fish. Unsaturates differ from saturates in that one or more of the links in the fatty acid chain is missing a hydrogen atom; the unattached bond or linkpiece doubles back on itself thus creating a double bond.
Monounsaturates are unsaturated fatty acids with only one double bond. Olive oil contains large quantities of monounsaturates. Monounsaturates seem neither to raise nor lower blood cholesterol; they are therefore neutral.
Polyunsaturates (often referred to by their acronym, PUFAs) are unsaturates with two or more double bonds. Soya and sunflower seed oil contain large quantities of polyunsaturates. PUFAs help to reduce cholesterol in the blood, but only by half as much as saturates raise them. PUFAs are found mainly in vegetables, cereal grains and fish. However, not all vegetable oils are rich in unsaturates. Lean meat can also provide useful amounts of polyunsaturates.
"Cis" form of fatty acids The double bonds of unsaturated fatty acids are naturally kinked – called the "cis" shape. The proportion of fats that remain in their "cis" shape after margarine manufacture is sometimes declared on the labels of polyunsaturate-rich margarines.
"Trans" fatty acids During some food manufacturing processes the folded chains of unsaturated fatty acids are straightened out. Although the fatty acids retain their double bonds, they do not behave chemically in the same way as the natural "cis" form.

It is possible for the kinks in polyunsaturates to be straightened out by getting rid of the double bonds. This sometimes happens during certain food manufacturing processes such as during the production of margarine and synthetic creams, when hydrogen is used to force the double bonds apart. This process is called hydrogenation and a hydrogenated fat is a saturated fat and so also promotes the synthesis of cholesterol.

Some medical researchers advise that we eat more polyunsaturates on two counts. First, they feel that there is sufficient evidence to suggest that polyunsaturates help to lower blood cholesterol, and second because they realize that patients find it easier to swap one kind of fat for another – such as butter for margarine – than to eat less of all fat. But at the moment the government medical advisers in the UK do not feel that the evidence is strong enough to warrant an

> *At the moment the government medical advisers in the UK do not feel that the evidence is strong enough to warrant an unequivocal recommendation to eat more polyunsaturates.*

unequivocal recommendation to eat more polyunsaturates.

For the most part, saturated and hydrogenated fatty acids make fats that are hard or solid at room temperature, whereas polyunsaturated fatty acids form liquid oils. Unfortunately, the hardness or softness of a fat is not a reliable guide to choosing which fats or oils to buy. Modern food technology and a few quirks of nature mean that some common oils are composed of saturated fatty acids and some solid fats are, in fact, excellent sources of polyunsaturates. Nor do saturates and polyunsaturates slot into a neat division between animal and vegetable fats, as may be seen in the chart below.

PROPORTIONS OF FATTY ACIDS CONTAINED IN SOME COMMON FATS AND OILS

	Saturates %	Monounsaturates %	Polyunsaturates	
			Essential Fatty Acids %	Other %
Butter, cream and milk fat	61	36	3	—
Beef fat	48	48	2	1
Bacon and pork fat	42	50	7	1
Chicken fat	34	45	18	2
Fish oil	23	27	7	43
Coconut oil	89	8	2	—
Olive oil	14	73	11	1
Palm oil	45	45	9	—
Corn oil	14	31	53	2
Soya oil	14	24	60	—
Sunflower seed oil	12	33	58	—
Margarine, hard (average)	40	45	15	—
soft (average)	30	40	30	—
polyunsaturate (average)	23	22	52	1

As can be seen from the chart, coconut oil is even more saturated than butter or cream. But coconut oil, palm oil and soya oil are usually the cheapest food oils and for this reason they are much used in food manufacture. The manufacturer's choice of oil will depend on price and availability in the world markets, and under such changing circumstances the oils are not usually named on the label of the finished product, but are included under the umbrella terms "vegetable oils" or "vegetable fats". As a result, the customer is often unable to tell whether

The manufacturer's choice of oil will depend on price and availability in the world markets, and under such changing circumstances the oils are not usually named on the label of the finished product, but are included under the umbrella terms "vegetable oils" or "vegetable fats". As a result, the customer is often unable to tell whether the label is describing a highly saturated product or one that is a good source of polyunsaturates.

the label is describing a highly saturated product or one that is a good source of polyunsaturates.

FATS AND HEALTH

Knowing the amount of saturates or polyunsaturates in a product has important implications for health. Saturated fatty acids increase the quantities of cholesterol in the blood, and raised levels of blood cholesterol are known to be a factor in coronary heart disease. On the other hand, polyunsaturates reduce the amount of cholesterol in the blood while monounsaturates seem to have little effect either way but may reduce cholesterol. Because all fats in food contain mixtures of fatty acids it is more important – and effective – to eat less of all fats rather than simply to swap rich sources of saturates for foods rich in polyunsaturates. Both measures together will, however, help to lower the saturates in the diet.

Recently, it has been shown that taking small quantities of specially enriched fish oils or fish itself, which contain some highly unsaturated fatty acids, will reduce the tendency of the blood to form clots in the arteries of patients being treated for heart disease. Further studies are needed to see whether these supplements might prevent heart disease and whether they pose any other risks to health. But in the meantime, eating oily fish such as herring and mackerel once or twice a week seems to make good sense.

ESSENTIAL FATTY ACIDS

Essential fatty acids (EFA) is the term used to describe those fatty acids that the body is unable to manufacture itself and therefore has to obtain from food. There are two families of essential fatty acids, one produced from linoleic and the other from linolenic acid, and we probably need both. Both families of polyunsaturated fatty acids are vital to health in the same way as vitamins are. Indeed they used to be known as vitamin F. These two essential fatty acids are the basis from which all the fats that help to make up the shape and structure of cells in the body can be made. They are found in any food that is rich in polyunsaturates, such as certain vegetable oils, wheat germ and fatty fish. Vegetable oils and wheat germ contain most of their EFA as linoleic acid, whereas fish contain most as the linolenic family fatty acid.

RECOMMENDED INTAKES

The recommended amount of EFA needed to avoid any deficiency disease is 2-5g a day (the amount that can be obtained from the quantity of a polyunsaturate margarine spread on two slices of bread). This is well below the ½oz (8-15g) that most people eat from Western-type diets. As far is is known, EFA deficiency has never been diagnosed in people eating normal foods. This is because it is almost impossible to construct a diet that has so little fat in it unless it is also short in many other nutrients.

A true deficiency in adults has come to light only in a hospital patient who had to be fed a highly artificial diet by tube. The

> **❛**
> *Because all fats in food contain mixtures of fatty acids it is more important – and effective – to eat less of all fats rather than simply to swap rich sources of saturates for foods rich in polyunsaturates.*
> **❜**

patient developed a scaly dermatitis, which cleared up once EFA was added to the diet. In the 1950s it was reported that a group of babies with eczema had been cured with supplements of EFA. It was subsequently discovered that the babies did not have eczema but EFA deficiency as a result of being fed fat-free milk (at that time skimmed milk was the standard feed for low-birth-weight infants). In the meantime, many infants with eczema were dosed quite uselessly with vegetable oils as the result of an over-hasty conclusion being drawn.

> *Most people in Western countries take about 40 per cent of their diet as fat, and in Britain it is recommended that fat should provide no more than 35 per cent of a diet. In countries such as Sweden and Canada even lower proportions of fat have been recommended. Most recently, in 1987, the European Atherosclerosis Society has recommended that only 30 per cent of the energy in the diet should come from fat.*

The evidence is not yet good enough to enable separate recommendations to be made for amounts of the fatty acids of the linoleic and linolenic families needed. Some scientists have argued recently that coronary thrombosis is a deficiency disease caused by too little of the essential fatty acids (in much the same way that scurvy is caused by a deficiency of vitamin C). It has been suggested that the recommended intake should therefore be increased to 10 per cent of the calories in the diet – i.e., approximately 1oz (20-30g) a day. Although experts on heart disease are beginning to think that we should perhaps be eating more than ½oz (8-15g), not all would advise a large increase as a general recommendation. Instead the opinion is that it is more important to concentrate on getting people to eat less of all types of fat, rather than to eat more polyunsaturates. Most people in Western countries take about 40 per cent of their diet as fat, and in Britain it is recommended that fat should provide no more than 35 per cent of a diet. In countries such as Sweden and Canada even lower proportions of fat have been recommended. Most recently, in 1987, the European Atherosclerosis Society has recommended that only 30 per cent of the energy in the diet should come from fat.

—ALCOHOL—

Alcohol can be a rich source of calories in the diet, providing 7kcals per gram (slightly less than fat but considerably more than protein or carbohydrate). Despite the fact that alcohol accounts for 5-6 per cent of the average person's daily intake, it has been strangely ignored by nutritionists. This may be because nutrition as a science has for most of its existence been concerned with deficiencies of nutrients. No one has yet seriously tried to claim that alcohol is in any way an essential nutrient! It may also be because alcohol is a drug and therefore its effect on the body is not simply that of a nutrient. However, now that nutritionists have become more concerned about excesses of nutrients –

> *Now that nutritionists have become more concerned about excesses of nutrients – including calories – they can no longer afford to neglect alcohol.*

Women can usually tolerate only half the alcohol that men can.

including calories – they can no longer afford to neglect alcohol.

Although alcohol provides calories, it differs from fats, carbohydrates and proteins in the way in which it is metabolized. Despite being rapidly absorbed into the bloodstream, it is broken down in the liver at a fixed rate. Some people's livers break down alcohol more quickly than other people's, so the rate can vary a bit from one individual to another. The usual rate is for 100mg of alcohol for each 2lb (1kg) of bodyweight to be broken down each hour, although the rate may range from 60-200mg an hour. Big people tend to break down alcohol more quickly than small people, and regular heavy drinkers can tolerate more alcohol than those who drink only occasionally. The rate is also affected by hormones and women can usually tolerate only half the alcohol that men can. Thus, on average, a 10-stone (65-kg) man drinking 2½ pints (1.4 litres) of beer (40g alcohol) will take 6 hours to break down the alcohol, and after an hour his blood alcohol will be 80mg per 100ml, which is just above the legal limit for drivers.

The absorption of alcohol into the blood can be delayed if it is drunk slowly with a meal. The peak blood level of alcohol can be almost halved in this way. The higher the concentration of alcohol the more rapid its absorption, so that one double whisky will have a quicker effect than a pint of beer, although they both contain the same quantity of alcohol. The sugars in sweet drinks also retard absorption, while the fizz of soda or mineral water will accelerate it. Strong, black coffee does nothing to increase the rate of alcohol breakdown and a glass of milk is no substitute for a meal as it has very little effect on the rate at which alcohol is absorbed from the stomach.

Small amounts of alcohol – the equivalent of 8-18 units of alcohol a week for men and 4-9 units a week for women – are probably harmless. (The table on page 22 shows how many units of alcohol are contained in various common drinks.) Some researchers have even gone so far as to maintain that small amounts of alcohol may help to protect against heart disease. On the other hand, one drink a day or so has been claimed to increase the risk of late miscarriages, and any woman who is planning to have a baby is well advised to avoid alcohol altogether until it is possible to work out the quantity that is safe. The risk of pancreatitis and strokes is believed to be increased in people who drink moderately during the week but who binge at weekends. The risk of cirrhosis of the liver and other diseases associated with alcoholism rises steeply once alcohol intakes reach the equivalent of 80g a day – i.e., the amount obtained from 5 pints of beer, 10 glasses of wine or 5 double measures of spirits. But if the health consequences of moderate and heavy drinking seem rather far off, the psychological effects – such as insomnia, depression, anxiety and increasing forgetfulness – may well be noticed sooner.

Strong, black coffee does nothing to increase the rate of alcohol breakdown and a glass of milk is no substitute for a meal as it has very little effect on the rate at which alcohol is absorbed from the stomach.

Once absorbed into the blood, alcohol acts as both a stimulant and a depressant.

It stimulates the heart to beat a little faster, it widens the blood vessels, causing flushing and a feeling of warmth, and it stimulates the flow of gastric juices, so acting as an "appetizer". But alcohol has the opposite effect on the brain and the nervous system. It depresses the parts of the brain that control behaviour by impairing the senses and interfering with bodily co-ordination. It also interferes with the ability to judge distances and with memory, judgement and concentration, and generally slows down the drinker's reaction time. A little alcohol can thus help ease feelings of awkwardness and tension as the drinker becomes less inhibited, more carefree – and careless. Unfortunately the effect of even a little alcohol will often convince the drinker that he is performing better and this inevitably encourages further drinking.

In fact moderate or "social" drinkers (men who drink 21-50 units and women who drink 16-35 units of alcohol a week) account for the majority of alcohol-related problems seen in our society.

In the case of young drinkers, binges are common and drunkenness causes death, not so much from alcohol poisoning as from the greatly increased risk of accidents, particularly on the roads. Few people would disagree that "heavy" drinkers are a risk to themselves and the rest of society. But since only about 6 per cent of men and 1 per cent of women come into this category, most people who would describe themselves as moderate drinkers find it hard to believe that alcohol-related problems are any concern of theirs. In fact moderate or "social" drinkers (men who drink 21-50 units and women who drink 16-35 units of alcohol a week) account for the majority of alcohol-related problems seen in our society. Although the experienced drinker is often able to take in more alcohol without becoming obviously intoxicated, he or she does not necessarily remain completely sober. This tolerance may be interpreted as an ability "to hold one's drink" when what in fact has happened is that the individual has learned to control the outer signs of too much drink. Social drinking and not just heavy drinking can cause the body to become used to – and dependent on – regular inputs of alcohol, which can permanently affect certain organs like the liver, heart and brain.

The currently recommended "safe" level of intake is a maximum of 18 units of alcohol a week for men and 9 units a week for women, with no more than two or three drinks at each occasion.

ALCOHOL PROBLEMS CHECKLIST*

Health problems
Stomach upsets?
Sickness, vomiting?
Difficulty sleeping?
Easily upset?
Depressed?
Indigestion?
Diarrhoea, loose bowels?
Tiredness/difficulty concentrating?

Social problems
Arguments at home about drinking?
Arguments at home made worse by drinking?
Family member threatened to leave because of drinking?
Been asked to leave pub/party, etc. because drunk?
Money worries because of drinking?
Problems with police because of drinking?

Accidents/work problems
Trouble at work because of drinking?
Absence from work because of drinking?
Been in accident because of drinking?

Symptons of developing tolerance
Unable to keep a drink limit?

Difficulty preventing getting drunk?
Restless without a drink?
Trembling after drinking the day before?
Drinking in the morning?

*(Taken from Royal College of General Practitioners report on alcohol, 1986)

UNITS OF ALCOHOL*

Type of Drink	Quantity	No. of Units
BEERS AND LAGERS		
Ordinary strength beer or lager	½ pint	1
	1 pint	2
	1 can	1½
Export beer	1 pint	2½
	1 can	2
Strong ale or lager	½ pint	2
	1 pint	4
	1 can	3
Extra strength beer or lager	½ pint	2½
	1 pint	5
	1 can	4
CIDERS		
Average cider	½ pint	1½
	1 pint	3
	quart bottle	6
Strong cider	½ pint	2
	1 pint	4
	quart bottle	8
SPIRITS		
1 standard single measure in most of England and Wales		1
1 standard single measure in Northern Ireland and parts of Scotland		1½
	1 bottle	30
TABLE WINE (including cider wine and barley wine)		
	1 standard glass	1
	1 bottle	7
	1 litre bottle	10
SHERRY AND FORTIFIED WINE		
	1 standard small measure	1
	1 bottle	12

These figures are approximate.
*(Taken from Health Education Council, 1983)

——CARBOHYDRATES——

The majority of carbohydrates are made from a single constituent – glucose. Glucose on its own is a sugar or, to use its technical term, a saccharide. Carbohydrate is a term used to cover a whole spectrum of substances from simple sugars at one end, through complex starches, finally ending up with the highly complex fibres at the other end. Sugars may consist of one or several saccharide units strung together. Starches like cornflour, on the other hand, are made up of much longer, often branched, chains of many glucose units called polysaccharides. Fibre is made from highly complex chains of glucose units and other substances.

From the physiological point of view, sugars and starches share more similarities than differences. Once broken down to glucose, both are equally good at supplying the body with energy. However, although physiologists working in a laboratory will tend to lump sugars and starches together under the general term carbohydrate, when it comes to assessing their role in the diet sugars and starches should be considered separately. The reason for this is that sugar is one of only two substances (the other being alcohol) that is often eaten on its own – as sweets or in sweet drinks – rather than as part of a whole mixture of other nutrients. Starches, on the other hand, are nearly always eaten as integral components of nutritionally varied foods.

SUGARS

Several single sugar units – called monosaccharides – exist in nature. The most common are glucose, fructose and galactose. Various combinations of these make up other simple sugars. The sugar bought in packets is called sucrose, and it is a compound of two single sugar or saccharide units. During digestion it is broken down to its two basic constituents – glucose and fructose. In addition to sucrose, lactose (the sugar of milk) is made up of one unit of glucose and one of galactose; and maltose (the sugar of malt extract) is made up of two glucose units strung together. Other more complicated sugars exist, and these are generally less sweet than the simple sugars. Of particular interest are stachyose – a component of beans on which certain bacteria in the gut feed, so generating quantities of gas – and glucose syrup, which is a common ingredient in many manufactured foods.

Glucose syrups account for about one-sixth of all the sugars eaten in the UK. They are very versatile ingredients that can be modified in a number of ways, and for this reason they are much favoured by the food industry. A whole range of syrups or powders can be made varying in sweetness according to how far the breakdown process is taken. Because they are less sweet than sucrose, they can be used in larger quantities without making food sickly. Glucose syrups are sometimes described as corn syrup – indicating the source of starch from which the syrup is made. Potato, rice and cassava starch can also make good glucose syrups.

SOURCES OF SUGAR

The three major sources of sugar in the diet are sugar added at table to food and drink, soft drinks and sweets. For some people biscuits and cakes are the major sources – particularly if they do not take sugar in tea and coffee and do not eat sweets. Sugar is also added to a wide range of other foods, including tomato soup, baked beans and some meat products, but these sources contribute relatively trivial quantities to the diet. In the UK most people eat between 14 and 26 per cent of their diet as sugar. This is an

In the UK most people eat between 14 and 26 per cent of the diet as sugar. This is an extraordinarily large proportion to be accounted for by a single nutrient.

extraordinarily large proportion to be accounted for by a single nutrient.

SUGAR CONTENT OF COMMON FOOD

Type of Food	Teaspoons of Sugar
1 chocolate digestive biscuit	1
1 plain digestive biscuit	½
1⅔-pint (330-ml) can cola drink	7
1 glass lemon squash	2
1 glass undiluted apple juice	4 (intrinsic, not added)
1 glass fresh orange juice	3 (intrinsic, not added)
2 tsps jam, honey, marmalade	2
2 tsps reduced-sugar jam	1
1 bowl Cornflakes or Weetabix	trace
1 bowl sugar-coated cereal	3
1 currant bun or doughnut	1
1 piece fruit cake or plain sponge	3
1 fruit yoghurt	4½
1 portion ice cream	2
1 small can fruit in syrup	10
1 small can fruit in juice	5 (intrinsic, not added)
1 portion baked beans or sweet corn	¾-1
1 1¾-oz (50-g) bar milk chocolate	5½
1 Mars Bar	9½
1 4-oz (113-g) packet peppermints or boiled sweets	20

SUGARS AND HEALTH

Sugar provides only calories and no other nutrients, which has earned it a bad reputation. These extra calories, which can displace more nourishing foods in the diet, and the special role of sugars in causing tooth decay are the principal ill-effects of sugars. They do not have a special role in the development of diabetes nor in heart disease, except through obesity. Overweight can, of course, result if too much of any food is eaten – whether it be cheese, beer or sugar. This can lead to diabetes and, in conjunction with a high fat intake, to heart disease. But although any food can lead to an increase in weight if it raises the calorie intake over the required amount, sugars can be a particular pitfall. Their very sweetness makes them attractive, and most people can still find room for a chocolate, even after the largest meal. The proportion of sugar in a diet is often indicative of the quality of it. For example, diets high in sugar are also often high in fat, as well as low in fibre. The very old and the young may also be at risk of mineral and vitamin deficiency if they have only small appetites and fill up on sugary foods. But except for the role of sugar in causing tooth decay, it is the quantity of sugar eaten that causes the problem, rather than there being anything intrinsically harmful about sugars themselves.

> *Except for the role of sugar in causing tooth decay, it is the quantity of sugar eaten that causes the problem, rather than there being anything intrinsically harmful about sugars themselves.*

SUGARS AND TEETH

Teeth are living tissues, like bones, and as such they have some ability to repair themselves, although rather slowly. They can repair dents and cracks in the enamel if they have enough time between intakes of sugary foods, if fluoride is available and if the teeth are kept free of acid. Acid is produced by the bacteria that inhabit the mouth. In order to grow, these bacteria need a simple, easily digested food – and sugars provide just that. As they multiply, bacteria make a soft, sticky layer which builds up around the teeth, particularly at the gum margin and in any crevices. If this layer, called plaque, is not regularly removed, it hardens, shielding the acid inside which will then eat into the enamel. The bacteria take only a couple of minutes to produce the acid and so the majority of damage is done to the teeth within about three minutes of a sugary or acid food being eaten – far too quickly for most people to use a toothbrush in time. The acid in the mouth can, however, be neutralized by saliva – if enough is produced. Some protein foods, like cheese, milk and nuts, are good at stimulating the flow of saliva, so a sticky pudding will not do as much harm to teeth if cheese or nuts are eaten immediately afterwards. The teeth can recover from a few bouts of acid production during the day but, unfortunately, dentists do not yet know how many can be tolerated. However, we do know that most people in the UK suffer from dental caries, and since we also know that the average person eats or drinks at least six times during the day, the "safe" number of occasions on which sugary foods and drinks can be consumed must be less than six. In the meantime, the best advice is to avoid drinking sugary drinks or eating sweet foods between meals; to keep sweet puddings to a minimum; and to brush the teeth thoroughly, at least twice a day, with a fluoride-containing toothpaste.

> *The bacteria take only a couple of minutes to produce the acid and so the majority of damage is done to the teeth within about three minutes of a sugary or acid food being eaten – far too quickly for most people to use a toothbrush in time.*

RECOMMENDED INTAKES

Although a large number of reports by expert groups have recommended a reduction in sugar intake, few have said by how much. Where quantities have been recommended, a 50 per cent reduction in average consumption has been suggested, so that sugar would provide no more than 10 per cent of the total calories. But this is a rather crude recommendation when you remember that it is the frequency, rather than the total amount of sugars consumed, that is critical in causing dental caries.

One report that did make this recommendation qualified it by saying that sweets, biscuits, soft drinks and other sugary snacks and drinks should be restricted so that no more than half the suggested sugar intake was consumed in this form. On the other hand, if people manage to keep their weight down and virtually cut out sugary snacks and drinks between meals, the suggestion for a 50 per cent cut could be relaxed. So a slim, healthy adult who is not putting on weight and whose teeth are in good condition probably need not cut sugar intake by as much as 50 per

> *It is the frequency, rather than the total amount of sugars consumed, that is critical in causing dental caries.*

cent. However children, whose teeth are particularly vulnerable, need to keep sugars to a minimum, particularly between meals.

KEYWORDS

Dextrins are small chains of sugar units obtained during the industrial breakdown of starch which are halfway between sugar and starch. They are a common component of glucose syrups. Dextrins are not overly sweet and are used on their own in glucose drinks and tube feeds as they are easily absorbed by patients who are seriously ill.

Glucose is one of the simplest of sugars. All starches and most sugars are eventually broken down to glucose during the course of digestion. Glucose supplies the brain and muscle with the energy they need. All surpluses are converted to fat.

Glucose or corn syrups are manufactured from the partial breakdown of starch. A whole range of syrups or powders varying in sweetness can be made depending on how far the breakdown process is taken. About one-sixth of all the sugars eaten in the UK are in the form of glucose syrups.

Fructose is another simple sugar found alongside glucose and sucrose in fruits. It is converted into glucose or fat by the liver.

Honey is 20 per cent water and 75 per cent sugars. Although honey does contain traces of vitamins and minerals, the amounts are too small to be useful.

Invert syrup is a syrupy mixture of glucose and fructose in equal parts. Its composition is much the same as honey although it does not have the compounds that give honey its flavour. It is sweeter than sugar (sucrose) syrup and is much used in the food industry.

Lactose is the sugar of milk. It is less sweet than the other simple sugars. The proteins in milk seem to counteract the potential damage to teeth from the lactose. However, milk *may* cause dental decay if small amounts are constantly in the mouth.

Malt extract Malt is traditionally produced during the brewing of beer when the newly sprouted grains are heated. Maltose is the name of a particular sugar which can be extracted from the dried malt. It is used for its characteristic flavour.

Saccharide is a sugar unit. Monosaccharides are single sugar units (e.g., glucose and fructose); disaccharides are double sugar units (e.g., sucrose and lactose) and polysaccharides are many sugar units strung together as in starch and fibre.

Sucrose This is the familiar sugar in the home. It is a natural component of fruits and vegetables and large quantities can be extracted from sugar beet and sugar cane. Sucrose accounts for about three-quarters of the sugars eaten in the Western diet.

Sugar The sugar bought in packets is sucrose. Although sucrose is the commonest sugar eaten, all sugars behave in the same way in the body. There is no advantage in eating glucose or fructose instead of sucrose. Varieties of sugar described as "brown" (whether demerara, muscovado, etc.) are extracted forms of sucrose, which have almost, but not quite, completed all the stages of refinement. The principal differences between brown and white sugar are those of texture and taste. From the point of view of health there is no real difference between brown or white sugars or honey.

——*STARCHES*——

The polysaccharides, or complex carbohydrates, are found principally in plant foods where starch is the plant's energy store and fibre is the polysaccharide packaging of the plant cell wall that creates the toughness and shape of the plant.

Starch, like sugar, has a bad reputation whereas fibre has recently been hailed as the answer to all ills. But looking at starch in such black and white terms is unhelpful. Although highly refined starches, like cornflour or arrowroot, may be little different nutritionally from sugar; starch-rich foods, particularly if they retain much of their natural fibrous matter, are very different.

Starch-rich foods such as bread, flour, rice, pasta, beans and potatoes are also good sources of protein and of a wide range of vitamins and minerals. If the external layers or skin of the grain or vegetable are eaten, they can also be rich sources of fibre. In fact, the potato is the nearest to a complete food on which an adult could survive – provided he or she could muster the appetite to eat 7-8lb (about 3.5kg) a day.

> *In fact, the potato is the nearest to a complete food on which an adult could survive – provided he or she could muster the appetite to eat 7-8lb (about 3.5kg) a day.*

In cultures where a lot of starchy foods are eaten, the staple – usually a cereal such as rice or maize – is used as the basis or foundation of a meal. Sauces using meat, fish, vegetables or oils and side dishes of vegetables, pulses and fruit are added to the bland staple to give flavour and interest. They also improve the nutritional quality of the meal, even if the cook is not always aware of this. Starchy staples like these usually require fairly healthy appetites as they make quite bulky meals. For this reason, very young children (who don't always have the heartiest appetites) can become undernourished. They need relatively more of the nutritionally complementary sauces or side dishes and less of the bulky, filling staples until their appetites increase. Another important characteristic of the cultures whose cuisine is based on starchy staple foods is that the people usually work the land and so are physically much more active than those who live and work in towns and offices. So, how much the difference in health between peasant farmers and Westernized city dwellers is due to differences in their levels of physical activity, or to the amount of starch, fibre or fat that is eaten is extremely difficult to determine.

STARCH IN THE UK DIET

In the UK the starchy staples we eat most of are bread, flour and potatoes. But over the years appetites have grown smaller (or weight consciousness has grown more widespread) and the consumption of bread and flour, in particular, has gone down markedly. In the last thirty years or so we have virtually halved our consumption of bread and flour, with consequent repercussions on the balance of all the other nutrients in the diet. The downward trend in bread and flour consumption started a long time ago. It can be traced back to about 1880, at the time of a rapid increase in the growth of cities and a huge shift in the population from the country to the towns with all sorts of changes in lifestyle (see also Chapter 5).

At the moment carbohydrate makes up about 45 per cent of the UK diet; of this almost half comes from sugar and the rest from the complex carbohydrates like the starch and fibre found in bread and flour. There is at the moment no recommended intake for starch, although if people eat less fat and sugar, complex carbohydrates would have to fill the gap,

> *How much the difference in health between peasant farmers and Westernized city dwellers is due to differences in their levels of physical activity, or to the amount of starch, fibre or fat that is eaten is extremely difficult to determine.*

in which case their contribution to the calorie content of the diet could rise from 25 to between 35 and 40 per cent.

——FIBRE——

Fibre is an umbrella word for several different substances that help to make up the supporting structures of plant cell walls. The term also includes some non-carbohydrate substances combined with them. In most diets throughout history fibre has been almost as inevitable a component as water. It was not, therefore, a substance that excited much interest. Indeed many people in this country used to long for a less chewy, less gritty diet. Not surprisingly, poor people, who must often have been physically tired from hard work and sick from debilitating infections before the days of antibiotics, yearned for the wheaten "white" bread of the rich. Indeed, fibre was taken so much for granted that when a national diet was composed during World War II it was virtually forgotten. At the time this did not matter because large quantities of bread made from less refined flour ended up increasing the quantity of fibre in the diet without any special provision having to be made.

However, fibre continued to be ignored by the majority of nutritionists until the late 1960s and early 1970s when it was discovered that fibre in the diet could help in the treatment of certain diseases of the gut. Since then research into fibre has increased rapidly, although so far raising more questions than answers. Knowledge of the types of fibre that exist and the different effects that each has on the body is still in the relatively early stages of research.

The chemistry of dietary fibre varies from plant to plant and is affected by the growing conditions and age of the plant. At the moment fibres are roughly divided into six groups – celluloses, hemicelluloses, lignins, pectins, gums and mucilages. Fibres not only vary in their physical state, from the dry gritty nature of bran to the soft gel-like texture of pectins and mucilages, but they also behave differently. For example, the dietary fibre found in fruit, and more particularly in beans, delays the absorption of glucose and certain drugs from the intestine. This characteristic can be of particular use in the development of diets for diabetics. By helping the retention of moisture and gas, so making the stool softer and bulkier, bran can also be a very effective cure for constipation, as well as having the effect of generally improving the action of the bowel.

But we do not eat whole plants like cattle and sheep eat grass; we chop, grind, sieve and cook our food. All these processes can have a marked effect on the properties of fibres. For example, the particle size of wheat bran and whether it is cooked or raw will affect its ability to relieve constipation.

Although laboratory analysis can provide a certain amount of information about individual fibres, such information is not necessarily a particularly helpful guide when it comes to working out what happens when fibrous foods are eaten. For example, lignins are very good at mopping up bile acids and so they might be expected to help lower blood cholesterol. Yet bran – which is very rich in lignins –

> *Fibre was taken so much for granted that when a national diet was composed during World War II it was virtually forgotten.*

does not produce this effect once it has been eaten, whereas certain gums and pectins do. There is also a difference between eating bran when it is extracted from wheat and eating it as an integral part of the cereal grain. Not only may the quantity of bran be much greater than that naturally present in food, but if it is raw there will be other substances like phytate present, which can affect the absorption of certain minerals. The phytate in bran, which, if it was consumed as bread, would normally be inactivated by the action of yeast, can also bind minerals like calcium, iron and zinc so that the body absorbs less of the them. This is unlikely to cause much of a problem in young, healthy adults who seem able to adapt to large intakes of bran, but it could cause problems in an old person who eats little but takes as much as 1-2 tablespoons (18-35ml) of bran a day in order to keep the bowels "regular". The diet on to which bran may be sprinkled is also likely to be very different from a diet made up of wholemeal bread, brown rice, vegetables and fruit, i.e., adding bran to cornflakes and to a fried breakfast will not convert low fibre foods into a high fibre diet.

> *We do not eat whole plants like cattle and sheep eat grass; we chop, grind, sieve and cook our food. All these processes can have a marked effect on the properties of fibres.*

FIBRE IN THE DIET

It is fibre-rich diets rather than large quantities of fibre by itself which are believed to be associated with less heart disease and fewer digestive diseases like cancer of the bowel. A diet that is rich in wholegrain cereals, beans, vegetables and fruit will differ in many ways from a diet made up of highly milled or refined foods, such as white flour and sugar, or foods naturally low in fibre, such as meat, milk and cheese. Societies that eat a lot of fibre are generally the same as those that eat a lot more starch and, as discussed in the section on starches, they are also usually much more active. There are also many other differences between developing and industrialized populations. For all these reasons, it is difficult to draw firm conclusions about the effects on health of fibre.

In the UK, the average amount of fibre eaten each day has been estimated as approximately ¾oz (20g). Newer methods of analysis have suggested an even lower figure of ½oz (13-14g). Two studies of vegetarians in the UK have shown that they eat roughly 1-1½oz (33-40g) of fibre a day (which happens to be the amount eaten during World War II), whereas in parts of Africa, the fibre intake can be extremely high, reaching 5oz (150g) a day. Practically all foods of plant origin are useful sources of dietary fibre. Sugar is a notable exception as it is a highly purified extract from cane and beet. On the other hand, white bread which may be made from highly milled flour does have some fibre – about 3 per cent or the same amount as that obtained from fresh fruit and leafy vegetables. The richest sources of fibre are wholemeal bread and flour, peas, beans, dried fruit and nuts.

> *It is fibre-rich diets rather than large quantities of fibre by itself which are believed to be associated with less heart disease and fewer digestive diseases like cancer of the bowel.*

Most people who change to a high

fibre diet soon notice they are passing much larger quantities of faeces more often, as fibre not only increases the bulk but also the rate at which the bowel contents are passed through the gut. However, changing to a high fibre diet should be done slowly as a sudden change can cause diarrhoea, pain and severe wind from the large amounts of gas suddenly produced. Although extra wind can be a problem, the effect is usually temporary as the individual adapts to larger quantities of fibre.

RECOMMENDED INTAKES

There are no official recommended intakes for dietary fibre, although most medical authorities concerned with diet are agreed that we should eat more of it. A comprehensive report by the Royal College of Physicians in 1980 recommended that extra fibre should be eaten, particularly in the form of "foods which are closer to the natural grain, vegetable or fruit than the highly processed and refined products which now form a large part of our food".

KEYWORDS

Bran consists of the fragmented outer coats of the grain, plus some starch. It is a byproduct from the manufacture of white flour and contains 40-50 per cent fibre.

Bran breakfast cereals are not all bran but contain variable amounts of wheat, sugar and salt as well as added vitamins and minerals. Their fibre content varies from 15 to 27 per cent.

Brown breads have a fibre content that is somewhere between white and wholemeal bread, depending on how highly milled the flour is, and how much extra bran has been added. In the latter case the bran content may be more than that normally found in wholemeal bread.

Fibre is composed of highly complex polysaccharides in plant cells, which are undigested by human enzymes. A little, however, may be digested by bacteria in the colon and absorbed into the body. Dietary fibre includes substances such as gums, cellulose, lignin and pectin.

Modified starches are food additives made from chemically altered starches. Some varieties may contain residual amounts of the chemicals used. They are used to provide texture, to thicken, to stabilize emulsions and to protect finished foods during storage and distribution.

Pectin is a gel-like form of dietary fibre found in variable amounts in fruit. Pectin enables jam to set.

Starch is usually found together with fibre in plants. It forms the main storehouse of energy for the plant. It was once thought that all starches were digested and absorbed but at a slower rate than sugars. Recent research is revealing a much more complicated picture. Some starchy foods are absorbed very quickly, others much more slowly and a certain amount is not digested at all but passes into the colon where it may be digested by bacteria.

White bread is made from flour containing only 72 per cent of the grain that is made whiter with the use of various bleaching agents. White bread contains about 3 per cent fibre.

Wholemeal bread is made from flour containing 100 per cent of the grain. The fibre content is 8.5 per cent.

——*VITAMINS*——

The term "vitamins" is the name given to a rag-bag of body chemicals that have very little in common. Like hormones, the primary function of vitamins is to help regulate the chemical processes that go on in the body, but, unlike hormones, they cannot be made in the body and so must be obtained from food. The amounts of these vitamins that are needed each day are so small that some can barely be seen with the naked eye.

The reason that such a miscellany of chemical compounds with quite different physiological functions are grouped together is an accident of history. Until the beginning of the 20th century vitamins were unknown. It was thought that pure fats, proteins and carbohydrates and a

Like hormones, the primary function of vitamins is to help regulate the chemical processes that go on in the body, but, unlike hormones, they cannot be made in the body and so must be obtained from food.

few minerals were all that was needed to sustain life. However, when it was discovered that rats died when fed an artificial diet made up of ingredients like lard, sugar and milk protein which were thought to provide all the necessary fats, carbohydrates and proteins, the hunt began to find what were then called the other "accessory food factors" needed to help them thrive. The speed with which these accessory food factors were discovered was dramatic. Between 1915 and 1945 over fifty were identified and, for easy reference, they were distinguished by letters of the alphabet.

However, many of these so-called vitamins were subsequently found to be known biological substances or compounds that the body can make for itself. Now out of the original 50, only 13 – and some would argue 12 – remain. This explains some of the gaps in the alphabetical and numerical lists. For example, although there are vitamins A, B, C, D, E and K there is no F, G or H and the intervening numbers between B_6 and B_{12} remain blank. Confusingly, there are also some vitamins, like niacin and folic acid, that are known just by their names and have no letter or numbers to distinguish them.

The substances that are recognized as vitamins are listed in the table on page 41, with their alternative names where they exist. You can safely assume that any so-called vitamins not on this list are not vitamins because the body makes its own supply and so does not need to obtain them from food. Some of the names you may come across on bottles of so-called vitamin and diet supplements are vitamin P (bioflavinoids), carnitine, inositol (vitamin B_{13}), orotic acid, para-amino benzoic acid (PABA), vitamin B_{15} (pangamic acid) and vitamin B_{17} (laetrile). In some cases these substances belong to the remaining 37 compounds originally thought to be vitamins but found not to be so. Three other vitamins – biotin, pantothenic acid and choline (or lecithin) – are so widespread in foods that they can be ignored.

VITAMIN A

Vitamin A can be obtained in two forms from food. Either as vitamin A in animal foods or as carotenes (which give carrots their colour) in some vegetables. The body can convert these carotenes into vitamin A.

Function and Deficiency Vitamin A plays a particularly important role in the structure of skin and mucus-secreting tissues. Without vitamin A a child's growth is slowed down because new cells cannot develop properly. Perhaps the best-known consequence of vitamin A deficiency is its effect on the eyes. At first vision at night becomes difficult and then the loss of mucus causes damage to the corneas, eventually leading to blindness. Vitamin-A-related blindness – or xerophthalmia –

Vitamin A-related blindness – or xerophthalmia – is estimated to cause half a million new cases of blindness each year in parts of the Third World.

is estimated to cause half a million new cases of blindness each year in parts of the Third World. Other mucus-secreting tissues, like the lungs, are also affected by a lack of vitamin A and this can make children vulnerable to chest infections and the like.

Although vitamin A deficiency is rare in Western countries (very occasionally it occurs in patients unable to absorb a wide range of foods), small supplements of vitamin A are often routinely given to babies in vitamin drops. This is just a precaution at a time when a child is growing very rapidly and may be at risk if his weaning diet is particularly unbalanced. The most important vitamin in vitamin drops is vitamin D – vitamins A and C are added for good measure, as it were.

It has been suggested recently that vitamin A and/or carotene might help protect against cancers, particularly those that arise on the surface of tissues such as those lining the insides of the lungs, breast, intestines, stomach, bladder and skin. The evidence is not clear-cut, but the US National Research Council's committee on diet, nutrition and cancer has recommended that people should eat more vegetables and fruit. This would help to increase the amount of carotene in the diet in a safe manner without the risk of harming health from an over-enthusiastic use of vitamin A in tablet form.

Toxicity Vitamin A is soluble in fat, which means that it can be easily stored in the body. The principal storage site for vitamin A is the liver, and most British adults have one to two years' supply in their liver alone. Because vitamin A can be stored, it is relatively easy for someone to overdose themselves; so far at least 500 cases of vitamin A poisoning have been reported. Taking a daily supplement of 10mg of vitamin A (10 times the recommended daily intake) can cause liver damage, dry itchy rashes and tender growths on the bones. Larger doses can bring on headaches caused by pressure from an increased level of cerebrospinal fluid, peeling skin, loss of appetite, hair changes, depression, confusion and even death. Large doses of vitamin A have also been shown to damage the developing foetus. On the other hand, high intakes of carotene from food do not appear to be harmful. They can cause the skin to turn an orangey colour but, as far as is known, that is all.

Synthetic forms of vitamin A, which are safer than the natural forms, have been, and are continuing to be, developed as vitamin A in large doses is occasionally used in the treatment of acne and certain other skin conditions. However, it should only be taken under medical supervision and should never be prescribed for girls or women who have a chance of becoming pregnant.

The principal storage site for vitamin A is the liver, and most British adults have one to two years' supply in their liver alone.

For all these reasons, the safest way to take in extra vitamin A is from food and not as a supplement.

Food Sources Carotenes are found in carrots, dark green leafy vegetables (e.g., spinach and broccoli), apricots, melon and pumpkin. Vitamin A is found in liver, cod liver oil (and other fish oils), kidney, milk, butter, cheese and eggs. Margarines are usually fortified with vitamin A, as are baby milks and many baby foods. If a food is fortified, the presence of vitamin A will be declared on the label.

In Britain about one-third of the vitamin A we eat comes from liver, one-quarter from vegetables and one-seventh from milk and milk products.

> *Without thiamin, carbohydrate, alcohol and – to a lesser extent – protein become useless as sources of energy. The body usually stores about a month's supply.*

VITAMIN B₁ (THIAMIN)

Function Thiamin plays a part in the metabolism of carbohydrates, alcohol and certain of the amino acids in protein. It is needed to enable a steady release of energy from these foods. Without thiamin, carbohydrate, alcohol and – to a lesser extent – protein become useless as sources of energy. The body normally stores about a month's supply of thiamin. The amount needed corresponds to the proportions of protein, carbohydrate and alcohol in the diet. On the whole, a diet that is rich in protein and carbohydrate usually has a reasonable supply of thiamin, so that thiamin deficiency is highly unlikely to occur in people eating a mixed diet.

Deficiency Thiamin deficiency can, however, occur when the diet consists of large quantities of alcohol or refined carbohydrate and very little else. For this reason, diets consisting mainly of polished white rice, as eaten in parts of Asia, can cause beriberi. Theoretically, a diet containing large amounts of sugar – a highly refined carbohydrate without any accompanying vitamins – could also give rise to thiamin deficiency. However, thiamin deficiency does not appear to be a problem in Britain, despite our large intake of sugar, so we presumably obtain enough from other foods. A deficiency of thiamin – along with many other vitamins and minerals – may well occur if someone suffers long periods of starvation or goes on a semi-starvation diet. Supplements of thiamin and other vitamins may also be advised as a precaution for patients suffering persistent vomiting or those (like kidney patients) who regularly receive blood dialysis.

Toxicity Because the B vitamins are soluble in water, only small amounts can be stored in the body and any surpluses are usually passed into the bladder and out of the body within a couple of hours. For this reason, large doses of thiamin are unlikely to be harmful. It is, however, possible for people who dose themselves with large amounts of thiamin to become physiologically dependent on these doses. The body becomes "lazy", as it were, about using and replenishing its own stores of thiamin as it adapts to a high intake. Withdrawal symptoms are therefore a risk when someone who previously took extra doses of thiamin stops doing so.

Food Sources Wheat germ is a particularly rich source of thiamin. Other good sources are wholemeal bread and flour, yeast and yeast extract, peas, beans, nuts, pork, duck, oatmeal, cod's roe, milk, potatoes, other vegetables and fruit.

> *Because the B vitamins are soluble in water, only small amounts can be stored in the body and any surpluses are usually passed into the bladder and out of the body within a couple of hours.*

In Britain almost half the thiamin in the diet comes from cereal foods.

There is also a legal requirement for all bread and flour (except wholemeal) to be fortified with thiamin to replace that which is lost during the milling of flour. In Britain almost half the thiamin in the diet comes from cereal foods.

VITAMIN B₂ (RIBOFLAVIN)

Like thiamin, riboflavin is essential in order to convert food into energy. But unlike thiamin, there are no real stores of riboflavin in the body and for this reason nutritionists tend to keep a closer watch on riboflavin levels in the diet. Riboflavin deficiency is, however, rare among people who take milk and milk products.

Deficiency When Riboflavin deficiency has been induced, it gives rise to a rather unexpected range of symptoms, which seem to bear little relation to the biochemical function of the vitamin. This may be because it is difficult to induce riboflavin deficiency without causing deficiencies of other nutrients. The specific signs include sores at the corner of the mouth and a smoothing of the surface of the tongue. However, since symptoms like these can arise as a result of a number of other conditions, including cold sores, badly fitting dentures and iron-deficiency anaemia, it would be jumping to over-hasty conclusions to assume that sores in the area of the mouth and nose are due to riboflavin deficiency, except in very special circumstances.

Toxicity Surplus riboflavin, like thiamin, is quickly passed out of the body and so toxicity is unlikely.

Food Sources Riboflavin is widespread in the diet, particularly in animal foods. The richest sources are liver and kidney followed by yoghurt, cheese, yeast extract, eggs, meat, wheat germ, wheat bran and mushrooms. Breakfast cereals are usually fortified with riboflavin and, if so, this is declared on the label. In Britain milk supplies one-third of the riboflavin in the diet. Ultraviolet light destroys riboflavin so bottles of milk should be taken indoors as soon as possible and not left to stand in sunlight.

NIACIN

Niacin, like thiamin and riboflavin, is also involved in the chain of biochemical processes by which energy is released from food. Although niacin can be obtained directly from food, the body is also capable of converting the amino acid tryptophan, which is present in all protein, into niacin.

Deficiency A deficiency of niacin gives rise to a specific disease called pellagra. Patients with pellagra develop dark, scaly patches of skin on areas exposed to sunlight. They may also have diarrhoea and eventually, if untreated, they develop a form of dementia. Pellagra mainly occurs in certain African countries where a lot of maize, but little milk or eggs, is eaten. Niacin is present in maize but is chemically bound up and so unavailable. Interestingly, pellagra does not occur in

In Britain milk supplies one-third of the riboflavin in the diet. Ultraviolet light destroys riboflavin so bottles of milk should be taken indoors as soon as possible and not left to stand in sunlight.

Central and South America where maize originated. This is because the making of tortillas traditionally requires maize to be soaked in lime-water, which has the effect of releasing the niacin from its chemical bonds. Pellagra does not occur when milk and eggs are regular items of the diet, as these foods contain abundant supplies of the amino acid tryptophan, which can be converted into niacin.

> *Very large doses of niacin have also been associated with peptic ulcers, itching, hair loss, liver damage, low blood pressure and heart beat disturbances.*

Toxicity Supplements of niacin are sometimes prescribed as part of the treatment of certain diseases, such as some forms of hyperlipidaemia (where levels of cholesterol and other fats are raised in the blood) and even chilblains. Large doses of 3g or more can inhibit the breakdown of fat from the fat stores in the body, which is why it is useful in the treatment of some hyperlipidaemias. Side-effects are common, however, and can start with doses as small as 100mg – only 5-6 times the recommended intake. In large quantities niacin can cause flushing of the skin due to the release of histamine. Histamine is a substance released by the body when it goes into a form of shock, such as that brought on by an allergic reaction. Histamine also stimulates gastric secretion and can cause a drop in blood pressure. Very large doses of niacin have also been associated with peptic ulcers, itching, hair loss, liver damage, low blood pressure and heartbeat disturbances.

Food Sources Niacin is found in much the same foods as riboflavin: liver, kidney, meat, fish, yeast extract, brewer's yeast, peanuts, bran, peas and beans, wholemeal bread and flour, fortified breakfast cereals, vegetables and milk.

VITAMIN B₆ (PYRIDOXINE)

Vitamin B_6 is the name given to a group of five closely related substances involved in the metabolism of amino acids – including the conversion of tryptophan into niacin. It is also necessary to help make the haemoglobin in blood.

Deficiency Deficiency of B_6 is very rare, mainly because it is found in so many foods. However, although deficiencies are rare, there have been claims that extra B_6 can help relieve both depression caused by the contraceptive pill and premenstrual tension. There is no physiological explanation why vitamin B_6 should do this. In many ways, the pill mimics pregnancy and it is known that pregnancy can cause the most extraordinary changes in blood levels of certain nutrients without any danger to health, so a low level of B_6 in the blood does not necessarily mean a deficiency. Thus, whether B_6 really is of help in either of these disorders will remain debatable until research involving larger numbers of women gives a clearer answer.

There are a few other disorders which respond to pharmacological doses of vitamin B_6. These include certain genetic disorders, some forms of anaemia and radiation sickness.

> *There have been claims that extra B_6 can help relieve both depression caused by the contraceptive pill and premenstrual tension.*

Toxicity Although B_6 is soluble in water, like the other B vitamins, several cases of B_6 poisoning have been reported in the United States. In almost all cases the patients were dosing themselves with very large doses (between 5 and 10 times the pharmacological dose and as much as 160 times the recommended dose) in an effort to relieve premenstrual symptoms like water retention. These doses caused numbing and even loss of muscular co-ordination. The body can also become dependent on regular large doses of vitamin B_6 in the same way as it can on regular large doses of thiamin.

VITAMIN B_{12}

Vitamin B_{12}, like vitamin B_6, is a mixture of several related compounds. It is needed by rapidly dividing cells, such as those in the bone marrow from which blood is formed. It is also needed for the structure of nerve cells. Normally the liver can store about 1,000 times the amount of B_{12} the body needs.

Deficiency Deficiency of B_{12} – pernicious anaemia – is usually secondary to some forms of intestinal disease that inhibit the absorption of B_{12} from the diet. However, because B_{12} is found only in animal foods, vegans (who eat only plant foods and no animal products) are theoretically at risk of deficiency. It is therefore customary for vegans to drink plant "milks" or yeast extracts that have been fortified with B_{12}.

Toxicity There are virtually no known toxic effects from vitamin B_{12}. One of the few occasions when very large doses are necessary is in the treatment of pernicious anaemia.

Food Sources Liver is the richest source of B_{12}, followed by kidney, sardines, oysters, heart, rabbit, other meats, eggs, cheese and milk. Although vitamin B_{12} is believed to occur only in foods of animal origin, there have been claims that B_{12} has been obtained from seaweeds. But the most probable explanation is that some B_{12} is present as a result of microbial contamination from manure or sewage.

FOLATE

Folate has several functions and, like vitamin B_{12}, it is needed by rapidly dividing cells, such as blood cells.

Deficiency Anaemia caused by folate deficiency is relatively common. It can occur simply as a consequence of a poor diet – particularly one that is low in fruit and salad vegetables – but it usually develops as a result of intestinal diseases, which can often hinder the absorption of nutrients.

There is also an increased requirement for folate during pregnancy, and folate deficiency has been suspected of causing spina bifida and other related neural tube defects. One of the drugs used in the treatment of leukaemia destroys folate and is known to cause neural tube defects in animals. Women who have given birth to babies with spina bifida have also been shown to have low levels of folate in their blood at the beginning of pregnancy. Some small-scale trials do suggest that giving women a small vitamin supplement containing folate around the time of conception will help prevent neural tube defects. Studies involving much larger numbers of women are currently under way.

Giving women who might have a spina bifida baby small extra doses of vitamins seems a harmless precaution. Indeed, it appears to be highly reasonable in the

> *Women who have given birth to babies with spina bifida have also been shown to have low levels of folate in their blood at the beginning of pregnancy.*

short term. However, there are dangers if such a practice is accepted without first being thoroughly evaluated. If extra vitamins prove not to be the answer, vital research would be held up unnecessarily. Equally plausible arguments were made in the past linking coal fires and blighted potatoes with the incidence of spina bifida, and both theories were subsequently disproved. If vitamin supplements are definitely proved to be effective, it will also be important to determine the size of dose that is both effective and safe.

Toxicity No serious toxic effects from moderate doses of folate are known, except the possibility of masking B_{12} deficiency. In such cases the anaemia clears up but the degeneration of the nerve cells continues.

Food Sources Folate occurs in many foods but is especially rich in liver and raw green leafy vegetables. Other sources include kidney, spinach, broccoli, lima beans, beetroot, bran, peanuts, cabbage, lettuce, avocados, bananas, oranges, wholemeal bread, eggs and some fish. Folate is easily destroyed during cooking, which is why it is important to include raw salads and fresh fruit as regular items of the diet.

Vitamin C (Ascorbic Acid)

Vitamin C has a number of functions, which include keeping the structure of connective tissue healthy and enabling iron in food to be more easily absorbed. Vitamin C also inhibits the formation of nitrosamines – a group of cancer-causing agents made from common substances in foods. A good intake of fruit and vegetables that contain vitamin C is believed to be the reason why the incidence of stomach cancer is relatively low in this country.

Deficiency A deficiency of vitamin C causes scurvy. In this disease connective tissue starts to break down, causing bleeding from small blood vessels, and wound healing is slowed. Eventually widespread haemorrhaging follows, together with the re-opening of old wounds. Only very small quantities of vitamin C are needed to prevent scurvy and it can take several months on a diet deficient in vitamin C before scurvy develops. Deficiencies are uncommon in Britain, but can sometimes occur in babies who are given cow's milk instead of formula milk and in the elderly – particularly widowers – who eat a very poor diet with virtually no fruits or vegetables.

In the UK the quantity of vitamin C recommended to be taken each day is still determined by the amount needed to prevent scurvy in a healthy adult with a threefold safety margin – 30mg or the equivalent of about half an orange. In the United States and Canada the recommended intake is twice this amount. Some nutritionists believe that the UK should increase its recommended intake to take into account the other functions of vitamin C, such as its ability to improve the absorption of iron from food and to aid recovery from illness.

An intake of 30mg is certainly not enough for hospital patients who have undergone surgery. This dramatically increases the body's needs for vitamin C, which helps to regenerate the protein needed to repair bones and to make scar tissue. A number of drugs and smoking are also known to increase the body's needs for vitamin C, and some authorities have suggested that hospital patients – particularly those who have undergone major surgery – should have 250mg a day. This is almost 10 times the recommended daily intake for a healthy adult and is the equivalent of 1¾ pints (1 litre) of orange juice or 13½lb (6kg) of grapes – grapes are a poor

> *Grapes are a poor source of vitamin C and so are not the best gift for a hospital patient!*

source of vitamin C and so are not the best gift for a hospital patient!

There have also been much-publicized claims that people should take massive doses of vitamin C – from 1 to 10g a day – in the belief that this will prevent many diseases, including the common cold. So far there have been over thirty research trials to investigate this. Three-quarters have not proved that vitamin C helps to prevent or cure colds, and in the remaining studies the results suggested only that extra vitamin C might help a very small number of individuals. So scientists, by and large, are not convinced of the benefits of large intakes and, indeed, have expressed concern at the real possibility that massive doses could be harmful.

Toxicity Very large intakes of vitamin C – a gram or more a day taken for long periods of time – have a number of disadvantages. Although the vitamin is soluble in water and the excess is normally excreted in the urine, large quantities can cause an increase in the amount of oxalate (a calcium compound) in the urine. If an individual has a tendency to form stones, all the extra calcium from the oxalate can form stones in the bladder. Very large quantities of vitamin C can also lead to iron overload and too much iron causes anaemia, just as too little iron does. Indigestion, diarrhoea and a number of other discomforts have also been reported by people taking massive doses of vitamin C.

Taking larger doses of vitamin C than the 30mg currently recommended in the UK may well be sensible, but doses so large that they need to be taken in tablet form are excessive and potentially harmful, except perhaps as a temporary measure after illness. If you are seriously worried about the level of vitamin C in your diet, the best course is to eat more fruit and vegetables, thereby getting the benefit of all the other vitamins and minerals that are naturally present too.

Food Sources Rich sources of vitamin C are blackcurrants, guavas, rosehip syrup and green peppers. Oranges, lemons, cauliflower, broccoli, sprouts and cabbage are also good sources, provided the vegetables are only lightly cooked and served immediately. Vitamin C is easily destroyed by cooking and when food is kept warm. In Britain one-fifth of the vitamin C eaten comes from potato chips. Potatoes are not a particularly concentrated source of vitamin C, but because they are eaten as large servings they make a substantial contribution to the diet.

VITAMIN D

Vitamin D is not a vitamin but a hormone. It is found in only a few foods and is principally obtained by the action of ultraviolet light (from the sun) on the skin. If everyone bared some skin to the sun sufficiently often, D could probably be one more "vitamin" that could be struck off the list. However, vitamin D deficiency can still be a problem where the skin is little exposed to sunlight. In northern climates, the

> *In Britain one-fifth of the vitamin C eaten comes from potato chips.*

groups of the population most likely to be at risk are babies, the housebound and dark-skinned people who have only recently come to live in the UK, and in southern climates, those who keep their skin permanently covered – such as women in purdah – may also develop vitamin D deficiency.

Vitamin D is needed to transport calcium from the blood into the bones and back again. A steady level of calcium is needed in the blood for a number of reasons: it is essential for the action of muscles like the heart, several enzymes need it and so do the nerves in order to function properly. It is also necessary for the normal clotting of the blood.

> *Rickets used to be known as the "English disease" because it was once so common in the cities when smog and crowded buildings effectively kept out what little sunlight there was.*

Deficiency Too little vitamin D causes the bones to weaken and eventually soften as calcium is worn away and not replaced. The weight of the body then causes the characteristic deformities of the legs and hips seen in rickets. It is very difficult to correct these deformities. Rickets used to be known as the "English disease" because it was once so common in the cities when smog and crowded buildings effectively kept out what little sunlight there was. The biggest contribution to the prevention of rickets was undoubtedly the introduction of legislation to help clean the air and remove the smog that used regularly to develop in cities.

Vitamin D is stored in the body. The surplus made during the summer, when people generally wear less clothing and are out of doors more, is usually plenty to last even the worst winter. Babies who are born in winter usually have sufficient stores laid down before they are born, but if the mother was deficient during pregnancy, then her baby may well need supplements. Rickets is no longer a problem in English children but it occurs among Asian women and children, particularly those living in the north. Quite why this section of the population is particularly vulnerable remains a mystery, but it can easily be prevented with vitamin supplements.

Toxicity It is very easy to overdose with vitamin D from tablets or drops. The amounts of vitamin D that were required to be added to infant foods had to be lowered when it was found that a few babies fed fortified milks, fortified weaning foods and vitamin drops were being made ill as a result. Doses of only five times the recommended intake can cause hypercalcaemia – too much calcium in the soft tissues – in susceptible children. Hypercalcaemia causes symptoms of thirst, loss of appetite, nausea and vomiting, and eventually hardening of the soft tissues as well as raised blood pressure.

Food Sources Fish liver oils such as cod liver oil are really the only naturally concentrated sources of vitamin D. Fatty fish such as sardines, herring, mackerel, tuna, salmon and pilchards are reasonable sources, and eggs, liver and butter provide a little. Some foods are fortified with vitamin D and margarine is the most important of these. Anyone who is at risk of vitamin D deficiency should be encouraged to expose some skin to sunlight every day, even if it is only sitting by an open window, and to eat margarine and fatty fish.

Baby milks and some infant foods are

> *Doses of only five times the recommended intake can cause hypercalcaemia – too much calcium in the soft tissues – in susceptible children.*

> *Guinea pigs, fruit bats and man are about the only animals that need vitamin C. Other species are capable of manufacturing it for themselves.*

also fortified with vitamin D and welfare vitamin supplements are also available for babies and young children if they need them.

VITAMIN E

Vitamin E is a name given to a group of related compounds of which the most active is α-tocopherol. Vitamin E performs a remarkably diverse range of functions in different animals. In rats it is essential for normal fertility; without it male rabbits, dogs and some monkeys are effectively castrated; cows and horses develop muscular dystrophy; turkeys haemorrhage; and chicks develop inflammation of the brain. However, a vitamin that is essential for one species can be of much less importance in others. For example, guinea pigs, fruit bats and man are about the only animals that need vitamin C. Other species are capable of manufacturing it for themselves and man is reasonably well protected from niacin deficiency since it can be made from the amino acid, tryptophan, in protein. So the effects of vitamin E deficiency on other animals will not necessarily be duplicated in humans.

Vitamin E has been described as a vitamin in search of a disease and, indeed, scientists have found it very difficult to create vitamin E deficiency in man. The two exceptions to this are premature babies and patients with diseases that seriously interfere with digestion.

Vitamin E seems to have a role in protecting the essential fatty acids from the destructive effects of oxygen. There is no proof yet to support claims that extra vitamin E improves sex life or promotes better health in general. In one study where some people were given vitamin E and others given an identical-looking capsule without vitamin E, no subsequent differences were found between the two groups.

Vegetable oils – which are the main source of essential fatty acids in the diet – are also rich sources of vitamin E, so deficiency is unlikely.

Deficiency True vitamin E deficiency has been identified only in people who have diseases that interfere with the absorption of fat and in premature babies. A mild form of anaemia may develop as well as muscle weakness and the loss of reflexes in the tendons. Newborn premature babies seem to have small reserves of vitamin E. If the baby has to have oxygen, these limited stores may be used up, resulting in a form of blindness caused by an excessive growth of fibrous tissue behind the lens in the eye.

> *Vitamin E has been described as a vitamin in search of a disease and, indeed, scientists have found it very difficult to create vitamin E deficiency in man. The two exceptions to this are premature babies and patients with diseases that seriously interfere with digestion.*

New research is suggesting that vitamin E may prevent some neurological side-effects that accompany digestive diseases, such as cystic fibrosis, and in patients who have undergone extensive surgery of the gut.

Toxicity Vitamin E, like vitamin C, is a vitamin that some people take in large doses. As far as is known, this is quite harmless.

Food Sources The richest sources of

vitamin E are vegetable oils, followed by margarine, eggs, butter, wholegrain cereals, wheatgerm and broccoli.

VITAMIN K

Vitamin K comes in two forms – one is found mainly in vegetables and the other produced by bacteria in the gut. It is necessary for the normal clotting of the blood.

Deficiency Because vitamin K can be manufactured in the gut and because it is so widespread in vegetable foods, deficiency is rare. It can of course occur in people who have diseases that make them unable to absorb much of the food they eat, or in those who have to take prolonged doses of broad-spectrum antibiotics (which can kill off the bacteria in the gut as well as germs in other parts of the body). The other section of the population requiring particular attention are newborn babies. Some babies, particularly those who have a low birth weight or have had a difficult delivery, have a risk of haemorrhaging in the first hours and days after birth. Some hospitals therefore have a policy of injecting all babies with vitamin K; other hospitals treat only those babies at particular risk.

Toxicity A synthetic form of vitamin K in use at one time was found to cause jaundice and anaemia of the newborn and so is now no longer prescribed.

VITAMIN CHART

Recommended Name	Other names	Deficiency	Toxicity	Approximate daily requirement in Adults
Vitamin A	Retinol	Common in developing countries	Yes	1mg
Thiamin	Vitamin B_1 Thiamin hydrochloride	Occasional in alcoholics	Rare	1mg
Riboflavin	Vitamin B_2	Rare in UK	Rare	1.5mg
Niacin	Nicotinic acid Nicotinamide	Pellagra mainly in parts of Africa	Rare but possible	15-20mg
Vitamin B_6	Pyridoxine Pyridoxine hydrochloride	Unlikely	Yes	3mg
Folate	Folacin Folic acid	Possible	Unknown but can mask B_{12} deficiency	200 microg
Vitamin B_{12}	Cobalamin Cyanocobalamin Hydroxycobalamin	Possible in vegans	Unlikely	3microg
Vitamin C	Ascorbic acid	Occasional	Possible	30-60mg
Vitamin D	D_2 and D_3 (ergo) calciferol	Yes – in Asians particularly	Yes	3-10 microg
Vitamin E	α-tocopherol	Unlikely	Unknown	10mg
Vitamin K	Vitamin K_1	Occasionally in newborn babies	Possible	100microg

—MINERALS—

Traces of a large number of mineral salts have been discovered in the body but only twenty or so have so far been found to be essential to humans in the way that vitamins are. Some of the other minerals present – such as lead and mercury – enter the body as a result of pollution, although it is possible that more than twenty may eventually be discovered to be essential nutrients. Research in this field is making rapid advances and scientific knowledge is constantly changing.

Most mineral salts cannot be dissolved in water, so making them difficult to absorb. For this reason, once inside the body they are not easily excreted, unless there is an excessive loss of body fluids, as from a haemorrhage or severe diarrhoea. There are a few exceptions to this rule: sodium and potassium salts and iodide and fluoride are easily absorbed.

On the whole a deficiency of minerals is much less of a problem than a deficiency of vitamins. The only mineral that is commonly deficient is iron, although some experts argue that since woman has been in existence long enough to have adapted to the inevitable losses from menstruation and pregnancy, perhaps iron-deficiency anaemia is less of a problem than is commonly supposed.

Animals, unlike humans, often show signs of mineral deficiency because they are more likely to eat deficient diets. Either the soil of the land they graze on may be deficient in a particular mineral or the animal feed – which is an artificially devised mixture of nutrients and foods – may turn out to have too little of a vital component. In human beings the only analogous situation arises in patients who have to be fed artificial diets by tube or in those who live entirely on home-grown foods in an area with a deficient soil. Most of the scientific knowledge about minerals comes from research done on animal nutrition where mineral deficiencies and excesses are much easier to observe.

MINERALS IN BODY FLUIDS

The body is bathed in fluid. All cells contain water and all cells are suspended in water. However the water outside the cells has important differences compared with that inside. Water outside the cells is salty because it contains sodium chloride (the same as common table salt), as can be tasted from sweat, whereas water inside the cells is rich in potassium. Maintaining a careful balance between the water inside and that outside the cell is a key metabolic activity performed by the kidneys.

The only mineral that is commonly deficient is iron, although some experts argue that since woman has been in existence long enough to have adapted to the inevitable losses from menstruation and pregnancy, perhaps iron-deficiency anaemia is less of a problem than is commonly supposed.

Deficiency Deficiencies of either sodium, potassium or water are unusual as the diet normally contains plenty of each. Occasionally, isolated episodes of excessive sweating can cause an undue loss of sodium, causing muscle cramps. Substantial tissue wastage, as occurs in starvation, serious injury and diabetes, or a loss of considerable amounts of water from severe diarrhoea can cause a marked loss of potassium. The immediate result is extreme muscle weakness, which can be fatal if the heart muscle or circulation is affected.

Toxicity Healthy kidneys excrete potassium and sodium quite easily. An excess of sodium usually causes thirst which encourages more fluids to be drunk in order to dilute the extra sodium. Very ill people occasionally get an excess of sodium and potassium after an intravenous infusion. Babies – whose kidneys are immature – have difficulty maintaining a balance between sodium and water and so are at much greater risk of dehydration. Salt added to weaning foods and larger quantities of sodium from over-concentrated milk feeds can easily cause an excess of sodium to build up. Too much salt is also believed to be a factor in the development of high blood pressure in some people (see Chapter 4).

Food Sources Adults need less than 3g of salt a day, yet their daily dietary intake can be anywhere between 5 and 20g on average. Most foods (except fats, oils, sugar and alcohol) are good sources of potassium. Most foods are also naturally low in sodium. However, a large proportion of processed foods have salt added so that the more of these that are eaten, the saltier the diet. Throughout history salt has been much prized, perhaps not surprisingly when one considers how monotonous large bowls of porridge or bread must have been without some added flavour or stimulant, whether in the form of salt, sugar or alcohol. Moderate intakes of these flavourings are harmless and may even be beneficial if they help to make dull food palatable. However once they become a habit, it is all too easy for these useful substances to be abused as the tastebuds gradually accustom themselves to increasingly greater quantities.

The main sources of sodium in the diet are salt (and anything to which salt or brine is added), bread and cereal products, meat products and milk and dairy products. The main sources of potassium are vegetables, meat and milk. Fruit and fruit juices contain only moderate amounts of potassium but they can be very useful if consumed in large quantities.

SODIUM AND POTASSIUM CONTENT OF SOME FOODS
(amounts of the minerals measured in mg per 100g of food)

	Sodium	Potassium		Sodium	Potassium
Milk	50	140	Peas	3	190
Cheddar cheese	610	120	Canned peas	380	150
Butter (salted)	780	15	Oranges	2	180
Margarine	800	5	White bread	525	110
Eggs	140	136	Wholemeal bread	560	230
Beef	70	330	Cornflakes	1160	99
Pork	65	360	Wheat breakfast cereal		
Chicken	75	290	biscuits	360	420
Sausages	760	160	Yeast extract	4500	2600
Bacon	1245	183	Soy sauce	5720	270
White fish	120	300	Tomato ketchup	1120	590
Smoked haddock	1220	290	Tomato purée (no salt)	20	1540
Potatoes	8	360	Tomato purée (with		
Crisps (ready salted)	550	1190	salt)	420	890

MINERALS IN BONES AND TEETH
Most of the minerals in the body are found in the bones where they make up about

> *Minerals give bones their strength and hardness – without them bones would be like lengths of rubber.*

half the weight of the skeleton, the remainder being composed of protein, water and a little fat. Minerals give bones their strength and hardness – without them bones would be like lengths of rubber. The commonest mineral in bone is calcium. But phosphorus is also important, together with small amounts of magnesium.

CALCIUM

A baby is born with about 25mg of calcium. By the time a child has stopped growing he or she will have laid down a further 1,200mg or so. Children lay down about 180mg of calcium each day in their bones and during growth spurts, like those of adolescence, the amount can be as much as 400mg. However, calcium deficiency is not usually a reason for inadequate growth. In poor countries where children do not grow so well, it is because of a general shortage of protein and calories. This slows down cell growth in the skeleton so that consequently less calcium ends up being deposited. It is thus the extra protein in milk, rather than the calcium, which seems to encourage growth in children who are undernourished. Nor does it have to be milk protein, mixtures of vegetable protein can promote growth equally well. The main advantages of milk over other foods are that it is a nutritious food and children generally find it easy to consume. Perhaps it is also fair to say that it is a food that researchers have found particularly easy to measure and hand out, so giving it rather more than its fair share of attention.

From about the age of forty, the skeleton begins to shrink until, by the age of about eighty, it is only 70 per cent of its height as a young adult. Although the bones may shrink, they do not automatically lose a disproportionate amount of calcium. It is common for bones to thin and weaken, particularly after the menopause in women and in old age generally. This weakening is called osteoporosis, and it is the main reason why falls can so easily result in broken wrists, hips and thigh bones in middle-aged women and the elderly.

The cause of osteoporosis is currently being researched, and it may well be that it results from several interrelating factors. For example, it is known that hormonal insufficiency can cause calcium loss as can too little exercise. Both crash diets and chronic gastrointestinal diseases seem to lead to calcium loss, while a high consumption of alcohol, coffee, meat, bran, salt and cola drinks make it more difficult for calcium to be absorbed from food. Interestingly, although people in the Third World do not grow as tall as Western people, they suffer less from osteoporosis. Whether supplements of calcium would delay the progress of osteoporosis is being researched.

> *Both crash diets and chronic gastrointestinal diseases, seem to lead to calcium loss. While a high consumption of alcohol, coffee, meat, bran, salt and cola drinks make it more difficult for calcium to be absorbed from food.*

Although 99 per cent of the calcium in the body is used by the skeleton, the remaining 1 per cent performs a vitally important function elsewhere. Between 5 and 10g are essential for triggering muscle contractions, including those of the heart muscle; for nerve function; for the activity of several enzymes; and for the normal clotting of the blood. The amount of calcium in the blood is regulated by several hormones, including those of the thyroid, and by vitamin D, which transports calcium to and from the bones. If there is a serious shortage of calcium in the diet – which is unlikely – the hormones are able to take calcium from the skeleton in order to replenish the blood. When a deficiency of calcium does occur it is, as far as is known, always secondary to a deficiency of vitamin D, or as a result of extensive surgery on the thyroid gland.

> *Phosphorus is much more widely distributed in food than calcium. The amount of phosphorus consumed is well above what is needed and deficiency as a result of an inadequate supply from food is virtually impossible.*

Recommended Intake Because 70-80 per cent of the calcium in food is passed out of the body, the recommended daily intakes are about three times higher than the amount actually needed. In the UK – as in other milk-drinking populations – the amount of calcium consumed is usually way above that which is required. The body seems to be capable of absorbing a larger proportion of the calcium in food, if it needs to. For instance, the absorption of calcium increases during pregnancy as the body lays down extra stores during the early months to meet the needs of the rapidly growing foetus in the last three months before birth. Breastfeeding places even greater demands on a woman's stores of calcium, but again her body is able to adapt, providing she is healthy, eats well and does not have a rapid succession of pregnancies.

Food Sources Good sources of calcium are milk, yoghurt, cheese, canned fish (when the bones are eaten), hard water, dried figs, green vegetables, peanuts, bread and flour. In the UK all bread and flour, except wholemeal, is fortified with extra calcium.

PHOSPHORUS

Phosphorus is found mainly in the bones but some is also needed for the chemical reactions whereby energy is released from food. Phosphorus is much more widely distributed in food than calcium. The amount of phosphorus consumed is well above what is needed and deficiency as a result of an inadequate supply from food is virtually impossible. On the other hand, deficiency as a result of medication has been reported in people taking large quantities of antacids containing aluminium hydroxide, which prevents the phosphates in food from being absorbed, causing muscle weakness and bone pains. Too much phosphorus in unmodified cow's milk can also harm newborn babies as it inhibits the absorption of calcium. This was one reason why it used to be so important for bottlefed babies to follow a rigid feeding schedule. Nowadays modified milks, in which the mineral levels are manipulated to approximate the amounts found in breastmilk, permit a more relaxed approach.

Food Sources The main sources of phosphorus are milk and milk products; bread and cereal products; and meat and meat products. About 10 per cent of the phosphorus in the diet is obtained from food additives, as phosphates, which have emulsifying properties, are often added to foods such as dessert mixes, sausages

Bran also contains phytate and anyone who regularly adds large spoonsful of bran to their diet could develop zinc and iron deficiency.

and cheese spreads. They are also an important component of baking powder, in which they are needed for their acidic properties.

MAGNESIUM

Besides being found in the bones, magnesium is necessary for a number of enzymes. Magnesium is widespread in foods, particularly in vegetable and cereal foods. A deficiency can very occasionally follow prolonged and severe cases of diarrhoea, when a number of other minerals may be lost at the same time.

ZINC

The body contains about 2g of zinc, most of which is found in the bones. Elsewhere zinc is found in the eye, prostate and skin (where it can play an important part in wound healing). Zinc is also a component of over fifty enzymes.

Deficiency A characteristic sign of severe zinc deficiency is hair loss and the eruption of pustules and boil-like swellings all over the skin. This has occurred in some babies born with a congenital disorder affecting zinc metabolism and in some hospital patients put on an incomplete tube-feeding regime. Symptoms arising from mild zinc deficiency are hard to diagnose, since it is difficult to suffer from zinc deficiency without having a deficiency of many other nutrients too. It has been suggested that zinc deficiency may be contributory to stunted growth in some parts of the world, such as the Middle East, where large quantities of unleavened bread are eaten. Phytates, found in cereals, bind metals like iron and zinc, making it impossible for the body to absorb them. Yeast, used for raising dough, destroys phytate, which is why this problem does not occur in the West. Bran also contains phytate and anyone who regularly adds large spoonsful of bran to their diet could develop zinc and iron deficiency.

Food Sources About 20 per cent of the zinc in food is absorbed and, like iron, the best sources are meat and meat products. Beans, wholemeal bread and other wholegrain cereal products are good sources while oysters are very rich in zinc.

FLUORIDE

Fluoride is mainly found in bones and teeth. Fluoride adds considerably to the strength of tooth enamel, and children who live in areas of the country where the water supply contains at least one part per million of fluoride (that is 1mg per litre, which adds up to 1-3mg a day) – whether naturally present or added – usually have much stronger teeth than those who live in deficient areas. Parts of India, China, Argentina and Africa contain as much as 10 parts per million of fluoride in their water supplies, which may add up to 10-30mg a day – an amount that is harmful. Sea fish is a good source of fluoride and adults often obtain 1mg fluoride from tea alone each day. For children who live in an area where the water does not supply sufficient quantities of fluoride, the most important source comes from toothpaste that is swallowed. Although fluoride in

Adults often obtain 1mg fluoride from tea alone each day.

the diet or painted on the teeth is beneficial to children who are particularly likely to suffer from tooth decay, this can still mean that babies may go short and it is in babyhood that the permanent teeth are being formed in the gums. Fluoride supplements in the form of drops or tablets are often advised for babies until at least the age when they are getting fluoride from toothpaste that is swallowed.

Toxicity Although fluoride is easily excreted in the urine, poisoning from too much fluoride is possible. In the parts of the world where the rocks (usually volcanic) naturally contain large amounts of fluoride, fluorosis does occur. The first sign is mottling of the teeth and eventually thickening and deformities of the bones. In this country fluoride poisoning is most likely to result from industrial pollution, for example among those who have to handle fluoride-containing minerals, such as the cryolite used in aluminium smelting.

Food Sources Sea fish, tea and occasionally water are the main sources of fluoride. There is no obvious source for babies, particularly those who are breastfed, in which case supplements are the only sure way of making up the deficiency.

——OTHER MINERALS AND TRACE ELEMENTS—

IRON

About half the iron in the body is found in haemoglobin in the blood; the other half in muscle tissue. Haemoglobin is needed to carry oxygen from the lungs to the rest of the body. Although the body recycles the iron from worn-out haemoglobin cells, some iron is lost whenever there is bleeding and from the gradual wearing away of the tissues lining the intestines. If these losses are not replaced, anaemia results.

Deficiency People with anaemia easily become tired. If they do anything strenuous, they quickly become breathless and giddy, the eyesight may be affected, headaches are more common, as well as insomnia, palpitations, poor appetite, digestive disturbances and pins and needles in the fingers and toes. The skin is usually pale and the tongue is shiny and smooth.

The groups that are most at risk of anaemia are children and adolescents who are going through growth spurts, pregnant women, women with heavy periods and people who have chronic bleeding (for example, from piles or as a result of gastrointestinal diseases). Where anaemia is diagnosed, iron tablets are the most efficient treatment until the haemoglobin is restored to normal. Thereafter, a diet containing plenty of iron and vitamin C should be sufficient. Sometimes iron tablets can cause nausea and constipation, in which case the dose or type of tablet may have to be changed.

Toxicity Iron pills are second to aspirin as a cause of accidental poisoning in young children who help themselves to Mummy's pills. The child has to be given a stomach pump as well as medicines to prevent as much of the iron as possible from being absorbed. In some parts of Africa and elsewhere all food and alcohol is prepared in iron vessels and iron poisoning has been caused when iron has leached into food from iron cooking pots. Heavy drinkers of cheap wines which are

> *Iron pills are second to aspirin as a cause of accidental poisoning in young children who help themselves to Mummy's pills.*

> *Other sources of iron are dried apricots, curry powder, soy sauce, chocolate and red wine.*

often rich in iron can also get a form of anaemia.

Food Sources On average, about 10 per cent of the iron present in a mixed diet is absorbed. Liver, meat and fish are the best sources. In these foods up to 25 per cent of the iron can be absorbed compared with less than 5 per cent of the iron in eggs, vegetables and cereals. The quantity of vitamin C found in a glass of fruit juice will enhance the absorption of iron from the poor sources, whereas tea will further hinder iron absorption. Other sources of iron are dried apricots, curry powder, soy sauce, chocolate and red wine. Potatoes, vegetables and cereal products can also make an important contribution if they are eaten in sufficient quantity.

IODINE

Iodine is present in high concentrations in the thyroid gland where it is an essential component of the hormones produced there. Unlike many other minerals, iodine is easily absorbed.

Deficiency A deficiency of iodine affects about 400 million people in the world and causes goitre – the swelling of the thyroid gland in the neck. This is most frequent in developing countries where there is little in the way of a food distribution system and where the food is grown on deficient soil. Soil deficiencies are most likely in mountainous regions. In England goitre was once known as "Derbyshire neck". An underactive or overactive thyroid gland is not due to imbalances in the hormonal system and has nothing to do with a deficiency or excess of iodine.

Toxicity Because the thyroid will happily absorb any iodine present, including radioactive iodine, iodine supplements are sometimes given to those who live in areas that have been exposed to large doses of radiation. This is done to saturate the thyroid with normal iodine in order to prevent it from absorbing iodine from food or water that has become radioactive. The absorption of radioactive iodine is therefore one of the few harmful effects of radiation that can be avoided.

Food Sources The amount of iodine in food largely depends on the amounts present in the soil where the vegetables and cereals are grown. In the UK the food distribution network is such that people usually eat very few locally grown vegetables. Seafood is the most reliable source of iodine, whereas cabbage and other brassicas contain substances that prevent its absorption. In this country milk is the main source of iodine – simply because it is commonly added to animal feeds.

COPPER

Copper is needed for a number of enzymes. Deficiency can occur in premature babies who have not built up adequate stores before birth. It is also poisonous in large quantities and the concentrations in drinking water have to be controlled. Cirrhosis of the liver in several young children has been diagnosed in parts of India and is believed to be caused by cop-

> *The absorption of radioactive iodine is therefore one of the few harmful effects of radiation that can be avoided.*

per poisoning as a result of food being cooked and stored in copper utensils.

Food Sources Shellfish and liver are particularly rich, but meat, bread, other cereals and vegetables can provide useful amounts. Children may get extra copper from swallowing the water in swimming baths where copper sulphate is often used to help keep the water clean.

COBALT

Cobalt is part of vitamin B_{12} and this is the only form in which it is used in man.

CHROMIUM

Chromium is present in most foods and although it is an essential nutrient, it is not yet clear what role it performs in human physiology.

MANGANESE

Manganese deficiency can cause poor growth and deformities of the inner ear. Tea is the richest source, but wholegrain cereals, leafy vegetables, beans, nuts and spices are also good.

SELENIUM

Selenium can behave very much like vitamin E in helping to prevent the oxidation of essential fatty acids, and sometimes the two are interchangeable. But unlike vitamin E, selenium is toxic in high concentrations. The main food sources are cereal products, fish and meat.

CHAPTER 2

WHAT DOES THE BODY NEED?

——WATER——

Humans need water more than they need food. Without it they survive for only a few days, whereas they can survive without food for several weeks. About half the water consumed comes from food; the other half from drinks. Most people drink far more than they actually need. The wide variations in the amounts drunk by young children provides a good illustration of this. Some children will drink excessively (and empty their bladders at a corresponding rate), particularly when drinks, usually sweetened, are used as a comforter. Others, who have not yet acquired the social habit of accepting drinks, will drink almost nothing (often to the consternation of their tea-drinking mothers) without getting dehydrated. If children were made to drink only water, then their "thirsts" would probably be more evenly matched.

A little water is produced as a result of the metabolic processes in the body. This metabolic production goes largely unnoticed unless there is a sudden change in diet, particularly from a high to a low carbohydrate one. This can cause great excitement to slimmers when they find they have lost 3lb (1.4kg) in three days. But this is mainly the result of a temporary water loss caused when the body's small stores of carbohydrate in the form of glycogen (the animal form of starch) are used up. For every gram of glycogen, 3-4g of water are lost. After the first week the weight loss may be only ½-1lb (0.2-0.5kg), which can be disheartening but is a much truer record of fat loss.

Adults need approximately 2 pints (just under 1 litre) of water a day. In healthy people thirst dictates when they need to drink more. However, the sick and the elderly do not always take in as much fluid as they need. Those with a fever lose salt as well as water, through sweating, and so do not feel particularly thirsty, while elderly people can have difficulty in going to the lavatory in the middle of the night and may therefore deliberately cut down their fluid intake during the latter half of the day.

——INDIVIDUAL DIETARY REQUIREMENTS——

When in good health, children and adults will automatically eat enough to satisfy their calorie needs. Provided they choose from a selection of nutritionally varied foods, like bread, cereals, fruits, vegetables, beans, milk, fish, etc., they will get enough of all the nutrients they require.

But modern life is not always so straightforward. Most people don't exercise enough, and they have access to an enormous range of foods. Many modern processed foods, such as fats, oils, sugar, sweets, chocolate bars, cakes, biscuits, crisps, ketchups, sauces, instant puddings and a whole range of instant snack foods, are not shining examples of nutritional variety. If eaten occasionally and in only small quantities, this type of manufactured food can add interest and flavour to regular items of the diet; but nowadays the roles are often reversed. Too often "taste" has become the overriding consideration, at the expense of nourishment. Instead of a little salt, sauce and fat being used to make a plate of potatoes tasty, a few thin slices of potato carry large quantities of salt, oil and flavours (which, as often as not have been nowhere near the food they are supposed to mimic) as crisps. Likewise, bread, which used to be eaten in large chunks, often plain but sometimes with a little dripping or treacle to improve its taste, has now for many dwindled down to a couple of slices a day – and those slices are probably only there in order to support thick quantities of butter and marmalade!

Nor do we have to do much preparation of our food. If we want fruit juice, we don't have to eat four apples; we can buy it ready squeezed. Nuts are available ready shelled and we don't have to cook our own biscuits and buns. It is so much easier to eat more now, when previously one might otherwise not have bothered.

So it is clearly important to establish some kind of guidelines for our diet. But unfortunately, finding out just what the fundamental dietary guidelines should be is not a straightforward matter. There are nutritional recommendations and they are often made by government-appointed expert committees in many countries the world over. On the whole, though, their recommendations are not intended for the general public. Although they publish tables known as "recommended intakes of nutrients" or "recommended daily allowances", these are mainly intended for use by government officials in ministries such as those concerned with agriculture and health, to help to assess whether a nation's food supplies are likely to be meeting the nutritional needs of the population as a whole.

These recommended figures may also be used to assess the adequacy of diets of particular sections of the population, but again the figures are concerned more with assessing the average diet than with identifying individuals with particular needs. Up to now, too, the majority of official surveys have been concerned with checking that people are not going short of certain nutrients, rather than whether they may be taking too much. These tables of recommended intakes can therefore offer only very rough guidelines to individuals and in some cases the figures can be highly misleading.

For example, if a group of mothers were to try to work out how many calories their babies were taking in from milk, although the babies as a whole would prob-

> *If eaten occasionally and in only small quantities, this type of manufactured food can add interest and flavour to regular items of the diet; but nowadays the roles are often reversed. Too often "taste" has become the overriding consideration, at the expense of nourishment.*

In order to cover the needs of the majority – particularly those who require a bit more than the average – the quantities recommended are in fact usually a bit higher than the amounts actually needed by the average person.

ably be taking in the average recommended amount, some infants would be taking considerably less than this while some would be taking considerably more. But this would not necessarily mean that any individual babies were on the verge of either undernutrition or of obesity. Babies vary considerably in their energy needs and these needs will also vary constantly depending on how active a baby is being and on whether he or she is in the middle of a growth spurt or recovering from an infection.

The precise amount of a nutrient each person needs is thus wholly individual. Because it takes years of experimental research to work out one person's requirements, this procedure can be embarked on only in very rare cases, such as, for example, when a child has to be given a highly artificial diet because of a congenital metabolic defect, or when an adult has to be tube-fed for very long periods.

──*RECOMMENDED DAILY ALLOWANCES*──

The procedure whereby a national committee makes recommendations concerning the amounts of nutrients that should be eaten began in the UK in the 1930s, a time when undernutrition was of greatest concern. The medical experts were then anxious to ensure that vulnerable groups of the population did not become deficient in nutrients. A similar aim to prevent deficiencies has also shaped the efforts of advisory groups in other countries.

The amounts of nutrients recommended by expert committees are based on the average quantities that need to be eaten each day by people in normal health. In order to cover the needs of the majority – particularly those who require a bit more than the average – the quantities recommended are in fact usually a bit higher than the amounts actually needed by the average person. The principal exception to this rule is the number of calories recommended (see the table on page 53). In this case the average is given because no one wants to suggest that people should eat a few more calories in a country like the UK where obesity is a common problem.

Although obesity and the more general problem of eating too much of nutrients like fats, alcohol and sugar has been recognized for many years, the idea of giving the recommendations a range with a maximum and a minimum recommended level of intake has been much slower to gain acceptance. Some countries started to tackle the problem of preventing overnutrition as well as undernutrition in the early 1970s. Sweden and Norway were two such pioneers. The UK, on the other hand, has been much slower to come round to the idea of recommending maximum safe limits. Instead government committees and the like have opted for more cautious and imprecise advice – such as "to eat less salt might be beneficial" (see the government booklet *Eating for Health*, HMSO, 1978) – without giving any indication of how much is already eaten and what degree of reduction is likely to be beneficial! It was not until 1984 that a government publication tackled (head on) the problem of too much of certain nutrients by recommending that the calorie intake from fat should be no more than 35 per cent of total calories. Although there is still no official advice in this country about how much sugar, fibre, salt or starch is advisable, a number of other expert groups in the UK and elsewhere have made recommendations to try to fill in the gaps in official advice.

All nutritional recommendations – whether official or unofficial – are judgements made on the best available evidence by a selected group of scientists and doctors. They are therefore bound to vary and none is sacrosanct.

All nutritional recommendations – whether official or unofficial – are judgements made on the best available evidence by a selected group of scientists and doctors. They are therefore bound to vary and none is sacrosanct. National diets differ, the illnesses and diseases that are most common also vary from one country to another and, of course, nutritional knowledge expands as research techniques are refined and new light is thrown on old problems. For all these reasons, nutritional recommendations are bound to alter over time.

For most nutrients, there is a considerable range of intake over which health remains stable. Below and above this range health can deteriorate rapidly (see the diagram on page 54). When the intention is to avoid deficiency diseases, the amount recommended is usually towards the bottom end of the middle range. In such cases the recommended amount is closer to the safe minimum so that most people will be healthy if they eat this amount or a bit more of the nutrient. Nutrients that come into this category are usually minerals and vitamins. On the other hand, when the intention is to avoid an excess of a nutrient such as fat, the recommended amount is closer to the safe maximum – or top end of the optimal range – so that most people will be healthy if they eat this amount or a bit less. Recommendations for energy and protein intake come somewhere in the middle of the optimal range.

CALORIES
The table below gives the recommended amounts of calories that are needed on average according to age and sex.

UK RECOMMENDED DAILY AMOUNTS OF FOOD ENERGY (IN KILOCALORIES)

Age	Males	Females
12 months	1200	1100
2 years	1400	1300
3-4 years	1560	1500
5-6 years	1740	1680
7-8 years	1980	1900
9-11 years	2280	2050
12-14 years	2640	2150
15-17 years	2880	2150
Young adults	2510 (3350 if very active)	2150 (2400 if pregnant) (2750 if breastfeeding)
Middle-aged	2400 (3350 if very active)	1900 (2500 if very active)
Over 75	2150	1680

HEALTH AND THE RANGE OF NUTRIENT INTAKE

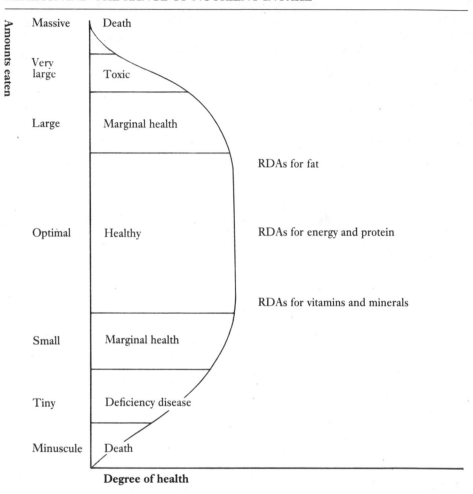

Degree of health

It may be calculated from the table that in a family of two adults and three children aged 12 months, 9 years and 12 years, the baby may eat about half as much food as his father or mother and the two older children will probably be eating as much as or more than their parents. Huge appetites at a young age are common but can sometimes catch parents unawares. Dishing out a larger portion of food to Dad rather than the twelve-year-old may help explain obesity in adults and the seemingly "bottomless" appetites of children, particularly when they reach puberty!

PROTEIN
In the UK, the recommended amounts for protein correspond to 10 per cent of the calories. This is well above the minimum safe level needed and is about the size of the quantities normally eaten in the UK. These recommendations for protein requirements are therefore acknowledged to be purely arbitrary.

VITAMINS AND MINERALS

The table below illustrates the quantities of a few of the vitamins and minerals needed at various stages of life. Those vitamins and minerals not mentioned are assumed to be so easily available in the British diet that any special recommendation is unnecessary.

UK RECOMMENDED DAILY AMOUNTS OF VITAMINS AND MINERALS

	Baby	Child	Adult
Vitamin A	450microg	300microg	750microg
Thiamin	0.3mg	0.7mg	1mg
Riboflavin	0.4mg	0.9mg	1.5mg
Niacin	5mg	10mg	18mg
Folate	50microg	200microg	300microg
Vitamin C	20mg	20mg	30mg
Vitamin D	7.5microg	10microg (if insufficient access to sunlight)	10microg
Calcium	600mg	600mg	500mg
Iron	6mg	10mg	10-12mg

From this table it can be seen that the UK recommendations for nutrients like the B vitamins and iron are in proportion to the size of the baby, child or adult. On the other hand, babies have relatively large needs for vitamins A, C and D and all children need proportionately more calcium than adults. Although women who are pregnant or breastfeeding need more vitamins A, C and D and calcium and iron, healthy women should be able to get these extra amounts from a combination of the larger portions they eat and the metabolic changes in the body during pregnancy which help to build up the nutrient stores.

Portions of food that would provide adult quantities of the recommended nutrients are shown below. Unless stated, in each case the weights refer to the uncooked ingredients.

VITAMIN A: 750 micrograms
4g (¾ teaspoon) liver
390g (14oz) eggs (8 standard eggs)
125g (4½oz) dried apricots (5 portions)
75g (2¾oz) butter (enough for 11-15 slices of bread)
95g (3¼oz) margarine (enough for 14-19 slices of bread)
112g (4oz) sweet potato (1 portion)
37g (1¼oz) carrots (1 large carrot)
75g (2¾oz) cooked spinach (a large portion)
270g (9½oz) Cheddar cheese

VITAMIN B$_1$ (THIAMIN): 1mg
2 litres (3½) pints milk
250g (9oz) liver
200g (7oz) pork
33g (1¼oz) yeast extract (enough for 11 slices of bread)

55

60g (2¼oz) breakfast cereal (2-3 bowls)
1kg (2¼lb) oranges (10 medium-sized)
300g (10½oz) wholemeal bread (11 slices)
555g (19½oz) white bread (20 slices)
300g (10½oz) peas

VITAMIN B₂ (RIBOFLAVIN): 1.5mg
0.9 litres (1½ pints) milk
35g (1¼oz) liver (1 small piece)
300g (10½oz) cheese
600g (21¼oz) beef (5 helpings)
300g (10½oz) eggs (6 standard eggs)
100g (3½oz) breakfast cereal (4-5 bowls)
14g (½oz) yeast extract (enough for 5 slices of bread)
350g (12½oz) mushrooms (13 portions – raw)
75g (2¾oz) kidney (2½ lamb's kidneys)

NIACIN: 18mg
200g (7oz) beef (2 small portions)
2kg (4½lb) potatoes (22 medium potatoes)
1kg (2¼lb) wholemeal bread (36 slices)
200g (7oz) chicken (2 small portions)
64g (2¼oz) instant coffee (enough for 21 cups)
300g (10½oz) white fish (3 small portions)
800g (1lb 12½oz) white bread (29 slices)
85g (3oz) peanuts (3 handfuls)

FOLATE: 300mg
110g (3¾oz) cooked liver
300g (10½oz) cooked broccoli (1 small portion)
210g (7½oz) cooked spinach (3 large portions)
1½kg (3¼lbs) peeled bananas (10 medium)
800g (29oz) peeled oranges (8 medium)
770g (1¾lb) wholemeal bread (27½ slices)
270g (9½oz) peanuts (9½ handfuls)

VITAMIN C: 30mg
330g (11¾oz) new boiled potatoes (6 medium)
600g (21¼oz) old boiled potatoes (10 medium)
15g (½oz) blackcurrants (1 dessertspoonful)
30g (1oz) green peppers
60g (2oz) oranges (½ peeled)
150g (5¼oz) boiled cauliflower or cabbage (2 portions)
50g (1¾oz) raw cauliflower or cabbage (2-3 salad-sized portions)
300-600g (10½-21¼oz) apples (amount depends on variety and most vitamin C is
in the peel) (3-6 medium)

VITAMIN D: 10 microgs, if little access to sunlight
5g (1 teaspoon) fish liver oils
125g (4½oz) margarine (enough for 18 slices of bread)
125g (4½oz) canned sardines (10 medium-sized sardines)
180g (6½oz) canned tuna (3 portions)
550g (19½oz) eggs (11 standard eggs)
2kg (4½lb) liver (22 portions)
80g (2¾oz) canned salmon (1½ portions)

CALCIUM: 500mg
0.56 litres (3 glasses or nearly 1pt) milk
250g (9oz) plain yoghurt (1⅔ small cartons)
500g (18oz) white bread (18 slices)
1kg (2¼lb) wholemeal bread (36 slices)
65g (2¼oz) Cheddar cheese
90g (3¼oz) canned sardines if bones are eaten (7 medium sardines)
880g (2lb) cabbage (10 large portions)
800g (28¼oz) peanuts (27 handfuls)
220g (3¾oz) watercress
2 litres (3½pts) unboiled hard water

IRON: 10-12mg
530g (19oz) beef (9 portions)
125g (4½oz) liver (1½ portions)
2kg (4½lb) white fish or chicken (16 portions)
300g (10½oz) dried apricots (10 portions)
40g (1½oz) curry powder (8 teaspoons)
500g (18oz) chocolate (2×½lb slabs)
250g (9oz) soy sauce (17 tablespoons)
1½ litres (2½pts) red wine
3kg (6¾lb) potatoes
160g (5¾oz) kidney (5 lamb's kidneys)
850g (1lb 14oz) baked beans (2 large cans)

—SPECIAL DIET SUPPLEMENTS—

There is an astonishing range of diet supplements available commercially, ranging from the familiar vitamins and minerals to very unusual and exotic extracts of roots, seeds, etc., most of which are of dubious value. Taking a diet supplement implies either a belief that one's diet is deficient in some way or a belief that the supplement will have some special effect on the body (rather like taking a "tonic"). Supplements may be taken under the guidance of a practitioner of alternative or complementary medicine, such as an osteopath, a naturopath or the American equivalent, known as a "clinical nutritionist", a term that is becoming more widespread in the UK. This term should not be confused with other nutritionists, not normally described as clinical nutritionists, who rarely see patients and who are mainly research workers in universities and related organizations. Nutritionally qualified

> *Most food supplements on sale are probably harmless whether they do any good or not provided the instructions are followed and they are taken for only short periods. Taking "pot luck" in this way may not be any more silly than reading a horoscope, providing commonsense is not thrown out of the window.*

people who do have patients are dietitians and medically qualified doctors, in which case it is as dietitians and doctors that they normally describe themselves.

"Clinical nutritionists", on the other hand, may also describe themselves as practitioners of orthomolecular medicine or nutritional medicine and they may not necessarily be medically qualified. They are concerned with nutritional deficiencies caused by our modern environment and by modern methods of growing and preparing food. Their method of treatment invariably involves nutritional supplements.

So to whom does the lay person go if he or she suspects they have a health problem with an underlying nutritional cause? GPs are not trained in nutrition and may not be interested in it. They can refer patients to a dietitian at a hospital, but there are not that many dietitians and they are usually fully occupied looking after obese patients, patients with kidney diseases, diabetes and so on. Having drawn a blank with conventional medicine, some people may investigate remedies such as food supplements available from health food shops or at a chemist's. Most food supplements on sale are probably harmless whether they do any good or not provided the instructions are followed and they are taken for only short periods. Taking "pot luck" in this way may not be any more silly than reading a horoscope, providing commonsense is not thrown out of the window.

Nutritional supplements, often in the form of a multivitamin and mineral supplement, are usually bought for three reasons. First, for "insurance" purposes, so that the user knows he has taken at least the recommended intake. Second, larger quantities of supplements may be taken in the belief that they will help counteract stress – whether caused by work, emotional problems or bad habits like smoking, alcohol, too much coffee, etc. Third, and most controversial, very large doses of vitamins may be taken for their therapeutic or pharmacological action in treating or preventing diseases like heart disease, cancer, arthritis and so on. This last use of megadoses of vitamins, where the dose may be 10-100 times the physiological dose, is highly debatable.

Those who practise alternative or complementary medicine claim that their various therapies have been used successfully at one time or another and that the results have been published in medical and scientific journals. They point out, too, that if the patient feels better, this alone is justification. To be fair, a similar approach has also been used by less scientifically minded members of the orthodox medical profession who would probably acknowledge that faith in the physician has a very important role to play in any treatment.

However, much of medicine today – which includes nutrition – does undergo thorough research, which involves running a gamut of testing, retesting and criticism in order to expose any holes or flaws in the scientific method or argument. If the research "proves" itself, it then becomes part of the accepted body of evidence. A true scientist should not accept answers from an experiment as valid unless the results can be repeated at least once under similarly rigorous testing procedures. On the other hand, many of the therapies advocated by alternative or complementary practitioners (as indeed, it must be said, some of those offered by conventional medicine) have not undergone such rigorous scientific testing to prove their safety and their efficacy.

For these reasons nutrition scientists get somewhat irritated when they sometimes see out-of-date theories and the results of inadequate research being promoted as "fact". More seriously, orthodox doctors and dietitians have had to cope with the consequences of some highly dangerous "diets" and fads, which have been promoted quite irresponsibly.

A liquid protein diet combined with fasting was believed to have caused at least sixty deaths in the USA in the late 1970s, and a number of other slimming regimes have been equally criticized for advocating very unbalanced diets. Doctors may also genuinely fear that some seriously ill patients – such as cancer victims – may be playing Russian roulette if, by seeking alternative therapies, they end up rejecting conventional treatment.

For example, a liquid protein diet combined with fasting was believed to have caused at least sixty deaths in the USA in the late 1970s, and a number of other slimming regimes have been equally criticized for advocating very unbalanced diets. Doctors may also genuinely fear that some seriously ill patients – such as cancer victims – may be playing Russian roulette if, by seeking alternative therapies, they end up rejecting conventional treatment.

Unfortunately it is the patient who often has to try to resolve these differences of opinion if he or she feels that alternative therapies are worth a try. Many of those who practise alternative – or as they would prefer to call it complementary – medicines point out that their methods can be followed alongside orthodox treatments. But as many patients have discovered, few GPs, and even fewer hospital doctors, share such liberal views. When confronted with a sceptic, the patient may not tell the doctor what other treatments he or she is taking. But if the doctor is not told, for example, that large doses of vitamins or other nutritional supplements are being taken or that radical adjustments have been made to the diet and for what reason, an important clue in the diagnosis may be missed.

RELATING MEASUREMENTS OF NUTRIENTS IN THE BODY TO HEALTH

Logically, any dietary supplements should be tailored to any individual's needs. However, finding out just what these are is difficult.

Taking blood samples in order to measure the amount of nutrients present is the commonest method of assessing nutritional status, but interpreting these blood tests can be difficult as it is all too easy to have false positives and negatives. If only one sample of blood is taken, the blood level of certain nutrients may simply reveal what a person has recently taken in from food, rather than reflecting the state of the stores in the body. Blood tests are therefore more often used as a follow-up to confirm a diagnosis made as a result of a clinical examination.

In recent years, hair analysis has been suggested as a way of measuring nutritional status. But it is not much used in conventional medicine as the mineral com-

In the meantime, the art of hair analysis as offered by commercial organizations is crude and unreliable. In a survey reported by the American Medical Association, identical samples of hair from two healthy teenagers were sent to 13 commercial laboratories with the result that the same sample of hair was classified as low, normal or high on more than half the minerals analysed.

position of hair is easily affected by shampoos and its slow rate of growth makes hair a clumsy tool. However, since a sample of hair is so much easier and safer to get than a sample of blood, hair analysis is a possibility that is being explored by biochemists. In the meantime, the art of hair analysis as offered by commercial organizations is crude and unreliable. In a survey reported by the American Medical Association, identical samples of hair from two healthy teenagers were sent to thirteen commercial laboratories with the result that the same sample of hair was classified as low, normal or high on more than half the minerals analysed. In some cases the same laboratory gave two different interpretations on the same sample of hair that had been submitted twice under different names!

Anyone who is tempted to take larger than recommended doses of vitamins for long periods really needs expert guidance. If you cannot get a doctor to advise you and you want to find a practitioner of alternative medicine, then try to choose one who is registered with some overseeing body (such as the British Naturopathic Osteopathic Association), which is responsible for organizing training and maintaining standards. Failing this, at least seek the advice of a qualified pharmacist at a chemist as he or she will know where to find information about the side-effects of drugs, including vitamin supplements and the like.

As far as possible, extra vitamins and other dietary supplements should come from an improved diet. Finally, remember that vitamin supplements and tonics – like all medicines – should be kept out of reach of children who could easily consume toxic doses if the pills get eaten like sweets.

THE EVOLUTION OF TODAY'S WESTERN DIET

Homo sapiens has probably been around for about half a million years. During this time man has made a massive impact on his environment. We have only to compare the kind of world we live in now with that obtaining 10,000 years, 1,000 years, 100 years or even 10 years ago. But several hundred thousand years is only a very short

Remember that vitamin supplements and tonics – like all medicines – should be kept out of reach of children who could easily consume toxic doses if the pills get eaten like sweets.

period in evolutionary terms and not long enough for man's basic anatomy and physiology to have changed very dramatically. Because man is probably biologically much the same now as he was half a million years ago, it is useful to look at the sort of diet he has eaten for about 99 per cent of his time on earth in order to compare it with what we eat today. Throughout this time man lived by hunting and gathering – as a very few, and rapidly dwindling, aboriginal societies still do today. For the remaining 1 per cent of his time he has been a farmer growing most of his own food and in the last 0.00001 per cent of his history, man in Western societies has been living in cities.

The diets attributed to early man have ranged from the exclusively vegetarian to predominantly meat-eating. The debate about man's early diet is not simply of historical interest; it has coloured attitudes to such matters as the importance of meat in the diet, the significance of refined versus unprocessed foods and the whole question of the role of diet in disease.

> *These ape-like ancestors of ours who were alive between 10 and 15 million years ago possessed a remarkable ability to chew. Unlike modern chimpanzees and gorillas, who can only chomp up and down, they were able to chew food round and round – a much more efficient process.*

So far, archaeological evidence in the last twenty years or so has revealed that we previously had a rather chauvinistic and "macho" picture of our forebears. Maybe it suited our self-image to imagine them as highly organized hunters who invented weapons and dominated the animal kingdom. However the image that is now emerging from the archaeological evidence is rather less romantic.

THE DIET OF THE FIRST FEW MILLION YEARS

In order to understand the sort of diet man has eaten for most of his time on earth, we need to look at the creatures from which man developed. The primates from which man evolved were small, weak animals who lived in the woods and grasslands. Fossil remains of the teeth of these creatures show that they were scratched and worn down by a diet of coarse, fibrous foods like roots, tubers and seeds. These ape-like ancestors of ours who were alive between 10 and 15 million years ago possessed a remarkable ability to chew. Unlike modern chimpanzees and gorillas, who can only chomp up and down, they were able to chew food round and round – a much more efficient process. From this remote ancestor developed modern apes and ape-man known as *Australopithecus*. He was able to stand upright and was about the same size as a modern eight-year-old.

The fossil evidence also shows that rather than being a sophisticated, aggressive hunter it was often *Australopithecus* who was hunted – the quarry of leopards and other carnivorous animals. He was able to survive because he was intelligent enough to learn how to keep out of the way and because his unspecialized, and hence primitive, biology enabled him to live on a variety of different foods in different habitats. As far as we can tell, he lived the life of a scavenger eating whatever he could lay his hands on most easily. This no doubt included some meat – maybe from the remains of a carnivore's kill or as a result of catching a young or weak animal that strayed from the herd – but the amount of meat was probably small. The bulk of his diet seems to have been made up of nuts, berries, leaves and fruits as well as grasses, seeds, roots and tubers which he could pull or dig from the ground with the help of a sharp stick or bone. This ability to survive on such a wide variety of foods is one of the keys to man's evolutionary success.

──*THE DIET OF EARLY MAN*──

Much of the interpretation of the fossil evidence has depended on what is known about today's hunter-gatherers. These societies actually do much more gathering than hunting. For example, anthropologists studying the traditional Hadza of Tanzania found that they depended for the bulk of their food supply on the activities of the women who daily gathered nuts, berries, seeds, tubers, fruit, fungi, insects and grubs. While the womenfolk were so industriously employed, the men spent their time gambling for arrows, pipes to smoke and other trade goods at the same time as planning and discussing a future hunt. There is no reason to believe that these societies were always on the brink of starvation; indeed, they have been described as the "original affluent society". All in all, a nutritional profile of the diet that man has eaten during most of his evolutionary span would suggest that he was used to much larger quantities of fibrous foods than we eat today. He may well have had a much larger intake of certain vitamins and minerals from his predominantly vegetable diet. The greater proportion of protein in the diet would have come from vegetable rather than from animal sources, and he is likely to have had a much less fatty diet than we have today since wild animals are leaner than domesticated species and the fibrous matter of oily plants and nuts would have prevented a large intake of oils from this source. Although there would have been some sugars from fruits and honey, the diet would have been much less sugary than it is today. We have no real way of telling how much salt was in the diet, but societies that lived by the coast might well have used some sea water for cooking.

──*SHOULD WE ALL EAT A STONE-AGE DIET?*──

Interestingly, many of the current dietary recommendations, such as eating less fat and sugar and more unrefined foods, are in the direction of man's "stone-age" diet. However, it would be a mistake to assume that a "back-to-nature" diet would be the answer to all man's dietary ills. For a start, one of man's evolutionary advantages has been his ability to adapt and survive on almost whatever food is available. Second, we no longer lead the active lives of hunter-gatherers and, third, archaeological evidence tells us very little about how healthy our forebears were. We know they were smaller than us and this may well have been due to fewer calories – it is very easy to get bored with chewing quantities of fibrous food, however plentiful the supply. We do not know what they suffered in the way of digestive troubles and other more serious diseases as twenty to thirty years was not an uncommon life span. The privilege of living to a ripe old age is one of the advantages of living in a society in which there are others who are younger and stronger to look after the weak and the old.

──*THE ADVENT OF FARMING*──

The first big change in man's diet started about 10,000 years ago with the advent of farming and the establishing of permanent settlements. No doubt before that time there had begun the gradual domestication of animals and plants as some hunter-gatherers found a less nomadic existence was to their advantage in certain parts of the world. Eventually areas of particularly good fertility – notably those surrounding river deltas in the even climate of the Eastern Mediterranean – made it more sensible to stay in one place. Settled farming enabled people to develop the selective breeding of both plants and animals so that by about 5,000 BC the familiar wheat, oats, rye, maize, pigs, cows and sheep that we know today had developed.

> *Evidence and records from Egyptian times show that the diseases of affluence had already begun then. Among the rich obesity, arteriosclerosis, gallstones, dental caries, gout and diabetes were all known – as was drunkenness.*

Evidence and records from Egyptian times show that the diseases of affluence had already begun then. Among the rich obesity, arteriosclerosis, gallstones, dental caries, gout and diabetes were all known – as was drunkenness. The diet was still an extremely fibrous one as the state of their teeth reveals. The poor ate a reasonable variety of foods but were still liable to some nutritional deficiencies as a result of common chronic infestations with worms and other parasites, or because of famine as a result of occasional droughts.

Similar disparities between the diets and health of the rich and the poor have continued throughout history, with populations suffering the excesses of the wealthy side by side with the deprivations of the poor.

THE INDUSTRIAL ERA

Farming was the way of life for the majority of people – as it still is in many parts of the world – until the Industrial Revolution in the West in the 19th century. The subsequent urbanization and huge population growth caused another major change in the sort of foods people ate.

In the last hundred years or so the majority of people in the West have changed from growing and preparing their own food to eating a diet in which about three-quarters of the food they eat is grown in many different parts of the world and transported and prepared for them by, what is now, a highly specialized and sophisticated food industry.

Between 1801 and 1891 the number of people living in rural areas in Britain rose from 6½ million to just over 9 million. But this was nothing compared with the expansion in the towns from 2¼ million to almost 20 million. And in the hundred years or so since then the population has again more than doubled to 55 million.

The 19th century saw the increasing importance of food imports. No longer were there just a few spices, coffee, tea, sugar and exotic fruit – like oranges from the East – for the wealthy, but increasingly large quantities of staple cereals

> *In the last hundred years or so the majority of people in the West have changed from growing and preparing their own food to eating a diet in which about three-quarters of the food they eat is grown in many different parts of the world and transported and prepared for them by, what is now, a highly specialized and sophisticated food industry.*

THE AVERAGE DAILY CONSUMPTION BY AN ADULT OF SOME FOODS OVER THE LAST HUNDRED YEARS OR SO

	Bread	Sugar	Potatoes*
1860 Farm labourer	27 slices	6tsp (36ml)	5 small
1900 Working class	15 slices	12tsp (72ml)	2 small
1930s Low income	9½ slices	19tsp (114ml)	4 small
1944 Wartime rationing	8½ slices	7tsp (42ml)	5 small
1960 Average	6½ slices	14½tsp (87ml)	4 small
1980 Average	4½ slices	9tsp (54ml)	3 small

*does not include processed products

[1]Although the absolute amounts of fats have not increased much this century, their proportion in the diet has gone up considerably as bread has gone down.

such as wheat from across the Atlantic. Instead of spending most of their time growing their own crops, the poor worked for wages and spent about three-quarters of their income on food. Since then the proportion of money spent on food has gone down considerably and now accounts, on average, for 15-25 per cent of disposable income in the UK.

By the end of the 19th century people living in towns were crowded together in cramped living conditions. The landlords who owned the properties often did away with kitchens in order to reduce the risk of fire and provide more sleeping space. This meant that most people had to rely on cook-houses, bakeries and coster-mongers for the provision and preparation of their daily food. Costermongers were the original fast-food vendors with their eels, baked apples, meat pies, whitebait, milk, oranges, strawberries, pie and mash, and buns. The cities were also the place where drunkenness was a perpetual problem.

Cooking thus became a skill that was easily forgotten through lack of practice, and what cooking there was increasingly became of the more plain and simple sort. Staple foods like bread and potatoes were still the most important items of the diet, although from 1880 they began their decline as its major items. At the turn of the century one social reformer noted that for many poor families potatoes were an invariable item of the diet. If money was short, there might be no greens or butter and hardly any meat before potatoes were affected. When there was no money even for potatoes then dinner would consist of suet pudding and treacle. Alcohol was also a substitute for food because of the sense of well-being it gave "as after a good meal".

Since then, as wealth has increased, food habits have continued to change but more and more as a result of personal choice. People are now not only free of the

Milk	Meat	Fats[1]	Alcohol[2]
¼ pint (0.14 litre)	3 slices	¾oz (20g) dripping	1½ pints (0.85 litre) ale
⅕ pint (0.11 litre)	4½ slices	¾oz (20g) butter	2½ pints (1.42 litre) beer or 5 gins
¼ pint (0.14 litre)	4½ slices	1½oz (43g) margarine	1¼ pints (0.71 litre) beer
½-⅔ pint (0.38 litre)[3]	6 slices	1¼oz (35g) butter or margarine	1 pint (0.57 litre) beer
½ pint (0.28 litre)	7½ slices	1¾oz (50g) butter	1½ pints (0.85 litre) beer
½ pint (0.28 litre)	8 slices	1⅓oz (38g) butter or margarine	2½ pints (1.42 litre) beer or 5 glasses wine

[2]Cigarettes have increasingly used up some of the money spent on alcohol.
[3]The Welfare Foods Scheme, started during World War II, boosted the consumption of milk.

fear of crop failures but they no longer have to rely either on what is grown in this country or on the seasons. If we want to, we can eat tomatoes and bananas all the year round. But freedom of choice bears its own problems for we are also in a position to live on a diet of crisps and ice cream if that is what we choose.

Inevitably such a wide choice can lead to excesses, like a child let loose in a sweet shop, and history may well show that the 1960s were a peak period of self-indulgence. In the 1960s people ate as much as they could afford of the foods they liked, such as meat, sugar, butter and cream, and spurned the plain – and supposedly fattening – bread and potato, unless it happened to be made into interesting shapes and highly flavoured snacks such as chips and crisps. By the mid-1970s, one social historian was commenting that foods were increasingly being divided into two categories: those that were healthy and those that were just for fun. In both instances people had very different standards: in the case of the former people were demanding more quality and purity; in the latter they asked only that they be fun to look at, as well as having a nice taste and a good image.

The 1980s are seeing another change in consumer expectations as health considerations influence the sort of foods produced. Low fat, low sugar, low salt and high fibre foods and those free of additives are increasingly being found on the supermarket shelves alongside the old familiar highly coloured, salty, fatty and sugary alternatives. The 1980s are also a time of mass unemployment. How-

By the mid-1970s, one social historian was commenting that foods were increasingly being divided into two categories: those that were healthy and those that were just for fun.

ever, despite this poverty which brings its own problems, people in this country are still relatively affluent compared with those in the newly emerging industrial nations in other parts of the world. In the Third World the people are now experiencing the population changes the West went through in the last century, together with the problems of drought and famine brought about by a combination of natural, environmental and political upheavals.

In the UK today the main problems remain those of excess and of eating the wrong kind of diet. The move towards healthy eating has still a very long way to go, and Britain's naturally cautious attitude towards new ideas makes the UK slower to respond to the advice and warnings of nutritionists than many other Western countries.

CHAPTER 3

THE DIGESTIVE SYSTEM

D igestion is the process by which food is chemically broken down into its basic components which are small enough to pass through the lining of the intestine, carried in the blood to the liver and reassembled as needed. Before food can be broken down chemically, it must first be broken down into smaller lumps – beginning in the mouth.

—THE MOUTH—

When food or drink is taken into the mouth it is tasted by about 3,000 tastebuds – on the tongue, palate, back of the mouth, throat and tonsils. The tastebuds can detect four sensations: sweet and salt on the tip of the tongue, sourness or acidity at the sides and bitterness at the back.

The digestive process starts in the mouth when saliva mixes with the food or drink. The amount of saliva that is released depends on a number of things. For example, the more chewing a food needs, the more saliva will be secreted, and smelling or anticipating food helps the mouth to "water".

The main functions of saliva are to help lubricate the food so that it can be swallowed, and then to help clear the mouth of any remaining food by washing it out from the crevices between the teeth and neutralizing any of the acids that are produced as a result of the action of bacteria on the trapped food (see pages 24-5).

Saliva is nature's mouth rinse. But, as we saw in Chapter 1, it has a particularly difficult job with the sort of diet most people eat nowadays.

Saliva also plays an important role in our sense of taste. A reduced flow of saliva is probably the main reason why elderly people complain that food "doesn't taste as it used to". Ill-fitting dentures prevent proper chewing and this in turn slows down the saliva flow. Much of the pleasure of food depends on anticipation of good food, followed by leisurely, thorough chewing.

Saliva also starts the chemical diges-

> *A reduced flow of saliva is probably the main reason why elderly people complain that food "doesn't taste as it used to". Ill-fitting dentures prevent proper chewing and this in turn slows down the saliva flow. Much of the pleasure of food depends on anticipation of good food, followed by leisurely, thorough chewing.*

tion of food – though in a small way. It contains an enzyme ptyalin which starts the process of breaking down starch to sugar.

——THE OESOPHAGUS——

After swallowing, the food or drink is quickly squeezed down a long, hollow tube of muscle, called the oesophagus, by a series of rapid muscle contractions and relaxations, until it is pushed into the stomach. It takes about three seconds for each mouthful of food to reach the stomach after swallowing.

——THE STOMACH——

The stomach is a muscular bag which initially stores all the swallowed food. In the stomach the food is steadily churned and mixed with juices that give it a consistency of liquid porridge. The stomach acids or gastric juices are stimulated to flow in the same way as saliva. About 5 pints (3 litres) of this acid – which is sufficiently powerful to burn a hole in a carpet – are produced each day. The stomach has three main functions:
1. To bathe the food or drink in acid. This kills off many of the bacteria present in food and water.
2. To act as a storehouse for food. Food normally stays in the stomach for 2-4 hours.
3. To pass a steady flow of food into the small intestine where digestion principally takes place.

In this way the stomach liquidizes food, cleanses it and enables digestion to proceed at a fairly steady pace, despite the irregular nature of food consumption. However, although the stomach is of considerable help in aiding a smooth digestive process, it is not essential, which is why people can survive and still eat a relatively normal diet even after the stomach has been removed – for example in the treatment of gastric cancer!

Although most of the digestive processes are performed in the intestines, the breakdown of protein starts in the stomach with the action of an enzyme called pepsin found in the gastric juice. This juice also contains a substance called "intrinsic factor", which is needed to combine with vitamin B_{12} so that it can be absorbed later on. The stomach can also absorb small quantities of a few substances such as water, aspirin and alcohol.

The churning action of the stomach is caused by regular wave-like contractions of the muscle wall. When the stomach has recently been emptied of food, the contractions are very weak. As hunger develops they increase in intensity (sometimes making themselves heard as tummy rumbles) and then gradually calm down as food is eaten.

——THE SMALL INTESTINE——

The duodenum is at the upper end of another long tube of muscle called the small intestine. This section of the gut is 1-1½in (2-4cm) in diameter and about 10ft (3m) long. It is not a smooth tube but is highly corrugated with hair-like projections called "villi", making the total surface area somewhere between 215 and 430 sq ft (20-40 sq m) – the area covered by the floor of a large room.

In the duodenum more digestive juices are poured on to the food mixture, turning the porridge mixture into a soup. This soup gradually spreads out to cover the whole area of the intestine and the components of food are gradually separated and absorbed, like items off a conveyor belt.

This section of the gut is 1-1½in (2-4cm) in diameter and about 10ft (3m) long. It is not a smooth tube but is highly corrugated with hair-like projections called "villi", making the total surface area somewhere between 215 and 430 sq ft (20-40 sq m) – the area covered by the floor of a large room.

Three kinds of juice are mixed with the soup – bile from the liver, pancreatic juice from the pancreas and intestinal juice from the walls of the intestine. Bile acts like a detergent, enabling fat to combine with water so that it can be absorbed through the gut wall. The other two juices provide the enzymes that break down the fats, proteins and carbohydrates in food into smaller units, namely fatty acids, peptides (protein units) and disaccharides (two sugar units coupled together), which can then be absorbed through the gut wall. Human beings have a very comprehensive enzyme system. Because man is an omnivore, which means he is able to eat something from almost all types of food, he has a corresponding variety of enzymes to cope with his wide-ranging diet. Several enzymes are triggered into production only when they are needed. For example, the enzyme sucrase is produced only when sugar (sucrose) is part of a meal. A few enzymes, such as lactase, which digests lactose or milk sugar, will disappear unless they are regularly activated by the presence of milk in the diet. Very occasionally, a baby is born with an inability to manufacture a particular enzyme, which then means he or she has to be put on a special diet that excludes the food that cannot be digested.

Once these smaller units are absorbed through the gut wall, they are broken down still further by other enzymes. Peptides are broken down to amino acids and disaccharides down to the simplest sugar of all – glucose. These units are then carried in the bloodstream to the liver where the process of building them up into human tissue begins. In this way the proteins, fats and carbohydrates, which in different combinations make up the foods we eat, are broken down and absorbed in the fully developed digestive system of the adult.

Babies, on the other hand, are born with an immature digestive system. In the first few days after birth a baby's intestine can absorb whole proteins without destroying them in the course of digestion. In this way it is able to absorb valuable antibodies, which are made of protein, from the early form of breastmilk called colostrum. By the same token it is therefore also vulnerable to foreign proteins like those in ordinary cow's milk. For this reason it is thought that allergies can be triggered off in babies if they are fed unmodified cow's milk or are given certain protein-containing solids, such as

Bile acts like a detergent, enabling fat to combine with water so that it can be absorbed through the gut wall.

wheat cereals, too early. Because a baby's digestive system takes many weeks to develop, care has to be taken when introducing solids to babies under six months.

——THE LARGE INTESTINE——

Once the liquid mixture has been propelled through the small intestine and so gradually denuded of most of its nutrients, it passes into the colon or large intestine. This is about twice the width of the small intestine but only 3ft (1m) long.

The colon is inhabited by a large quantity of bacteria and for this reason the faeces are "dirty" and a potential source of disease once they come into contact with the outside world. But the bacteria do have an important function as they can synthesize vitamin K. In all, food takes about 12 hours from the time it is swallowed to reach the colon. Once in the colon, large quantities of water are absorbed back into the body so that the liquid mixture is able to solidify into a mass – the faeces. Faeces are about three-quarters water with variable amounts of gas (it is most probably the gas rather than variations in the water content that determines the softness of the stools). The remaining quarter is made up of bacteria, dead cells rubbed off from the internal surface of the colon and a little undigested food.

Once in the colon, the contents may take anything from another few hours to several days before they are excreted. The length of time it takes food to pass through the body is called transit time – and it is transit time that is thought to be principally affected by fibre. Very roughly, the more fibre in the diet, the shorter the time it takes for the contents of the colon to pass through. Faeces that are passed through quickly as a result of the presence of good-sized quantities of fibre are generally softer and more plentiful. The average person in the UK passes 3-6oz (80-160g) of faeces a day and an average vegetarian in the UK passes 8oz (225g). In parts of the world where fibre intakes are more than 10 times that of the UK, 1lb (0.5kg) of faeces are passed each day (five times the amount in the UK). At the moment the mechanical effects of fibre are thought to benefit the overall health of the large gut. Fibre is also believed to encourage digestion to take place throughout the whole length of the small intestine rather than concentrating it all at the top end of the gut as happens on a bland, low fibre diet.

——THE LIVER——

Although human beings can cope without the stomach, pancreas, gall bladder, colon and half the small intestine, they cannot survive without the liver. The liver is the place where all nutrients absorbed from digestion are first taken to. It is the largest gland in the body and in the adult weighs 3-4lb (1.3-1.8kg). When the body is at rest about a quarter of the blood supply lies in the liver.

> *The colon is inhabited by a large quantity of bacteria and for this reason the faeces are "dirty" and a potential source of disease once they come into contact with the outside world.*

The liver does a multitude of things and is responsible for about a quarter of the body's metabolic activity, of which the most urgent is keeping a steady concentration of glucose in the blood. Glucose is one of the two principal sources of energy from food, and a continuous supply of glucose is needed to keep the brain working. The liver has the responsibility for maintaining this supply of glucose. If necessary, it will break down protein – even breaking down the body's own muscle tissue – in order to supply the vital glucose needed by the brain.

In the liver, proteins, fat and glucose stores called glycogen are built up and many toxins – such as alcohol and drugs – are broken down while others are made.

The liver also produces bile. Bile performs two principal functions: first, it is a means by which old, worn-out blood cells are excreted and second, it contains bile acids, which emulsify fats so that they can dissolve and so pass into the bloodstream. About a pint (0.5 litre) of bile is produced each day. Most of it is discharged directly into the small intestine, but a small quantity is stored in the gall bladder – a small bag attached to the underside of the liver.

——*THE GALL BLADDER*——

Bile in the gall bladder is concentrated a little and, in the course of this process, deposits of cholesterol, blood pigments and bile salts may form. These solid materials may crystallize together to form lumps anything from the size of gravel to the size of a hen's egg. Gallstones are very common but by no means all cause problems. These occur when a stone rises up and blocks the neck of the gall bladder so that the bile cannot get out.

——*THE PANCREAS*——

The pancreas is an offshoot of the intestine and is the main source for the supply of digestive juices to the small intestine. These digestive juices contain a number of enzymes which help in the breakdown of fat, protein and carbohydrate. Apart from its role in digestion, the pancreas is also important for the manufacture of insulin and other hormones necessary for keeping the amount of glucose in the blood at a steady level.

——*THE KIDNEYS*——

Although not strictly part of the digestive system, the kidneys perform a number of functions which are of particular relevance to diet and health.

They regulate the amounts of water and the minerals sodium, potassium, calcium, chloride and phosphate that are present in the body fluids. They also are the principal route by which the waste breakdown products of proteins are passed out of the body, via the urine.

The average amount of urine produced by the kidneys each day is 3 pints (1.5 litres) but they are able to produce as little as 1 pint (0.5 litres) and as much as 35 pints (20 litres). The kidneys can not only alter the volume but also the concentration of the urine, as they excrete more of those elements that are surplus and reabsorb those that are in short supply. It is also the kidneys that make the active form of vitamin D from substances that are initially synthesized by the action of sunlight on the skin.

———INDIGESTION———

Indigestion is one of those all-embracing terms that can mean different things to different people. A food may be indigestible in the way that some people (and particularly small children who don't always chew food properly) can pass out sweetcorn and certain other foods in almost the same form as they went in. This does not necessarily, or even usually, give rise to discomfort. Fibre in food is indigestible too but rather than being considered a disadvantage, it is thought to be very important in maintaining gut health.

Indigestion can arise at any point in the gastrointestinal tract and includes heartburn, discomfort or pain in the stomach or gut, flatulence or nausea, which occurs as a result of eating food. Sometimes indigestion can be a sign of more serious conditions such as a gastric ulcer or gall bladder disease, but usually it is due to some interference with the normal working of the stomach. Bolting food, overeating, larger amounts of fat or fibre than usual, heavy smoking, too much alcohol or stress, particularly at mealtimes, can all cause bouts of indigestion. The best way to prevent occasional bouts of indigestion is to eat meals at regular times in a calm, unhurried atmosphere, which allows plenty of time for careful chewing. Some foods and drinks are particularly liable to bring on bouts of indigestion. These are listed below:

1. Alcohol, cola drinks, strong tea and coffee.
2. Hot, spicy foods such as pickles and curries and heavily salted foods.
3. Fried foods and gravy made with fat.
4. Tough, over-cooked meats and sausages.
5. Fatty fish.
6. Newly baked bread, wholemeal bread, pastry and fruit cake.
7. Rich, heavy puddings.
8. Excessive quantities of sugar or sweets.
9. Unripe fruit, dried fruits, nuts and pips, and fruit skin and peel.
10. Raw salad vegetables like celery, onions, cucumber, tomatoes and radishes.

CHAPTER 4

IN HEALTH AND IN SICKNESS

The average life span for someone reaching the age of forty-five in the UK is about seventy-five – a little less for men and a little more for women. As with all averages, there are many who live much longer and many who die well before seventy-five. Health education, contrary to some opinion, is not so much aimed at extending the average life span as at preventing early deaths or disability – particularly those occurring before retirement age – and at maintaining as good health as possible for those who do survive.

Being healthy means different things to different people. For some it may mean simply not being ill and being able to live to an old age. Others want actually to feel fit and some want more than this. They want to be not just "not ill" but positively healthy with feelings of vigour, peace of mind and fulfilment.

Health, therefore, has as much to do with the mind as with the body. It has to do with the relationships you have with other people and the opportunities that can help you to live the kind of life you want to, and the obstacles that may get in the way. Eating habits can have a profound influence on all these aspects of health. What you eat may improve your chances of better health or lessen them; the food you choose may be welcomed by your family and friends or it may cause friction; and what you eat needs to be an important source of enjoyment in your daily life, not an uncomfortable reminder of pleasures forgone.

These and many other factors have to be considered when thinking about making changes to your eating habits. But before a decision is made, you need to start with some basic information about how what you eat affects your health.

—OBESITY—

Most people would agree that overweight is bad for health. However, not all are agreed about how much surplus fat is too much. Teenage girls may drive themselves to distraction if they are even a few ounces above their desired weight; while young men, overweight from too much beer, will assure everyone that they are merely big-boned, if not actually "muscular". (If in doubt, well-developed muscles are hard, whereas fat is soft.) Although gaining a little extra weight as one gets older may be harmless, it can become excessive, though the individual, his family and the family doctor may not always notice it because the weight gain is so gradual. In these circumstances, the patient can find it difficult to see the connection between his excess weight and his general state of health. But with increasing weight goes an increasing severity of chest infections, and a greater the likelihood of developing gallstones, hernias, varicose veins and hypertension. The overweight person also has a greater chance of dying from cancer, accidents such as falls, strokes, heart disease and – most of all – diabetes.

There are times when people are particularly likely to put on weight such as during periods of enforced inactivity, for example after an illness or a change to a more sedentary job; giving up smoking encourages nibbling; and some people find they overeat during periods of anxiety and depression. After pregnancy many women also find it difficult to lose all the extra weight gained. Excess weight can also happen as a result of changes in metabolism, for instance during pregnancy or as a result of the natural slowing down of body metabolism with age. For all these reasons it is a good idea for everyone to weigh themselves once every six months or so in order to check that their weight lies within the acceptable range set out in the charts below.

GUIDELINES FOR BODY WEIGHT

The minimum level for diagnosing obesity is taken as 20 per cent above the upper limit of the acceptable weight range.

METRIC

Height without shoes (m)	Men Weight without clothes (kg) Acceptable average	Acceptable weight range	Obese	Women Weight without clothes (kg) Acceptable average	Acceptable weight range	Obese
1.45				46.0	42–53	64
1.48				46.5	42–54	65
1.50				47.0	43–55	66
1.52				48.5	44–57	68
1.54				49.5	44–58	70
1.56				50.4	45–58	70
1.58	55.8	51–64	77	51.3	46–59	71
1.60	57.6	52–65	78	52.6	48–61	73
1.62	58.6	53–66	79	54.0	49–62	74
1.64	59.6	54–67	80	55.4	50–64	77
1.66	60.6	55–69	83	56.8	51–65	78
1.68	61.7	56–71	85	58.1	52–66	79
1.70	63.5	58–73	88	60.0	53–67	80
1.72	65.0	59–74	89	61.3	55–69	83
1.74	66.5	60–75	90	62.6	56–70	84
1.76	68.0	62–77	92	64.0	58–72	86
1.78	69.4	64–79	95	65.3	59–74	89
1.80	71.0	65–80	96			
1.82	72.6	66–82	98			
1.84	74.2	67–84	101			
1.86	75.8	69–86	103			
1.88	77.6	71–88	106			
1.90	79.3	73–90	108			
1.92	81.0	75–93	112			

(Taken from the Royal College of Physicians Report on Obesity, 1983)

NON-METRIC

Height without shoes (ft,in)	Men Weight without clothes (lb)			Women Weight without clothes (lb)		
	Acceptable average	Acceptable weight range	Obese	Acceptable average	Acceptable weight range	Obese
4 10				102	92-119	143
4 11				104	94-122	146
5 0				107	96-125	150
5 1				110	99-128	152
5 2	123	112-141	169	113	102-131	154
5 3	127	115-144	173	116	105-134	161
5 4	130	118-148	178	120	108-138	166
5 5	133	121-152	182	123	111-142	170
5 6	136	124-156	187	128	114-146	175
5 7	140	128-161	193	132	118-150	180
5 8	145	132-166	199	136	122-154	185
5 9	149	136-170	204	140	126-158	190
5 10	153	140-174	209	144	130-163	196
5 11	158	144-179	215	148	134-168	202
6 0	162	148-184	221	152	138-173	208
6 1	166	152-189	227			
6 2	171	156-194	233			
6 3	176	160-199	239			
6 4	181	164-204	245			

(Taken from the Royal College of Physicians Report on Obesity, 1983)

HABITS NOT DIETS

Slimming can be hard work and there are many commercial organizations and others only too anxious to help slimmers find an "easy" method. Perhaps the most important thing to realize is that there is no reliable quick method of slimming and that the whole concept of "going on a diet" belongs to the past. Unfortunately only a few days, or even weeks, of drastically changing the diet will not produce a long-term cure in the case of those who have more than a few pounds to lose. Indeed, constantly going on and coming off diets can be harmful to health and can cause some people's metabolisms simply to adapt to smaller and smaller intakes of food so that they can survive on less with greater efficiency. Should they revert to their old eating habits their more efficient metabolism will now be able to do the same work using less energy and may end up making them fatter than when they began.

Instead would-be slimmers need to think about making permanent changes to their habits. This means taking exercise if they do little and finding new ways of keeping active once they grow too old for a young person's sport. It also means working out ways of making permanent changes to eating habits, taking particular care to cut down on the empty- and high-calorie foods, like sugars, fats and alcohol. Making changes slowly provides the opportunity to experiment and to enable the slimmer and his family to adapt

Perhaps the most important thing to realize is that there is no reliable quick method of slimming and that the whole concept of "going on a diet" belongs to the past.

75

'*A loss of 2-4lb (0.9-1.8kg) a week for the first two or three weeks and thereafter of 1-2lb (0.45-0.9kg) is an excellent target. This is the equivalent of 500-1,000kcals, less than would normally be eaten each day.*'

gradually. A loss of 2-4lb (0.9-1.8kg) a week for the first two or three weeks and thereafter of 1-2lb (0.45-0.9kg) is an excellent target. This is the equivalent of 500-1,000kcals, less than would normally be eaten each day.

Before going on any slimming programme, each person needs to ask himself or herself just why they are trying to lose weight; what weight they are aiming for; what their success at slimming has been like in the past and if the person who cooks the family meals is going to support them. Those who do their own cooking may need to ask someone else to do the shopping so that they are not tempted into buying foods such as biscuits, cream or snacks, which are often eaten just because they are there but are not missed when they are not available. Sometimes joining a good local slimming club can give the necessary moral support and companionship if the family is not particularly supportive. But if family and friends are not helpful, it is important to find out why. If they realize a slimmer is serious, they may be more prepared to share and help out with the experience rather than criticize the slimmer for being "different".

EXERCISE

Walking for an hour uses up the same number of calories as would be provided by about two slices of bread and butter. This may not seem much, but exercise should not be underestimated in any health or slimming programme. Dieting on its own can be rather depressing and can feel more like a form of self-punishment which deserves a few rewards every now and again. It can become all too easy either to give up or, once the weight target has been reached, to revert to old eating habits and start the whole process of putting on weight again. On the other hand, sensible exercise can do much to encourage a slimmer if it improves morale. It is therefore very important to choose a form of exercise that you enjoy rather than one that may use up more calories but is beyond your capabilities.

Exercise also has other benefits. First, those who are overweight, and so have a heavier body to move, use up more energy for the same amount of activity. Second, after exercising, the metabolic rate is raised for a few hours, so more energy is used up sitting or lying down immediately after exercise than would have been used up before. Third, when exercise is taken after meals, more of the energy in food is converted into heat than into fat.

EXAMPLES OF CALORIES USED UP DURING EXERCISE

Light exercise: 2½-5kcals per minute
Walking
General do-it-yourself such as carpentry, bricklaying, plastering and decorating
Most "exercise" classes
Golf
Bowling
Hatha yoga

Moderate exercise 5 – 7½kcals per minute
Hiking with a backpack
Digging in the garden
Tennis
Ballroom dancing
Cycling up to 10mph

Strenuous exercise 7½-10kcals per minute	*Very strenuous exercise 10kcals or more per minute*
Football	
Modern dance	Swimming lengths
Country dancing	Cross-country running
Swimming	Hill climbing
Jogging	Squash
	Rowing at speed
	Skiing

DRUGS

There are drugs available on prescription that help depress the appetite, but these are not normally prescribed unless a person is severely overweight as they can have unpleasant side-effects. Some may cause sleeplessness, nervousness, a dry mouth, palpitations and a rise in blood pressure and others may cause drowsiness, nightmares and diarrhoea. All are addictive and usually lose their effect after a couple of months.

——CORONARY HEART DISEASE——

Coronary heart disease is the leading cause of death in most Western countries. (The exception is Japan where strokes are the main cause of death.) In most Third World countries coronary heart disease is rare, although it is becoming a problem amongst the well-to-do as they become more and more "Westernized".

In the past in the West, coronary heart disease did occur, but it was uncommon until about 1925. Since then, it has increased steadily and it is still rising in Eastern Europe. In Western Europe coronary heart disease is now static and it is actually declining in the United States and Australia. In Britain 150,000 people die each year from coronary heart disease – which is a quarter of all deaths.

Dying of a heart attack in old age can sound a pretty good way to go, and if people only died of coronaries after they reached retirement age, then there might well be much less concern. However, between the ages of forty-five and sixty-four 1 in every 225 middle-aged men will die of coronary heart disease. When it comes to the figures for heart attacks – and the subsequent worry they frequently engender – the risk of a man having a heart attack before he is sixty can be anywhere between 1 in 16 for a healthy, relatively fit man, to 1 in 3 for an overweight, unfit man eating a bad diet or smoking. Women generally have a much lower risk, but even then, 1 in 50 women in the low-risk category will have a heart attack before they reach sixty and if they smoke and are on the pill at forty the risk increases to 1 in 4.

WHAT HAPPENS

The disease process underlying coronary heart disease is atherosclerosis. In atherosclerosis the walls of the arteries get thicker so that the space within the blood vessels gets narrower. The principal material that accumulates in the arteries is cholesterol. Cholesterol is carried in the blood from the liver where it is made. And the more fat, particularly saturated

In Britain 150,000 people die each year from coronary heart disease – which is a quarter of all deaths.

Even severely underweight people, like those with anorexia nervosa, can often have raised levels of cholesterol in the blood. Thus the kind of diet eaten to lose weight is probably as important as the actual weight loss itself.

fat, in the diet, the more is made. Like all surpluses, what the body does not need it either stores – if it has the facilities – or it tries to get rid of.

When there are large quantities of cholesterol in the blood it cannot all be dealt with and some inevitably will stick anywhere that the blood flow is interrupted. So scars in the arteries and joins where the blood vessels branch off are particularly likely to become silted up with cholesterol. Once patches of deposits occur, these attract yet more deposits so that the arteries get more and more clogged and the blood has a harder and harder job to push its way through an ever-narrowing tube. This process takes years to develop and so heart disease, like high blood pressure, gradually worsens with age if not checked. But not all forms of heart disease are gradual. If the inside of a blood vessel gets so furred up it actually closes, the result is a clot or thrombosis. Thromboses or clots may cause little trouble if they are in a blood vessel where there are plenty of alternative routes for the blood to flow, but if there are no alternative routes then that piece of body tissue will die and if the tissue is heart muscle the result is a heart attack. A furred-up artery, if detected soon enough, can be bypassed by means of surgery.

Thromboses in the veins of the legs or a clot in the lungs – known as a pulmonary embolism – are totally different conditions and are unrelated to heart disease.

DIET TO PREVENT HEART DISEASE

Repairing the damage is never likely to be as effective as preventing it from arising in the first place. It may be too late for middle-aged people to do this, and where the arteries are already likely to be furred up to some extent, the dietary advice needs to be geared towards preventing clots or thromboses from occurring. But it is not too late for young people who can be helped to stop their arteries from becoming clogged up. To some extent the advice is similar in both cases as a low fat diet is important for both prevention and repair.

DIETS TO LOWER PLASMA CHOLESTEROL

In the case of those who are overweight, eating less will often help lower the concentrations of cholesterol, but not always. Even severely underweight people, like those with anorexia nervosa, can often have raised levels of cholesterol in the blood. Thus the kind of diet eaten to lose weight is probably as important as the actual weight loss itself. A low fat diet, particularly one that is low in saturated fat, helps lower blood cholesterol, and eating more of certain types of dietary fibre like pectin and guar found in fruit and pulses respectively can also help to reduce cholesterol. Four portions of vegetables and fruit a day can reduce cholesterol concentrations by about 5 per cent.

Four portions of vegetables and fruit a day can reduce cholesterol concentrations by about 5 per cent.

DIETS TO AVOID THROMBOSES

People who already have coronary heart disease need additional advice aimed both at preventing the formation of a clot (thrombus) and at protecting already weakened heart muscle (the myocardium). Apart from stopping smoking and reducing weight, specialized dietary advice – other than that aimed more generally at lowering blood cholesterol – is not yet very clear. So far it looks as if the fatty acids found in fatty fish like pilchards and mackerel (and cod liver oil) may well help in preventing thrombus formation. And a high fish diet may partly explain why Eskimos eating their traditional diet used to be remarkably free from coronary heart disease, despite eating so many fatty foods. Other polyunsaturated fatty acids, like those found in soya, corn and sunflower oils, seem to have a similar, though much lesser, effect. There may be more foods which exert a protective effect: there have been occasional, isolated reports that foods like onions, garlic and red wine may be protective. At the moment there is not enough evidence to guarantee any specific benefit from these foods, but it seems to be a promising area for research.

A high fish diet may partly explain why Eskimos eating their traditional diet used to be remarkably free from coronary heart disease, despite eating so many fatty foods.

EXERCISE, BODY MINERALS AND HEART ATTACKS

Strenuous exercise has been blamed for causing sudden death from heart attacks. How this occurs is not clear, but it has been suggested that death may be caused by a sudden drop in body minerals brought about by changes in blood chemistry induced by exercise. During unaccustomed, strenuous bouts of exercise the heart muscle can become very short of the minerals potassium and magnesium. When this happens the weakened heart muscle is highly susceptible to injury. Although there is no suggestion that too little potassium or magnesium in the diet causes the deficiency, more potassium and magnesium in the diet may help when the body undergoes the stress of going into a potassium-losing state, such as occurs during and after strenuous exercise.

Exercise is not the only cause of severe losses of body minerals. A heart attack can be brought on in the same way in people who are on diuretics, those suffering prolonged severe diarrhoea, in patients with digestive diseases or in people experiencing starvation. Fats and sugars are virtually devoid of potassium and magnesium, so a diet rich in these foods is less likely to ensure reserve supplies of minerals than a diet of wholegrain foods, potatoes, pulses, meat, fish, fruit and vegetables.

WHAT ABOUT STRESS?

It has been suggested – and many people believe – that stress and strain encourage heart disease. On the whole, medical experts do not believe that stress on its own causes the narrowing of the arteries which underlies coronary disease. On the other hand, once coronary heart disease is established, emotion can trigger off clinical symptoms. So keeping stress under control can be an important way of preventing a coronary crisis. And obviously someone who is unable to relax will find it far harder to give up emotional props, like smoking and comfort foods, or to find time to allow him or herself to take more exercise. Stress undoubtedly can be a

79

If coronary heart disease is to be prevented, it requires a package effort involving giving up smoking, losing weight, eating less fat, eating more wholegrain foods, fruits and vegetables, taking more exercise and in the case of women over the age of thirty-five or so finding an alternative form of contraception to the "pill".

cause of much misery and may make it much more difficult for an individual to look after his or her health. But stress is probably not a direct killer, as it is commonly believed to be; just the last straw on the camel's back.

PREVENTION

It is important to remember that coronary heart disease is not inevitable and much of it is preventable. But there are no short cuts, either from drugs or from eating a single "tonic" food. If coronary heart disease is to be prevented, it requires a package effort involving giving up smoking, losing weight, eating less fat, eating more wholegrain foods, fruits and vegetables, taking more exercise and in the case of women over the age of thirty-five or so finding an alternative form of contraception to the pill.

A SUCCESS STORY

In North Karelia, a part of Finland, which once had the highest death rates from coronary heart disease in the world, the people asked the government to help them improve their health. A community programme was set up in the early 1970s which offered people medical check-ups as well as advising them on their diets and smoking habits. Within a few years the death rate from coronary heart disease had fallen by a quarter in men and halved among women.

——— HIGH BLOOD PRESSURE AND STROKES ———

High blood pressure – known as hypertension – substantially increases the risk of strokes. Strokes occur when the blood circulation to the brain is interfered with. They can be thought of as a "brain attack", caused in the same way as a heart attack, by an interference in the circulation of the blood. Both conditions are brought on by atherosclerosis, or narrowing of the arteries. A stroke may occur either when a weakened artery in the brain tears and bleeds into the surrounding brain tissue, or when a clot blocks an artery, causing a part of the brain to die from lack of oxygen. If high blood pressure can be brought under control, then this will do much to lessen the chances of a stroke.

Unlike coronary heart disease, which predominantly, though not exclusively, affects men, strokes affect men and women almost equally and are second to heart disease as a cause of death in those under sixty.

High blood pressure can be caused by a number of different, but interrelated factors. Although mental or physical stress can cause an immediate rise in blood pressure, the effect is usually only temporary, lasting a matter of hours or so. A persistently raised blood pressure, on the other hand, seems to be mainly caused by three things: heredity, obesity and a high sodium or salt intake. Women on the contraceptive pill are at risk of high blood pressure, too, and heavy drinkers also tend to have higher blood pressures than light drinkers.

Hypertension often runs in families and there is a theory that the enzyme which regulates the balance of sodium and potassium inside and outside the cells may be less effective in these people. It is known that the activity of this enzyme is genetically determined and differs in various ethnic groups. It may be that such people are sensitive to the large intakes of salt that are so characteristic of Western societies. Thin people as well as fat people can suffer from high blood pressure, but it is particularly common in the over-weight and usually falls as the weight goes down; overweight may therefore be a trigger in susceptible people.

> *A persistently raised blood pressure, on the other hand, seems to be mainly caused by three things: heredity, obesity and a high sodium or salt intake.*

Although most Western countries have a high salt intake, many non-industrialized communities do as well. For example, some Pacific islanders cook in sea water and parts of Africa have had plentiful access to salt in the past. However, in communities such as Alaskan Eskimos, some South American Indians and the Kalahari Bushmen of Botswana, which have a very low intake of salt – no more than 2-3g a day – there is no hypertension. As a nation's salt intake increases, so the incidence of hypertension increases proportionately. In northern Japan where the daily salt intake is about 1oz (25g), the number of those with hypertension is 40 per cent of the population.

Although there is a clear link between a nation's average salt intake (the biggest source of sodium in the diet) and the incidence of hypertension, this relationship is not always apparent in the case of individuals. Someone eating the equivalent of 2-3 teaspoons (10-15g) of salt a day does not necessarily have an abnormally raised blood pressure. A few people do show such a relationship and these people often have a family history of hypertension or are overweight.

It has been said that no single advance in community health would improve the quality of life more than the control of hypertension. Hypertension can be treated by drugs, which help by enabling more sodium to be excreted in the urine. Unfortunately these drugs can sometimes cause side-effects such as fatigue and depression. But a diet low in sodium can also have the same beneficial effect on blood pressure. In such cases no salt is allowed to be added at table or in cooking and only low salt foods are permitted. Since many processed foods are highly salted, the patient has to eat a diet of predominantly fresh, home-prepared foods.

In one particular study in Australia, a group of patients with mild hypertension were divided into two lots. All were given drugs to begin with and half were put on a low salt diet. The groups on the low salt diet ended up with more of its members having lower blood pressure and needing less in the way of drugs. This group also reported suffering less depression and needing fewer analgesics than those who had to rely solely on drugs. Another distinct advantage that can be achieved from

> *It has been said that no single advance in community health would improve the quality of life more than the control of hypertension.*

81

In the UK and in North America current estimates of the average salt intake are 9-11g a day. The World Health Organization has recommended that salt intake should be no more than 6g a day – the equivalent of a rounded teaspoon.

a change in diet rather than giving medication is that the whole family is likely to be affected (few cooks like to prepare separate dishes for individual members of the family), and less salt in the diet in early life may well help prevent the children, who may have inherited the susceptibility, from developing hypertension in later life.

In the UK and in North America current estimates of the average salt intake are 9-11g a day. The World Health Organization has recommended that salt intake should be no more than 6g a day – the equivalent of a rounded teaspoon. It may at the same time be beneficial to increase the amounts of potassium-rich foods, as potassium seems to be able slightly to counteract the blood-pressure-raising effect of salt and other sodium-containing substances.

Low to medium sodium foods:
Rice, oats, plain flour (self-raising flour usually contains sodium-based raising agents); matzos and pasta; fruit, vegetables and potatoes; fresh meat, poultry and fish; herbs and spices; salt-free bread, butter, margarine and breakfast cereals; Ricotta cheese and milk.

Moderate to high potassium foods:
Potatoes, vegetables, fresh fruit and tomatoes; dried fruit, nuts and fruit juices; pulses; coffee, beer and wine; milk; oats and bran-based breakfast cereals; fresh meat and fish; treacle.

—BOWEL AND RELATED DISORDERS—

DIVERTICULAR DISEASE

Diverticular disease of the colon did not seem to be known before the beginning of this century. It is a very common bowel disorder in the West, increasing with age and affecting about one in three of those over sixty. It does not necessarily cause trouble so many of those with the disorder may not be aware of it.

In diverticular disease the wall of the colon is considerably thickened and the lining of the colon is caused to balloon out through the wall at intervals. People who experience trouble may have symptoms of pain and constipation or diarrhoea and bleeding. Serious complications can arise if either the balloons or nearby blood vessels burst. It is thought that the disease may arise as a result of too little fibre in the diet causing the colon to work harder – which could explain the increased thickness of the colonic muscle – as it is made to push small, hard faeces.

At one time a diet low in fibre was recommended in the belief that less strain would be put on the colon. In the last ten years or so the treatment has been completely reversed and a high fibre diet, often in the form of supplement of bran, is now the standard medical treatment.

IRRITABLE BOWEL SYNDROME

People suffering from irritable bowel syndrome commonly suffer pain, together with alternating bouts of constipation and diarrhoea. Nobody really knows what causes the disease, although some people can find some relief from eating a high fibre diet.

PILES AND VARICOSE VEINS

Although there have been claims that varicose veins in the legs or anus (i.e., haemorrhoids, otherwise known as piles) do seem to be more common in Western countries, no really satisfactory explanation has been put forward. Some believe that because a low fibre diet can cause constipation, the subsequent straining on the lavatory puts pressure on the veins in the anus and legs. However, it is equally possible that obesity and lack of exercise are the causes – or maybe the fact that we sit on lavatories rather than squatting on the ground!

APPENDICITIS

Appendicitis is much more common in the West than in developing countries. Various theories have been put forward to explain the causes of appendicitis, though none has yet proved conclusive. A lack of dietary fibre does not seem to explain why appendicitis is common in developed countries. On the other hand, those that do not develop appendicitis seem to eat more greens and salads. Recently it has been suggested that appendicitis may be caused by alterations in children's immunity following improvements in sanitation and hygiene. Since diet can alter the nature of the bacteria that live in the intestines, a diet of green and salad vegetables may have a protective effect on the bacteria in the appendix.

GALLSTONES

The average woman has a fairly high risk of developing gallstones during her life time, whereas men are only half as likely to do so. But only about a third of the gallstones that do develop prove troublesome. The problems usually arise when a stone in the gall-bladder tries to get out and then gets stuck.

Most gallstones are made of crystals of cholesterol, which have clustered together with a few minerals like calcium salts picked up along the way. Cholesterol is normally kept in a liquid emulsion when combined with bile acids and lecithin in bile. However, if the concentration of cholesterol goes up, or that of bile acids and lecithin, goes down, then the cholesterol crystallizes out.

Gallstones occur as a result of a combination of factors. Female sex hormones stimulate the production of stones and so, not only are women more at risk, but the risk is increased in those who are pregnant or on the pill. A number of dietary factors also seem to have a link with gallstones, such as overweight, irregular meal-times, and alternate periods of fasting and bingeing (as with those – usually young women – who are forever putting themselves on strict diets and then giving up). A high sugar intake has also been linked with gallstones, but quite why sugar should have this sort of physiological effect has not yet been explained satisfactorily. If people who eat a lot of sugar also eat less dietary fibre, this may pro-

> ❝ The average woman has a fairly high risk of developing gall stones during her life time, whereas men are only half as likely to do so. ❞

> *Some people have a particular tendency to form stones and the commonest dietary association with all types of stones is a low water intake.*

vide part of the explanation, as dietary fibre seems to protect against gallstones. A little alcohol – about one to two glasses of wine a day – also seems to stop cholesterol from crystallizing out of the bile.

Once gallstones have started to cause trouble, they may have to be removed surgically or drugs can be given to dissolve the stones. Dissolving stones can take several months and during this time a low fat diet may be necessary, particularly if the gall-bladder is tender and inflamed. Small, regular meals are also helpful.

KIDNEY AND BLADDER STONES

Stones in the kidney and bladder may be made of calcium, oxalate or uric acid. Some people have a particular tendency to form stones and the commonest dietary association with all types of stones is a low water intake. Those at risk should drink plenty of water, particularly last thing at night and when the weather is hot. The next most common link is a high intake of protein. Other dietary factors that encourage the formation of calcium stones are high intakes of salt, sugar, vitamin D, calcium, alcohol, curry, spicy foods and Worcestershire sauce, as well as a low intake of fibre.

Oxalate stones are particularly likely to form if large tablet-sized doses of vitamin C are taken at the same time as a diet rich in oxalate foods:

beetroot	chocolate
currants	oranges
figs	carrots
rhubarb	green beans
spinach	turnip greens
tea	onions
soft berry fruits like blackberries,	cucumber
gooseberries, strawberries, raspberries	lemon peel.

CIRRHOSIS OF THE LIVER

Cirrhosis of the liver is a disease in which the normal soft tissue of the liver becomes infiltrated with tough scar tissue. Liver damage of this sort cannot be repaired, and treatment is aimed at preventing the disease from worsening. It is frequently caused by a high intake of alcohol and, generally, the higher the consumption of alcohol within a country, the greater the incidence of cirrhosis. But this relationship is not always apparent, and the UK has much less liver cirrhosis than might be expected from its rate of alcohol consumption. Liver cirrhosis can also arise as a result of other causes of liver damage, such as hepatitis B, which is responsible for about a third of the cases of cirrhosis in the UK.

Those who are most at risk of cirrhosis are heavy drinkers: i.e., men who drink 8 drinks or more a day and women who drink about half this. By no means all heavy drinkers develop cirrhosis while others with certain blood tissue-types are particularly susceptible. Once cirrhosis is established, the patient's health and prognosis can be improved if he gives up alcohol.

——DIABETES——

Diabetes affects about 1 per cent of the population. People with diabetes have a deficiency of insulin, either because too little is made in the pancreas, or because their body cells are unable to use insulin properly so that they need larger amounts than are normally made. If there is insufficient insulin, glucose accumulates in the blood. The kidneys then try to get rid of this surplus by excreting the sugar in the urine. In order to do this they require large quantities of fluid, so making the diabetic very thirsty. Excess glucose in the blood is relatively harmless; what matters is that the glucose is failing to be passed into the tissues that need it. Fat needs some glucose to complete the process of releasing its energy. If no glucose at all gets through (as happens in severe diabetes), the process stops halfway. At this stage, if the halfway breakdown products – called ketone bodies – are not metabolized, they start to build up and cause ketosis (also known as acidosis) and will eventually lead to coma and death.

There are two types of diabetes – one that requires insulin and one that can be treated by diet alone. The former is not caused by diet but the latter is a common complication of obesity and once obesity is 15 per cent or more above normal weight, the incidence of diabetes rises steeply. Obesity is not the only factor however, and it seems that there has to be an underlying genetic predisposition as well. Despite the presence of excess glucose – or sugar – in the blood and urine, the development of diabetes seems to bear no relationship to the amount of sugar eaten. In fact, a much closer relationship has been found with the amount of fat eaten.

Diabetes that develops in middle-aged overweight people is the commonest form of diabetes, accounting for about 90 per cent of all cases. It is usually much milder than insulin-dependent diabetes and can be treated simply by diet.

The kind of diet advised in the treatment of diabetes has changed considerably in the last eighty years or so. At the beginning of the century, before the discovery of insulin, diabetics had to be treated with a nauseous diet of 85 per cent fat and only 5 per cent carbohydrate. Since then the amount of carbohydrate allowed has gradually been increasing. By 1970, when drug treatment of diabetes was particularly favoured, the type of diet recommended was almost within the "normal" range but was still made up of 50 per cent or so fat. Since then, a low fat, high carbohydrate diet has been increasingly recommended as a result of better research and an attempt to lower the complications from the side-effects of the disease. For example, not only does diabetes predispose to arterial disease but a high fat diet and some of the drugs used to lower blood sugar also promote heart disease. A comparison between Asian and European diabetics has also shown that Asians who eat a high starch diet have fewer atherosclerotic complications and have better blood glucose control. It has been discovered too that some forms of dietary fibre – notably guar and pectin

> *Diabetes that develops in middle-aged overweight people is the commonest form of diabetes, accounting for about 90 per cent of all cases. It is usually much milder than insulin-dependent diabetes and can be treated simply by diet.*

One in four women and one in forty men are affected by osteoporosis and a fractured hip is a more frequent cause of death than several common forms of cancer put together.

from foods such as lentils and peas – improve diabetic control. The British Diabetic Association currently recommends that the diet should contain 55 per cent of the calories as carbohydrate, particularly the starchy, fibrous forms of carbohydrate, and only 35 per cent of the calories as fat. A high salt intake is also discouraged as salt probably affects the levels of glucose in the blood. Interestingly, these dietary recommendations are almost identical with the current dietary recommendations for general health.

But whatever the ideal diet in theory, the best one will be the kind that the diabetic is most likely to stick to most of the time. The balance between drugs, diet and insulin therefore has to be individually worked out. Fortunately the overweight diabetic does not have to wait for his weight to go down before the benefits are realized as his blood sugar will usually be under control within a few days of being on a calorie-controlled diet.

—OSTEOPOROSIS—

Osteoporosis is a thinning and weakening of the bones which, as far as is understood, is an almost inevitable consequence of old age. One in four women and one in forty men are affected by osteoporosis and a fractured hip is a more frequent cause of death than several common forms of cancer put together. The gradual loss of protein and calcium from the skeleton can, however, be hastened by certain hormone changes, which is why women are particularly affected after the menopause. Lack of exercise is another factor which encourages this type of bone wastage. A lack of calcium, vitamin D and fluoride may exacerbate the condition, and it has been suggested that they may actually cause it, although this theory is not generally agreed. There are other communities where, although less calcium is eaten, there is less osteoporosis. In the meantime it would seem prudent if middle-aged women and the elderly were encouraged to eat calcium-containing foods, to take regular exercise and to get out into the sunlight – in order to stimulate the manufacture of vitamin D in the skin – as much as possible. In some cases hormone therapy may be advised.

OSTEOMALACIA

There is another much less common, but related, disorder called osteomalacia which is caused by vitamin D deficiency. It is the equivalent of rickets in adults and can occur at any age. The cure is extra vitamin D.

—CANCER—

Cancer seems to be one of those diseases that is caused by several different factors acting together. We are exposed to carcinogens – cancer-causing agents – every day but only a few develop into cancer. Some of the factors that contribute to the development of cancer are known, but there are probably many more waiting to be discovered. Although heredity may play a small part in some cancers, environmental agents are believed to play a much larger role in as many as 80 per cent of cancers, either by inducing abnormal changes in the cells' genetic material or by weakening the body's defence mechanisms.

There are three ways by which foreign compounds can enter the body: through the skin, the lungs or the intestines. When looked at in terms of the surface area, the intestines have a million times greater chance of absorbing foreign compounds than the skin, and a thousand times greater chance than the lungs. However, the potential to absorb foreign compounds does not tell us definitely whether they are absorbed by a particular route or not. Likewise, the fact that a chemical can induce genetic changes in cells in a test tube in a laboratory does not prove that it is dangerous in the context of the human body. In order for these carcinogens to take a hold the circumstances need to be right and much will depend on the state of the body's defence mechanisms.

Epidemiologists – those who study where, when and how often diseases occur – have estimated that synthetic chemical additives in food account for less than 1 per cent of all cancers. On the other hand, the nutritional balance of the diet, such as how much fat, fibre, etc. is eaten, can have a considerable impact on the development of cancer, probably through its influence on the body's defence mechanisms, and is believed to account for a third of all cancers.

The cancers most clearly related to diet are those of the oesophagus, stomach and large bowel. But even these cancers are probably caused by a combination of different environmental agents from one country to another. For example, it is thought that cancer of the oesophagus in China is due to the presence of nitrosamines in mouldy foods, together with a deficiency of the trace element molybdenum in the diet. But in Iran, oesophageal cancer is thought to arise as a result of vitamin deficiencies and the taking of opium. In the Transkei, South Africa, mycotoxins from moulds together with deficiencies of zinc, niacin and other vitamins and minerals are thought to be responsible. And in Europe, alcohol – especially that derived from apples such as cider or Calvados – and tobacco are thought to be the associated factors.

Stomach cancer has been linked with a high consumption of dried, salted fish; pickled foods; cured meats; salt and the lack of refrigeration. Thus stomach cancer is more common in communities where few people have fridges and have to rely on perishable foods preserved by more traditional methods such as smoking, pickling and salting. In contrast, the incidence of stomach cancer has halved in Britain and other industrialized

> *Although heredity may play a small part in some cancers, environmental agents are believed to play a much larger role in as many as 80 per cent of cancers, either by inducing abnormal changes in the cell's genetic material or by weakening the body's defence mechanisms.*

> *Epidemiologists – those who study where, when and how often diseases occur – have estimated that synthetic chemical additives in food account for less than 1 per cent of all cancers.*

> *Cancer of the large bowel is particularly common in Western countries and is the second largest cause of deaths from cancer, after lung cancer in men and breast cancer in women.*

countries in the last twenty-five years and this is believed to have been brought about by keeping food in refrigerators and because of a possible protective factor in salads and citrus fruits.

Cancer of the large bowel is particularly common in Western countries and is the second largest cause of deaths from cancer, after lung cancer in men and breast cancer in women. In the case of bowel cancer, unlike cancer of the oesophagus, the dietary factors which are associated with it are much the same throughout the developed world. A high fat intake and a high meat intake are thought to play a part, whereas wheat fibre and vegetables like cabbage are thought to be protective.

In 1982 the United States National Research Council published some dietary guidelines which they felt might reasonably help protect against cancer. They recommended that Americans should eat less fat – preferably no more than 30 per cent of the diet as fat; more fruits and vegetables and wholegrain cereals; very little salt-cured, salt-pickled and smoked foods; and to drink only moderate amounts of alcohol.

—*FOOD POISONS*—

Although much attention is paid to environmental contaminants and the possibility that food additives are harmful, less notice is usually taken either of the many toxic substances that are naturally found in foods or of the real, sometimes long-term, risks to health from bacterial contamination and mould growth.

NATURALLY OCCURRING TOXINS

There are believed to be thousands of toxic substances naturally occurring in foods and a few are listed in the table below:

SOME POSSIBLE TOXIC EFFECTS OF FOODS

Food	Pharmacological agent	Effects
Most cheeses	tyramine	Raises blood pressure.
Almonds	cyanide	Prevents oxygen from being transferred from blood to the tissues.
Raw kidney beans	haemagglutinins	Damage red blood cells.
Broad beans	vicine	Anaemia in people of a certain blood type.
Potatoes, especially the green parts	solanine	Interferes with transmission of nerve impulses, causing headache and diarrhoea.
Olives, olive oil	benzo(a)pyrene	Cancer
Cabbage, radishes and watercress	goitrogens	Goitre
Shrimps	arsenic	Blood poisoning
Parsley, carrots	myristicin	Hallucinations
Bananas	serotonin	Heart lesions
Wholewheat, bran	phytic acid	Inhibits absorption of zinc and iron.

Most of the above toxins are quite harmless when eaten in the amounts normally found in foods. Some foods eaten either in particularly large quantities or in unusual circumstances may give rise to problems. For example, solanine is concentrated in the green parts of potatoes; some people taking drugs like monoamine oxidase inhibitors may have to limit their consumption of cheese; bran, if eaten raw and by the tablespoonful, may reduce the absorption of iron and zinc; and some people, particularly those from Mediterranean regions, are born with an enzyme deficiency that makes their blood particularly susceptible to vicine in broad beans.

The commonest form of food poisoning in the home is caused by the contamination of food with the bacteria, salmonella.

As far as small doses of these toxins are concerned, man like other animals has developed a number of biochemical mechanisms which either help to get rid of many of these toxins or to neutralize them.

NATURAL CONTAMINANTS

More important than the toxins found in foods are the toxins which may be added to food from contamination by moulds or bacteria. Cancers caused by aflatoxins and mycotoxins from moulds are a real problem in parts of the world where grains and nuts are stored under inadequate conditions.

In the developed parts of the world where there are efficient and sophisticated food industries, this sort of food contamination is very unusual. In the UK food poisoning is much more likely to be the result of inadequate hygiene and careless food preparation in canteens and kitchens.

FOOD POISONING

The commonest form of food poisoning in the home is caused by the contamination of food with the bacteria, *salmonella*. There are several species of *salmonella*, and although each can give rise to different symptoms, the species concerned can really only be identified by laboratory analysis. Gastroenteritis – that is, traveller's tummy or diarrhoea in babies – may be caused by a virus or by food or water that is contaminated with bacteria.

Depending on the type of bacteria or virus, the attack may take anything from a few minutes or a day or so to develop. Although most forms of food poisoning result in diarrhoea, vomiting and abdominal pain, some are characterized by such symptoms as fever – or lack of it – blood in the diarrhoea, sweating, a burning sensation, weakness or convulsions.

It is not usually possible to tell whether a food is likely to cause food poisoning or not as the food may look, smell and taste the same. The foods that are most likely to give rise to food poisoning are:

stews, casseroles and mince	milk and cream
poultry	eggs
cooked rice	seafood
meats (particularly if boned and rolled when the bacteria may be transferred to the centre of the meat)	coconut and chocolate
	dried foods and spices

FOOD ALLERGIES AND INTOLERANCES

The word allergy has a narrow technical definition, as well as a much broader, popular meaning. In its technical sense, an allergy means that the body's immune system reacts to certain harmless substances in the same way as it does to invading germs. A quick allergic response is caused by an inflammation due to an accumulation of histamine and other smaller substances. Histamine from body proteins is normally released in order to repair damaged or injured tissues, though in the case of allergies there are, of course, no injured tissues. Antihistamines may therefore help to relieve allergic symptoms like itchy rashes and a runny nose. Such symptoms are familiar side-effects when the body is fighting off germs like the measles virus or the common cold and, in the case of an allergic person, they can also be triggered off by normally harmless substances, like pollen, which causes hay fever, or wool next to the skin causing an irritating rash, or house dust mite in the lungs causing asthma, and so on.

"Allergy" in its wider, popular sense covers a whole range of sensitivity reactions to foods, and can include virtually any kind of food intolerance.

Most doctors feel they understand true allergies – in the sense of an abnormal immunological reaction – and they may be able to treat them by advising tests to identify the cause. However, when the term "allergy" is used in its broader sense – meaning any kind of food sensitivity – many doctors are at a loss. Trying to discover the offending item or items can be as exasperating as looking for a needle in a haystack; even more so when the symptoms are vague, like frequent headaches, a general feeling of "unwellness", depression, fatigue and so on. Sometimes a patient may claim he knows which foods he is allergic to and, sure enough, if he drinks orange squash – or whatever – he will develop characteristic symptoms. However, if the offending item is subsequently introduced in a disguised form, these symptoms are not necessarily evoked. The doctor may well conclude that the problem is a psychological one that is emotional in origin, and not a real sensitivity to food. It is well known that the emotions can play a large part in exacerbating allergic attacks like asthma and eczema, and an asthmatic child is much more likely to have an attack when either he or his parents are anxious. It is also known that anxiety can cause hyperventilation – rapid, shallow breathing which is often unnoticed by the patient – and this in turn can cause dizziness, nausea and a general feeling of being unwell. The sight of any food or drink that evokes anxiety can then set off a whole chain of physiological responses.

> **Trying to discover the offending item or items can be as exasperating as looking for a needle in a haystack; even more so when the symptoms are vague, like frequent headaches, a general feeling of "unwellness", depression, fatigue and so on.**

Depression, fatigue, lethargy, headaches and so on can all be caused by worry and stress, and no doubt have affected people in many societies throughout history. It has also been common to blame a wide variety of causes, which will vary from one age to another, according to popularity. For all these reasons, it is not surprising if a probably stressed, fatigued doctor responds unfavourably to patients with similar symptoms and dismisses the idea of an allergy being the cause as just another passing fad. However, not all doctors are so sceptical today and there has been much research recently into the causes and symptoms of allergies. There is also an increasing number of doctors who specialize in food and other sensitivities.

Since our knowledge of food sensitivity is accumulating rapidly, it is possible to summarize only some of the findings here. It is also important to realize that progress in this area of research is particularly likely to be along the lines of "two steps forward and one step back". As an example, cow's milk at one time looked as if it might be a definite cause of colic in some babies in the early weeks. Since then some studies have failed to find any connection and others have confirmed the link. Thus, at the moment the evidence is conflicting. It may turn out that only a few babies are sensitive, or it may be that the quantity of milk drunk by a breastfeeding mother is the key or, of course, it may turn out to be something totally different.

SYMPTOMS OF FOOD SENSITIVITY

Many symptoms of food allergy arise within a few minutes or a couple of hours of a food being eaten. Some may take a couple of days to develop, in which case the real culprit may be overlooked and an innocent food may mistakenly get the blame.

Common symptoms, the approximate time they take to develop and their causes are shown in the table below:

Symptoms Mouth tingling or lip swelling (a form of oedema)
Approximate reaction time Between 1 minute and 2 hours
Non-food causes Diseases of connective tissue in skin and joints; certain drugs; physical causes like a punch on the nose; and contact with dusts, etc.
Known food causes See gastrointestinal reactions (page 92)

Symptoms Itchy, blotchy rash like nettle stings (urticaria)
Approximate reaction time 1 to several hours later
Non-food causes Exercise; heat
Known food causes Acute reactions may be caused by small amounts of egg white, peanuts, fish, cow's milk and larger amounts of strawberries, shellfish, pawpaw, fruit, some wines, fermented cheeses and sausages. Chronic urticaria may result from salicylates in aspirin and those naturally occurring in high doses in foods like most soft fruit (such as strawberries and pineapples), tea, spices, mint, honey, liquorice and cucumber or from tartrazine (a yellow food colour E102) or the preservative benzoates (E210 to E219).

Symptoms Streaming nose (rhinitis)
Approximate reaction time 1 minute to 2 hours
Non-food causes Pollen, moulds, dust
Known food causes Same foods as for asthma.

Symptoms Asthma
Approximate reaction time If caused by food, any time between 1 hour and 2 days later
Non-food causes Inhaled irritants, infections, changes in the weather, exercise; emotional disturbances of parent or child.
Known food causes In adults food-sensitivity asthma is really caused only in those exposed to large quantities of dusty grain, flour, coffee, etc. In children eggs, fish, nuts and chocolate are believed to be common causes but there is little hard evidence for this. Some additives including tartrazine and benzoates can sometimes cause asthma, and sulphur dioxide (E220) and sodium metabisulphite (E223) can aggravate attacks. Sulphur dioxide may not necessarily be "declared" on a food label, and it can be present in a spray that is sometimes used on salads and fresh fruit salads in hotels and restaurants.

Symptoms Eczema
Approximate reaction time Usually 2-3 days after exposure but can develop within a few hours
Non-food causes Many – e.g., washing powders, soaps, wool, nickel next to the skin, etc.; emotional disturbances of parent or child; babies often develop an eczema-like condition which is frequently "grown out" of during infancy
Known food causes Milk, eggs, wheat are the most common causes as well as the early introduction of solids to babies.

Gastrointestinal reactions:
Symptoms Vomiting
Approximate reaction time Between a few minutes to 2-3 hours after food is eaten
Known food causes In children: cow's milk, egg white, nuts, seafood and some fruit are particularly common causes; in adults: wheat, dairy foods, maize, some fruits, tea and coffee are mostly responsible.

Symptoms Diarrhoea, bloating and constipation
Approximate reaction time 3-24 hours or so later
Known food causes In children: cow's milk, egg white, nuts, seafood and some fruit are particularly common causes; in adults: wheat, dairy foods, maize, some fruits, tea and coffee are mostly responsible.

Symptoms Migraine
Approximate reaction time An hour or two or several hours later
Non-food causes Tension, menstruation, bright lights can often precipitate migraines.
Known food causes Via pharmacological agents naturally present in cheese, chocolate, citrus fruits, wheat, some alcoholic drinks and fatty foods like cream and sausages. Also cow's milk, eggs, tomatoes and the additives benzoic acid (E210) and tartrazine (E102) have been shown to cause migraine in children.

Symptoms Arthritis of the gouty type
Known food causes Aggravated by alcohol, high protein diets and low fluid intakes.

Symptoms Hyperactivity (in children)
Approximate reaction time If caused by food allergy it seems to occur together with diarrhoea, urticaria, migraine or eczema
Non-food causes Brain damage, deafness and other health problems and handicaps can cause behaviour problems
Known food causes Only a few overactive children are affected by food. The foods causing symptoms seem to be individual to each child. In one study at Great Ormond Street Hospital, tartrazine and benzoic acid were top of the list, but soya, cow's milk, grapes, egg, wheat, oranges, peanuts and maize were commonly involved too.

DIAGNOSIS

Whenever a food allergy is suspected, the diagnosis should always be done with professional medical help, as it can take several weeks or even months, sometimes on unusual diets, to work out the cause of the problem. Professional help is particularly important in the case of small children who are more susceptible to food allergies than older children and adults. But the symptoms may be due to some other disorder and sometimes the method used to detect an allergy can cause more illness than the allergy itself. Paediatricians have recently reported seeing a number of children suffering from malnutrition as a result of inadequate diets when parents are believed to have markedly restricted the child's diet in an attempt to remove unsuitable foods. Unfortunately, it is all too easy for a parent, anxious to find a cure, to fail to be objective. Sometimes parents may be too emotionally involved and so can find it difficult to distinguish either a real improvement or a deterioration in health from the typical ups and downs that are in the nature of many disorders – including allergies.

The usual way to try to detect a food "allergy" is to make gradual alterations to the diet and to keep a record of any symptoms. If the allergic reaction is not particularly severe, the patient – or in the case of children, the parent – may be asked to keep a diary of all the foods eaten and to note any symptoms over a period of several weeks.

Alternatively, one or a very few selected foods may be removed from the diet for a week or two and any change noted. Cutting out nutritionally valuable foods is harmless provided it is done for only a short time, although in some cases a substitute may need to be introduced. For example, if a woman who is breastfeeding suddenly gives up all dairy products, she risks going short of calcium at a time when her calcium output is particularly high. Small children who obtain much of their nourishment from milk may go hungry when milk is suddenly cut out of their diet if they fail to eat correspondingly more of other foods.

Sometimes the patient may be put on an "elimination diet" for two to three weeks, and the suspected foods are then reintroduced one by one every three to seven days. A typical elimination is made up of the foods that are believed least likely to cause an allergic reaction. These are usually lamb, rice, peeled potatoes, carrots, lettuce, pears, a refined vegetable seed oil, water and sugar. However, elimination diets can cause nutritional deficiencies if they are not worked out and managed properly.

Sometimes a diagnosis may be confirmed by giving the patient capsules or disguised samples of various foods to see whether a reaction is provoked. In the most reliable tests neither the patient nor the tester is allowed to know which food or ingredient is being tested as this can prejudice the result. For example, typical symptoms may be unconsciously looked for and so "found", or a change in the manner of the tester may subconsciously alert the patient, which in turn may provoke a response.

If the allergy is thought to be due to an immunological defect, the patient may undergo a series of skin pricks or blood tests to test for allergies. But these are not infallible as both false positives and false negatives can be produced.

A SPECIAL NOTE ABOUT BABIES
Allergies are often inherited, not usually the same allergy as the parent but another kind of allergic response. In the case of

In the most reliable tests neither the patient nor the tester is allowed to know which food or ingredient is being tested as this can prejudice the result. For example, typical symptoms may be unconsciously looked for and so "found", or a change in the manner of the tester may subconsciously alert the patient, which in turn may provoke a response.

Allergies are often inherited, not usually the same allergy as the parent but another kind of allergic response. In the case of babies born into a family where one or both parents or a brother or sister is allergic, it is worth taking a number of precautions in order to try to lessen the chance of the baby developing an allergy, or at least to try to prevent it from being too severe.

babies born into a family where one or both parents or a brother or sister is allergic, it is worth taking a number of precautions in order to try to lessen the chance of the baby developing an allergy, or at least to try to prevent it from being too severe.

1. Keep dust (including talcum powder) to a minimum.
2. Avoid scented soaps, "biological" washing powders and wool next to the skin.
3. Breastfeed for at least the first four to six months.
4. When weaning starts, introduce one new food at a time, three or four or more days apart. This will help to identify any problem foods.
5. Delay the introduction of cow's milk, egg white, oranges, soft fruits, fish and wheat to at least 6 months. (Some of these foods should be left until 10 months or so.)
6. Avoid foods with additives. Commercial baby foods are not allowed to have colourings and other additives added to them (with one or two exceptions in the case of dried foods), so there is no reason why they should be fed other foods containing them.
7. Today's modified formula milks are not as allergic as cow's milk or the old-fashioned baby milks. Soya formula milks, which are often fed to babies in the hopes of avoiding allergies, can, in fact, cause an allergy if the baby is sensitive to soya protein. They are therefore mainly advised when the baby is known to be unable to tolerate cow's milk in any form, or is at high risk of being allergic to it.

Food allergies do not necessarily last for ever, and allergies in children are particularly likely to be outgrown during the early years. From the age of seven or thereabouts, allergies to foods are often "grown out of" and non-food agents like pollen, house dust mite, cat's fur, etc. are the commonest causes of any allergic reactions.

——POSITIVE HEALTH——

"Not feeling ill" is not the same as "feeling well". Many people who have tried to change to healthier lifestyles and eating habits have reported that they feel better straightaway. Although knowing that you are doing something to help yourself can be a tremendous boost to morale, the benefits are not just psychological. There are also clear physical gains: you can feel the difference extra fibre makes to your bowels; diabetics can improve their blood sugar levels after only a few days of a calorie-controlled diet; a low fat diet can produce a clinically measurable improvement in blood fats in a couple of weeks; and a low salt diet can help improve blood pressure after a few weeks.

To gain most from these benefits, it is important that any changes should be positive ones. Unfortunately, most doctors and nutritionists are too fond of giving people negative advice, telling them what they should not do or what they should eat less of.

To gain most from these benefits, it is important that any changes should be positive ones. Unfortunately, most doctors and nutritionists are too fond of giving people negative advice, telling them what they should not do or what they should eat less of. Cutting down and cutting out foods without any real idea of what can be substituted is not only hard, unrewarding work, but it can cause real feelings of anxiety, as many soon find out when they are coping with hunger at the same time as trying to find something acceptable to eat. Under such circumstances food can rapidly lose its pleasure and family relationships can be put under strain as they try to think of meals which can be served to a "difficult" eater.

Making a positive change, on the other hand, means deciding to eat more of certain foods and – unless you suffer from an insatiable appetite – this can often mean you eat less of other items. For example, eating more wholemeal bread, more boiled and baked potatoes, more crisp salads, more fish and chicken and more home-cooked foods most of the time can do much to improve the nutritional balance of your diet. If there are occasions when you have to – or maybe want to – eat a pile of greasy chips or an "instant" dessert, you can do so knowing they are playing a much smaller part in your diet than previously. Allowing yourself such foods, but at the same time limiting the number of occasions when you eat them, will help you to control what you eat. As you gradually gain confidence and by trial and error learn which sort of healthy foods you enjoy and which could become part of your everyday eating habits, you may gradually lose the taste for the foods you were formerly accustomed to.

Making changes on behalf of someone else – your partner or children – can also help you feel good. People who belong to families in which one member has to be on a special diet are able to do much to relieve the burden of "being different" by sharing the diet. Even if you feel it is too late or not worth the trouble to change your own diet, you may feel it is worth it for your children's sake.

Like taking up exercise, changing what you eat is best done gradually. This will not only give your digestion and physiology time to adapt but will also allow a breathing space to work out and make decisions about what *you* want in the way of health and not just what someone else wants you to do.

ACHIEVING BETTER HEALTH

The key changes to diet for better health can be summarized as follows:

Calories: Frequent regular exercise for everyone; those who are overweight should aim to lose about 1-2lb (0.5-1kg) a week, which will probably be achieved by going on a 1,200-1,500 kcalorie diet.

Protein: No special changes needed; a lower fat, more vegetable-based diet often results in a little more rather than less protein being eaten.

Fats: Should provide no more than one-third of all the calories in the diet; at present, fats account for about 40 per cent of energy. Of all fats saturated fats in particular should be reduced.

Sugars: At present, sugars account for about one-fifth of the calories eaten. From the point of view of dental health it is more important to reduce the number of times sugar is eaten during the day rather than the total quantity. However, reducing the frequency will very likely lower the total quantity eaten. Eating less sugars in this way could roughly halve sugar intake, which is important from the point of view of reducing surplus calories in the diets of those who have a weight problem.

Starchy carbohydrate: At the moment, starchy or complex carbohydrates account for about a quarter of the calories we eat. If less fat and sugar are eaten as recommended, more starchy carbohydrates would be needed to replace the missing calories so the quantity eaten might almost double.

Fibre: The average person in the UK probably eats ¾oz (20g) of fibre a day (although this figure may well change as methods of analysis change as well as the definition of just what dietary fibre is). There are no official recommendations for fibre though eating twice as much starchy carbohydrate as at present would be likely to double fibre intake and increase it still further if more wholemeal rather than white bread and flour were eaten. It has been suggested that fibre intakes should increase by 50 per cent, although a bit more would not matter. Fibre from fruits, pulses and vegetables is different from wheat fibre and also valuable.

Minerals and vitamins: With the exception of iron and vitamin D, deficiencies of minerals and vitamins are rare in Britain today. More vitamin C from extra fruit and vegetables would help the absorption of iron. Growing children and, possibly, the elderly and women after the menopause need extra calcium. More exercise in the open air would do much to encourage healthy bones as well as the synthesis of vitamin D in the skin.

Salt: We eat approximately 1½-2 teaspoonsful a day. This should be reduced to the equivalent of a slightly rounded teaspoonful. Although only a minority of people may need to make this change, it would not harm the majority to do so.

Alcohol: An excessive intake of alcohol has been described as the equivalent of 50 units or more of alcohol a week for men and over 35 units for women. 20 units of alcohol or less for men and 15 units or less for women a week are thought to be harmless, and, in the absence of better evidence about how much is "safe", women planning to start a baby or who are pregnant should preferably not drink at all (see page 20).

DIETS AROUND THE WORLD

Trying to work out what one-third of the total calories recommended as fat would look like in terms of food served up on a plate is difficult. However, if the target recommendations for change are compared with the nutritional patterns of rich and poor countries, it can be seen that they come roughly halfway between the two (see the chart on page 98). People in Third World countries generally rely very heavily on one or two staple crops such as rice or maize. Small quantities of oil, meat, pulses and spices are served together with vegetables as side dishes or relishes to moisten and flavour the staple. In rich Western countries, on the other hand, although potatoes and flour are still "staple" foods, much greater emphasis is placed on meat and its equivalent. In our culture meat is the focal point of the main course. When potatoes are served they are very often fried in some way, and the small quantities of flour that are eaten are frequently served as sugary cakes, biscuits and puddings rather than bread.

If the nutritional composition of the Italian diet is studied in more detail, it can be seen to bear a remarkable resemblance to the types of diet that are now being recommended in the US and UK.

But there are diets that come in between those of rich and poor countries. About twenty years or so ago it was noticed that Mediterranean countries like Greece and Italy not only had much less heart disease than countries such as the United States and the United Kingdom, but they also had a much smaller proportion of fats, particularly saturates, in their national diet.

If the nutritional composition of the Italian diet is studied in more detail, it can be seen to bear a remarkable resemblance to the types of diet that are now being recommended in the US and the UK. This is not to say that everyone should eat Italian food all the time, but a study of Italian and related cuisines can help give a number of clues to ways in which our eating habits could be adapted without sacrificing the pleasures of good food.

Describing Italian food as healthy may come as a surprise to some if thoughts of overweight Italians, greasy olive oil, spaghetti bolognese and veal cutlets are the only images conjured up. However, the popular view of Italian cuisine is based on fleeting impressions from restaurants and English versions of Italian recipes and also on a misunderstanding of the effects poverty can have on diet and physique.

In a country where a substantial proportion of the population is poor but where there is just enough food to meet their needs, it is not uncommon for adults to be given most of the food available and for children to be slightly underfed. Such children may be below average height but otherwise perfectly healthy, while the adults in such a country will tend to be short but, with a more plentiful food supply, they can very easily put on weight. This pattern of growth was common in the UK a few generations ago. In countries where the standard of living is higher and more equally distributed – as in Scandinavia – all the children tend to be taller and the so-called class differences in height are virtually non-existent. In wealthy countries where there is an excess of food the children are both taller and very often heavier, and in these countries children as well as adults may be both tall and obese.

Real Italian food can also be rather different from the sort of Italian food we eat in Britain. Most countries adapt foreign dishes to fit in with their own diets. We tend to favour dishes that look familiar and considerably modify the less familiar ones. The result can then often lead to disappointment for tourists who go in search of an authentic dish like a "real" spaghetti bolognese.

But if national food supply statistics rather than holiday impressions are compared a rather different picture of the Italian diet emerges. Compared with several other European countries, Italy has less meat (but of the meat supplied it has a very high proportion of poultry), oils and fats, milk and sugar but very large supplies of vegetables (except potatoes), cereals and fruit. The UK has middling supplies of most of these foods, except for a very high consumption of milk and a very low proportion of fruits and vegetables (except for the potato).

Although a comparison of national food supply data can be only a rough guide to what is actually eaten, there seems little evidence to support the belief that the Italian diet is a particularly fatty one. The myth may simply have arisen because the fat in the Italian diet is particularly visible, whereas much of the fat in the British diet is hidden in meat, meat products, milk and cakes. The distinctive taste of olive oil in Italian cuisine may also be partly responsible for making a memorable impression on conservative British palates!

Experimenting with and trying out different dishes around the world can not only be tasty but can also help give a greater understanding of cooking techniques so that familiar British dishes can be modified by adding and not sacrificing interest.

Any cuisine that uses little salt, sugar, fat, dairy products or meat and can make larger quantities of cereal foods, vegetables and beans tasty deserves attention. There are many other cuisines besides Italian cooking which can provide inspiration, such as those from the Middle East, Vietnam, Spain, Central and South America, India and China and elsewhere. Experimenting with and trying out different dishes around the world can not only be tasty but can also help give a greater understanding of cooking techniques so that familiar British dishes can be modified by adding and not sacrificing interest.

APPROXIMATE PROPORTION OF CALORIES (EXCLUDING ALCOHOL) FROM FAT, CARBOHYDRATE AND PROTEIN

Western Countries	Third World	Mediterranean	Recommended change for the UK
Fat 42%	Fat 13%	Fat 34%	Fat 33%
Starch 25%	Starch 70%	Starch 40%	Starch 45%
Sugar 20%	Sugar 7%	Sugar 15%	Sugar ?10%
Protein 12½%	Protein 10%	Protein 12½%	Protein 12½%

PART II

THE
FOOD
INDUSTRY

JOHN RIVERS

CHAPTER 5

THE PLOUGH AND THE COMBINE HARVESTER

THE GROWTH OF AGRICULTURE

Many people today feel that they have had the ill-luck to have been born into the generation that is destroying the traditional British countryside, farming methods and whole way of life. They point to the progressive disappearance of hedgerows, the arrival of strange crops like oilseed rape, to the increasing mechanization of crop growing and the use of intensive animal husbandry (more popularly called factory farming). This vogue for nostalgia has been taken over by the advertising industry which frequently portrays a rural utopia where "traditional" farmhouse values apply – "traditional", of course, being assumed to be a valuable quality, particularly of food.

Though it is true that some of the modern changes in farming are destroying centuries-old aspects of the countryside, much of our conception of farming traditions is totally false. In fact, traditional British agriculture and the traditional British diet, as we usually understand them, are less than two hundred years old and throughout that time both have been in a state of constant flux. Many of the changes that we see around us and that cause so much anxiety are not new but merely the continuation of a pattern of change. Many items in our diet, which we believe to be long-established and therefore safe, turn out to be historical newcomers. The potato, for example, arrived only in Elizabethan times, tea in the 18th century and wheat became the major cereal in our diet only in the 19th century. These "traditional" cornerstones of the British diet are, therefore, innovations, and their introduction part of the pattern of constant change that is still with us. These continuing changes are not necessarily improvements: nor should they be judged exclusively in nutritional terms.

> *In fact, traditional British agriculture and the traditional British diet, as we usually understand them, are less than two hundred years old and throughout that time both have been in a state of constant flux.*

There are many other criteria to consider when judging the success or failure of agriculture: economic, ecological and even ethical. But looking at the reasons behind these changes and perhaps explaining to what extent more changes are likely, will make it clear that trying to return to a largely imaginary rural past, rich in wholemeal dietary joy, is as futile and misguided as trying to pursue the end of a rainbow.

Trying to return to a largely imaginary rural past, rich in wholemeal dietary joy, is as futile as trying to pursue the end of a rainbow.

There is, of course, a traditional agriculture in Britain, but it is not the rustic 19th-century agriculture of Thomas Hardy; it is the pattern of farming practised in the Middle Ages, whose decline began with the Black Death in the 14th century. We cannot return to it now because it is quite incapable of supporting the population of our planet. And if we realized what it was like in reality, perhaps we would not, after all, wish to go back.

The agriculture of medieval England would look very strange to the modern eye. There were no fields as we now know them; rather each field was divided into strips, each farmed by a different peasant family. Likewise there were no farms, but a peasant would have a series of strips in different, often widely separated, fields. This system involved planting different crops in different years and leaving land fallow one year in every three or four, to maintain its fertility.

But perhaps the strangest aspect of agriculture would have been the fact that most of the land wasn't farmed at all. There were large expanses of relatively open ground, known as common land, on which no crops grew, land that nobody owned that was treated as common property, on which anyone could graze animals but that no one could take over for arable farming or building. The animals that were grazed were largely sheep, raised primarily for their wool, and pigs.

This system began to decay after the Black Death in 1348 made agricultural labour a scarce and expensive commodity. But its final demise came in the 18th century, when a revolutionary new notion, the idea of farming for profit, began to emerge. The impetus for this change came from the growth of the urban population, which, by the end of the 18th century, already comprised one person in five. This provided a market for food and the opportunity for the farmer to make large profits. But traditional agriculture did not produce enough surplus either to satisfy the landowner or to feed the growing population. So, in a series of Enclosure Acts, Parliament made it possible for the wealthy to take over much traditional common land and to use it for farming. Much of the new enclosed common land was used to grow wheat, or corn as it was then called, which for the first time replaced barley and rye as the major cereal. The Enclosure Acts created much of today's landed gentry and at the same time caused great suffering amongst England's rural poor.

Bigger fortunes became available to farmers who could now increase the scale of their operations, and here new technology came to their aid. For if the population's need for food provided the reason behind the enclosures, science and technology produced the tools. The improvements in roads and later the arrival of railways enabled food to be moved to market and made it possible for deeply rural areas to supply urban markets. Improvements in the design of ploughs allowed landowners to cultivate soil that had hitherto been too heavy, while the development of fertilizers meant they could farm more intensively, and without the need to let the land lie fallow. At the same time scientific experiments led to new strains of crops and animals being developed.

All these changes, of course, created the same mutterings of unrest as parallel ones in our own time have done, and critics of agricultural change prophesied the most dire consequences. Admittedly some historians do believe that these changes had an adverse effect on the nutritional value of the diet and that the 18th and early 19th centuries were a time of chronic malnutrition and sporadic severe food shortages, culminating in the Irish potato famine of 1845-6, which resulted in a million deaths and perhaps twice as many people emigrating to North America.

But although the diet of much of the population was dreadful, this was not caused by the Agricultural Revolution. Indeed, most people would have been worse off if there had been a change back to traditional agriculture, which would not have been able to produce enough food. Much of the suffering occurred because so few people could afford an adequate diet. Agriculture did produce food, but low wages only allowed most town dwellers to buy an extremely restricted diet. Even with the Agricultural Revolution, the country could not produce enough cheap food to feed its rapidly growing population adequately and indeed still cannot produce all the range of foods we eat, although Britain is more self-sufficient now than at any time since the beginning of the Industrial Revolution. The suffering became particularly acute in the 18th and early 19th centuries when the government imposed the Corn Laws restricting the import of cereal grains to protect British wheat growers from overseas competition.

——*IMPORTS AND THE BRITISH DIET*——

Cereals were among the few foodstuffs that it was feasible to import in the early 19th century, most others being too perishable. But two exceptions were already of great importance and their popularity had momentous consequences, not merely for the British diet but for the world.

The first of these imports was tea, which entered the British diet, along with coffee and cocoa, in the late 17th century. All three drinks quickly became the soft drugs of their time, the alternative to alcohol, smart drinks for the urban gentry who drank them for the "lift" they gave, and a source of moral indignation to many. They quickly became fashionable: in 1738 the composer J.S. Bach even wrote a piece of music, the "Coffee Cantata", inspired by the new habit of coffee drinking.

All three drinks quickly became the soft drugs of their time, the alternative to alcohol, smart drinks for the urban gentry who drank them for the "lift" they gave, and a source of moral indignation to many.

Like beer in our own time, a whole industry developed to serve these drinks in convivial surroundings and they were soon being consumed as much for the entrée to the fashionable places that served them as for their own sake. One well-known relic of this is Lloyd's of London, the insurance business, which was originally Mr Lloyd's coffee house, a meeting place for insurance underwriters.

The consumption of all three beverages spread from the fashionable élite during the late 18th and 19th centuries. At first tea, the cheapest of the three, was consumed in greater amounts – in 1800 tea consumption was almost 1½lb (0.7kg) a head a year when coffee consumption was only about 1oz (30g). But although the consumption of both increased in the 19th century, coffee became increasingly popular until by 1880 consumption had risen nearly fiftyfold, compared with a fivefold increase in tea consumption. Thereafter, as the price of tea tumbled, coffee declined in popularity and tea became the almost universal English drink. During the 19th century cocoa consumption increased about twentyfold, but its unfortunate side-effect of causing flatulence prevented it from becoming universally popular. Only in the 1880s was a method developed for removing the cocoa butter, which caused the problem, from the bean and then, although cocoa consumption rose, it was mostly consumed as a component of chocolate confectionery.

> *Sugar has been called white gold, and the metaphor is apt. When it first arrived in Europe from the Middle East and North Africa in the 14th century, an ounce (approximately 30g) of gold would buy only 30lb (14kg) of sugar; even by the 16th century it would buy less than 100lb (45kg). Today it would buy over 1,000lb (450kg).*

Throughout the late 18th and early 19th centuries the tea trade was in the hands of the first great British multinational, the East India Company. Originally it had imported tea from China, but it had proved difficult to maintain a reliable supply, and by the early 19th century the East India Company, effectively the rulers of India, had set up plantations in Ceylon and India to ensure its source of supply. Indian tea had a different flavour from Chinese tea, and each attracted its own adherents. Indian tea was the cheaper and so became the popular tea, while the more expensive China tea became "exclusive" and fashionable.

The second import of significance in the early 19th century was sugar. Sugar has always appealed to man's sweet tooth, although for centuries it was a minor item of diet. For most people in the past the major source of dietary sweetness was honey, and not much of that was available. It may seem difficult to believe, but 500 years ago sugar was a rare and expensive spice, imported from the Orient at great expense and costing ten times as much as honey. Sugar has been called white gold, and the metaphor is apt. When it first arrived in Europe from the Middle East and North Africa in the 14th century, an ounce (approximately 30g) of gold would buy only 30lb (14kg) of sugar; even by the 16th century it would buy less than 100lb (45kg). Today it would buy over 1,000lb (450kg). Sugar was too profitable a crop to ignore, and various attempts were made to introduce the cane to Europe or to the European colonies, of which the plantations in the West Indies were the most successful. Because the demand for sugar was apparently without limit, these plantations expanded and a steady stream of slaves was imported from Africa in the most barbarous conditions to grow the cane. Sugar production rose steadily at great cost in slavery: it has been estimated that one slave died for every one to two tons of sugar produced.

By 1833, when slavery was abolished, sugar consumption in Britain was already

> *When import duty on sugar was removed in 1845 consumption stood at 24lb (11kg), and as prices thereafter fell to very low levels, sugar consumption began its virtually uninterrupted rise, passing 80lb (36kg) per head by the end of the 19th century on its way to today's level of 110lb (50kg) a person a year.*

at an average level of 18lb (8kg) a person a year. When import duty on sugar was removed in 1845 consumption stood at 24lb (11kg), and as prices thereafter fell to very low levels, sugar consumption began its virtually uninterrupted rise, passing 80lb (36kg) per head by the end of the 19th century on its way to today's level of 110lb (50kg) a person a year.

The initial impetus for the importation of sugar was its popularity as a sweetener for drinks, but cheap supplies lead to the growth of an industry that used sugars in all sorts of other ways. First, it was added to condensed milk to form a thick paste called sweetened condensed milk that was, until the invention of the refrigerator, the most commonly available method for preserving milk. Sweetened condensed milk was cheap and popular both for putting in tea and for putting on bread. It was in fact one of the few ways available for making palatable a diet dominated by bread. Honey was too expensive for poor families to buy. Another spread was soon found with the marketing of golden syrup, a concentrated solution of sugar, which seemed, to the poor consumer, a good alternative to honey. Sugar was also used to preserve fruit, and thus jams and spreads became popular in the Victorian diet. The poor, indeed, lived largely on a diet of bread, jam and tea.

Above all, cheap sugar formed the basis for two new industries: the confectionery industry, founded in the mid-19th century by a handful of Quaker families, the Rowntrees, the Cadburys and the Frys, and the cake and biscuit industries, which grew up on the back of cheap flour and cheap sugar at the end of the 19th century. So the cornerstones of the British diet, or at least those parts that now cause so much anxiety, were the result of cheap sugar.

The other dominant factor in the shaping of the modern diet, cheap flour, did not arrive until after the repeal of the Corn Laws in 1846 in the wake of the Irish famine. Contrary to many landowners' expectations, agriculture did not suffer at first; rather it continued to expand, sustained by the demand of the rapidly growing urban population, which progressively increased from one in five of the population at the start of the 19th century, to four in five by its end. Agricultural decline set in only during the last three decades of the 19th century, when British farming sank into a slump that lasted more or less continuously until World War II, with more than 10 per cent of the rural workforce leaving the land each decade. The reason behind this slump, like that behind the earlier growth, was technological change, but this time the changes took place overseas.

The development of the railroads in the USA and Canada after the Civil War made it possible to ship grain from the prairies to the East Coast cities and hence to Europe. The scale of production was immense and the prices were low, and North American wheat imports soon dominated the British diet. By 1877 about 40 per cent of all wheat consumed came from the USA and Canada. By 1914 it was 80 per cent. It was this importation of wheat that set the pattern of British cereal consumption on its present path. First, as prices fell (and they fell by 50 per cent between

1873 and 1893) cereal consumption rose, and it was probably this that averted widespread starvation among the urban poor. Another beneficial change resulted from the fact that American wheat is different from the type grown in European countries. It is called hard or strong wheat, as opposed to soft wheat, and it

It was the importation of North American wheat that led directly to the British white loaf that has for so long been the subject of complaint.

makes better bread and has a higher protein content. This was particularly important to the Victorian poor for whom cereals were a major source of protein. On the debit side, it was the importation of North American wheat that led directly to the British white loaf that has for so long been the subject of complaint. The wheat was imported through only a few ports, which led to the centralization of milling facilities, the demise of the old watermills and windmills and the development of steam-powered mills. These used the new method of roller milling, flattening the wheat grain between rollers rather than grinding it between stones, which made possible the cheap production of a much whiter flour and enabled white bread to become a common component of the diet. With traditional milling the wheat grain was so finely broken that it was difficult to separate the bran and the germ and so white flour had been an expensive luxury. In the roller mill the bran and the wheat germ were flattened into a flake, and this and the bran could easily be sieved out, leaving a flour of hitherto unattainable whiteness, freely and cheaply available. Since everyone was being offered the chance to eat a rich man's bread, they quickly did so, and so the British diet was suddenly deprived of nearly all its cereal fibre content as well as all the B vitamins in the wheat germ. The miller, of course, found this attractive as the 30 per cent of the flour now rejected could be sold to the new industries providing feed for farm animals.

The small-scale millers, however, could not compete against the lower costs and great popularity of roller-milled flour, and the flour-milling industry rapidly became an oligopoly. In 1851 there were 37,500 independent millers: by 1935 the figure had fallen to 2,000, while today over 75 per cent of all milling and two-thirds of bread production reside in the hands of just two companies, Rank-Hovis McDougall and Associated British Foods (ABF).

Ironically, as white bread became the food of the masses, the more affluent developed a desire for brown bread or whole cereal instead. This was seen in the Hovis loaf developed in 1892 as a product of especial health value – its name comes from the Latin, *Hominis vis* (the strength of man) – and in the breakfast cereal, which was developed by W.K. Kellogg in 1906, giving commercial expression to the diet reform prescribed by his vegetarian doctor brother, who advocated more natural and therefore more healthy food. The millers soon saw these products as another outlet for grain, and, as their popularity grew, so did the involvement of the giant companies, so that today, for example, ABF is one of the major breakfast cereal manufacturers in the UK.

Faced with intense competition from imported grain, many British farmers switched from wheat to animal production but thereby gained only a short respite. Canned meat imports arrived from Australia about 1860, and from America in 1868. Such meat was not highly regarded, being of poor quality and sometimes a

'*By the late 19th century the British farmers who had grown rich from providing the food for the Industrial Revolution of a century before were being bankrupted by its success.*'

source of food poisoning. It was eaten because it was cheap compared with home-produced meat, but it never secured more than 20 per cent of the market for meat. However, in 1880 the first shipments of refrigerated meat from Australia arrived in the SS *Strathleven*, and with this technological advance the British meat farmer lost his protection. The same railroads that brought American wheat to the East Coast ports now brought cattle too, and the first cargo of refrigerated meat arrived from the USA soon after the first Australian cargo. New Zealand and Argentina soon followed suit, until by 1914 half of all meat eaten in the UK was imported. The same agriculture that had lost its market for wheat now suffered the erosion of its market for meat. Again, the British public benefited in the short term, and in the late 19th century as cheap meat arrived so consumption doubled.

But for the British farmer the outlook was bleak. Faster transport and better methods of preservation progressively eroded the profitability of all the alternative crops he might consider. Some fruit and vegetables could be grown at home, but fruit growing was always easier in hotter, sunnier countries, and as transport and preservation improved, not only could our own native fruits be imported more cheaply than we could grow them here, but new, more cheaply produced tropical and semi-tropical fruit, such as bananas, oranges and pineapples, became widely available alternatives.

For a brief period dairying became profitable because farm milk could now be brought to the cities by railway and also because the Victorians seemed surprisingly willing to eat somewhat rancid butter. But new technology soon eroded this market too. With refrigeration, butter and cheese from New Zealand and Australia became cheaper than home-produced alternatives, even after transport and preservation costs had been paid. By the late 19th century the British farmers who had grown rich from providing the food for the Industrial Revolution of a century before were being bankrupted by its success. Britain was the wealthy manufacturing centre of the world, but as its industry grew its farming declined. In the fifty years following the Great Exhibition of 1851 employment in the heavy industries, like mining, the iron and steel industries and ship-building, grew about fourfold but the number of farmers fell by nearly a quarter.

——*OUR MODERN DIET*——

Ironically, when British agriculture was booming the average Briton's diet was appalling, but as it slumped in the late 19th century so the diet improved. There can be no doubt about this improvement, for though white bread, more sugar, loss of fibre and more meat fat might now be seen as changes for the worse, they improved the lot of the 19th-century masses and offered an escape from malnutrition and poverty. The improvement in health that occurred during the 19th century is largely attributable to improved supplies of food. Not that all was well. Inadequate nutrition continued to be a problem at least until World War II, but the aggregate level of feeding slowly rose. Of course, as it did so, it brought with it a pattern of eating and food consumption that today many people see as actively harmful and very few believe to be desirable. Nevertheless it is difficult to see how a more healthy diet (by today's standards) could have been produced in the amounts needed with the technology available. Even such a brief look at the changes that occurred in the 19th century shows the fallacy of the belief that our present diet, with all its faults, is the result of the machinations of a malign food industry. Our present diet is simply the product of our history, and like so many historical processes must be seen as "the outcome of chance and necessity".

World War II introduced a new factor. Britain is extremely vulnerable to blockade and as our reliance on imported food grew greater, so did that vulnerability. Already, in World War I, we had suffered food shortages due to the U-boats' disruption of surface shipping. As World War II loomed, planners were determined to prepare for the same problems, rightly too, for the initial German victories left Britain isolated.

The wartime food policy was not merely intended to ensure equitable distribution of what food there was. The government took over the whole direction of food production, encouraging farmers to increase productivity, and dictating what should be grown or imported.

It was concerned not just with preventing any *deterioration* in the nation's health during the long years of the war, but also, since it was still bordering on nutritional deficiency, with *improving* it. There was no conception in these policies that excesses could be bad; the problem was to get rid of deficiency. So in the wartime posters fat and sugar were depicted as good. When, in order to waste less cereal, the milling practices were changed to produce a more wholemeal bread instead of white flour, nutritional experts, afraid that this increased fibre might reduce the absorption of minerals like calcium and therefore be harmful, stipulated that millers should produce a flour halfway between white and wholemeal. In another particularly tragic case, so much vitamin D was added to fortify infant milk that vitamin D poisoning claimed quite a number of infant lives.

After the war the system of rationing persisted until the 1950s but, more importantly, the system of directing agriculture was never dismantled. It became less draconian, but a complex system of subsidies developed to ensure that farming never again slid into a slump and that we would never again be so vulnerable. Through this system of price support, farmers were given relatively secure markets and began to invest heavily in the technology that would let them increase production even more. During the 1950s and 1960s British agriculture became both highly technological and highly profitable. The change that occurred when we joined the EEC is less than has often been supposed, for the Common Agricultural Policy (CAP), with its guarantees to producers, was not really so different from the pre-existing British system, except that the guarantees and subsidies were more generous. Most of the problems that the CAP has created come from the fact that it was designed, before the UK joined, by a

> Our present diet is simply the product of our history, and like so many historical processes must be seen as "the outcome of chance and necessity".

smaller EEC dominated by France and Germany, where it served to prevent the demise of the still existing peasant farming methods and preserve the countryside. In Britain the CAP met an agriculture that was already relatively mechanized and intensive. Instead of preserving the traditional rural life, it simply encouraged further intensification. The results – those infamous meat, butter and grain mountains, and milk and wine lakes – are a monument to the inability of a group of nation states to sacrifice their individual gain for the common good. Eventually they will have to do so, if only because the CAP costs too much to be maintained indefinitely. There are, indeed, some signs that this might be happening now. Some EEC grants are being given to farmers to encourage them to take land out of food production and use it for forestry, which may return some land to unspoilt countryside that we can again enjoy. But even if our agriculture is cut back to reduce the food surpluses, it will almost certainly retain most of its present characteristics: highly productive, highly profitable and highly intensive. It is this latter factor, the subject of so much debate, to which we will now turn.

——INTENSIVE FARMING——

Farmers who attempt to produce with what they call "maximum efficiency" are usually doing no such thing. To produce as much food as possible, greater stress must be laid on cereals and potatoes rather than animals or fruit. But such a strategy would be difficult to impose because we like the inefficient foods. During the last war, when government scientists tried to discourage the growing of onions, which have little nutritional value, to free land for more nutritious crops, public pressure forced them to drop the idea. Farmers today grow the foods we want to eat, not necessarily the ones we need, and when they talk of maximizing efficiency what they mean is maximizing economic efficiency – i.e., their profits.

To do this, farmers try to produce the foodstuffs for which they get good yields and high prices. The limiting constraints on what crops they can grow are to a large extent fixed by geography: for example, it would be a foolhardy farmer who tried to grow soft fruit in Yorkshire, while in the West Country the lush pastures make dairying an attractive option. Given the crops that can be grown, the farmer does not then necessarily grow the one which gives the "maximum" profit per unit of yield. Rather, he seeks to produce the largest total profit. It is, for example, more profitable to produce 100 tons of crop at a profit of £50 per ton than 60 tons at a profit of £70 a ton.

Whatever crop is chosen, the bigger profits come with higher yields, and since these are fixed ultimately by the amount of land that the farmer has, there is a tendency to seek the highest possible yields per acre. The farmer does this by growing or rearing as much as possible per acre and by reducing the time taken to get the crop, or animals, to the state at which they can be sold and the land reused.

This is the basis of the modern approach, known as "intensive farming".

> *Farmers today grow the foods we want to eat, not necessarily the ones we need, and when they talk of maximizing efficiency what they mean is maximizing economic efficiency – i.e., their profits.*

Its impact on arable farming can be seen in a variety of ways. With most crops there has been increased use of artificial fertilizers, pesticides and mechanized aids (such as greenhouses and irrigation for crops like lettuce). There have also been changes in the crop strains planted as well as the introduction of new crops which give big net profits, oilseed rape, with which vast areas of south-east England are now planted, being one spectacular example.

Similar intensive methods have been adopted in animal production. Meat animals are reared as rapidly as possible, weaned early and frequently kept inside to be fed high energy and high protein diets instead of being allowed to graze. In the attempt to speed up and maximize growth various chemicals, notably hormones and antibiotics, are used. The most extreme example of intensive animal production, called factory farming, has attracted special criticism. The much-quoted example of the unfortunate factory-farmed hen, caged in often impossibly cramped conditions and either required to lay eggs at a spectacular rate or intensively reared to produce cheap chicken for the supermarket, has become a notorious cause for widespread public concern.

This rise in the intensity of production is reflected in various statistics. Since the aim of intensive farming is to increase the amount of livestock that a given amount of land can support, we can, for instance, assess the intensiveness of pig production by the ratio of the number of animals kept to the number of piggeries. Between 1966 and 1976, while the number of separate piggeries on UK farms fell by 61 per cent, the total production of sows rose by 12 per cent, so that on average the scale of the pig-keeping increased almost threefold.

While intensive arable farming has attracted no criticisms on ethical grounds, intensive techniques in animal production have provoked a great deal of moral outrage. Undoubtedly such techniques are disturbing to see, and an increasing number of people have become vegetarians through disgust at the conditions under which such animals are kept. In reply, farmers' organizations claim that animals kept under these conditions of warmth, ample food and regulated daylight may in fact suffer less than free-range animals. But this controversial issue is really beyond the scope of this book.

Our concern here is with the effects that intensive production methods might have on the nutritional quality, and here there are four issues to consider.

The first issue is whether nutritional value declines because of a reduction in the nutrient content of the produce, which might make nutrient deficiency more likely. The second question is whether there might be a rise in possibly adverse nutrients such as saturated fat, which could mean that intensively produced food might predispose to the diseases of affluence. Third, many people believe that somehow intensively farmed foods have lost some of their flavour. The final area of concern is whether animal products produced intensively present a special risk because they contain toxic residues from such items as hormones and other growth promoters or antibiotics.

INTENSIVE PRODUCTION AND LOW NUTRIENT LEVELS IN FOOD

Many people question whether intensive production causes low nutrient levels in food. The short answer to this question is a qualified "no". It is remarkably difficult to produce animals or plants that are deficient in the nutrients they would normally

In spite of what many people believe, provided the nutrients are all present and in the right ratio, there is no difference in nutritional value between food from plants fertilized with "natural" organic fertilizers and those treated with "artificial" inorganic fertilizers.

contain. The nutrients that animals and plants contain are not there to make them more useful as foodstuffs; they are necessary to the life and health of the animal or plant. Nutrient-deficient plants and animals make no sense to the farmer because their growth is poor and their yields are low.

In the case of plants, the only nutrients the farmer can control are those provided in fertilizers. The plant makes everything else itself. The plant nutrients provided in fertilizers are nitrogen, minerals and trace elements. If these are not provided in the correct balance, the health of the plant will be affected and in some cases it will have a lower content of the missing nutrient. The farmer, of course, dislikes this because his yields, and hence profits, will be reduced, and fertilizers are, therefore, adjusted carefully to feed the crops to get maximal yields.

Claims that food is produced with "natural" or "organic" fertilizers are not uncommon. These include animal manures, which are contrasted with "inorganic" fertilizers, in which the minerals needed by the plant are present as simple chemicals, usually made in a chemical factory. In spite of what many people believe, provided the nutrients are all present and in the right ratio, there is no difference in nutritional value between food from plants fertilized with "natural" organic fertilizers and those treated with "artificial" inorganic fertilizers. One century-old experiment comparing the two types of fertilizers on wheat yields has yet to show any difference in the nutritional value between the two methods. If any difference did exist it would probably favour artificial fertilizers, since unmodified organic fertilizers are less likely to be well-balanced.

The ecological advantage, however, probably does lie with organic fertilizers, for the nutrients they contain are released only slowly as soil bacteria act on the manure, and they therefore do less ecological damage than the simple inorganic fertilizers, which can be rapidly leached from the soil and then pollute waterways. However, slow-release inorganic fertilizers are now available which should reduce this problem. Organic fertilizers also help to maintain soil structure, as does all organic material like compost (which has little value as a fertilizer).

The only way to deplete an animal of nutrients is not to include enough in its diet. Although the rapid growth that farmers try to achieve may increase the requirement for some nutrients, the farmers and the feed manufacturers have put a lot of effort into compounding diets that meet all the needs of the factory-farmed animal. For factory-farmed animals, like free-range ones, an early sign of most deficiencies is a reduction in growth. Since the economics of intensive farming depend upon getting animals up to marketable weight as quickly as possible, any growth failure will mean a reduction in profits.

The issue is, perhaps, less clear-cut if the end product is not the animal itself but a by-product, such as eggs or milk. It is now acknowledged that the high levels of productivity required of the intensively reared laying hen not only appear to upset some aspects of its metabolism, but lead to the production of eggs that are slightly lower in vitamins B_{12} and folic acid than free-range husbandry produces. These lower levels of vitamins are of little practical significance in any normal diet, but it is clearly important, for the sake of the hens as well as the consumer, to correct these imbalances and research is in progress to do this.

> *There are some other instances, however, where the nutritional value of food actually rises because of factory farming.*

There are some other instances, however, where the nutritional value of food actually rises because of factory farming. For example, the vitamin A and D content of milk from cows kept by traditional methods is higher in the summer than winter because when the animals are put out to pasture in the summer they consume more β-carotene (from which they make vitamin A) from the fresh grass and make more vitamin D in their skin from the sunlight than they do during the winter. Modern systems of intensive husbandry add high levels of both vitamins to the intensive feed and thereby largely obliterate this seasonal drop in the vitamin content of milk.

Although the body regulates the level of most vitamins, the fat-soluble ones (vitamins A, D, E and K) can be stored if fed at high levels. Levels of these vitamins therefore tend to be higher in intensively farmed animals, whose diets are richer in nutrients, than in free-range animals.

One common complaint is that eggs from factory hens have paler yolks. In fact, the darker colour in eggs from free-range hens is because the hens consume foods containing coloured pigments, like the carotenoids. These dissolve in the fatty egg yolk giving it a deeper colour. Factory-farmed animals, on the other hand, are given vitamin A itself, which is colourless, so their eggs have more vitamin A in them even though their yolks are paler. This particular fuss died down because as soon as the farmers realized that the colour of egg yolks mattered to the consumer they added carotenoids as well as vitamin A to the feed.

DOES INTENSIVE FARMING CAUSE DEGENERATIVE DISEASES?

The most important difference between factory-farmed animals and free-range ones is their difference in body fat. Intensively reared animals tend to be fatter than free-range ones. One way to obtain fast growth is to feed as much food as the animals will eat. Another way is to adjust the diet so that the propensity of the animals to fatten increases. For example, feeding barley to cattle gets high rates of growth, but at the same time the animal becomes fatter. This does not mean that barley is especially fattening to humans. Ruminants have a special fore stomach, or rumen, where the food they eat is fermented by micro-organisms. This fermentation process enables them to break down the dietary fibre in plants, which for them, therefore, is not indigestible roughage but a source of calories. But barley undergoes a peculiar fermentation in the rumen which encourages the animal to become fat.

Although fatness in farm animals is undoubtedly made worse by intensive feeding, factory farming did not cause fatness in our meat. It merely made a bad situation worse. Unfortunately, fattening animals has been an aim of British agriculture for over two hundred years. The selective breeding programmes, which began at the time of the Enclosure Acts, were intended to produce animals that grew fast and developed more body fat. Like humans, the bigger animals are, the fatter they tend to be. The production of animals that are as large as possible has always meant, therefore, the production of animals that are as fat as possible. So for two hundred years the fat content in the British diet was increasing.

Now that the public are responding to health advice by avoiding fat meat, the intensive farmer is being forced to plan his feeding schedules to cut down carcass fat, and intensively farmed meat with a lower carcass fat can now be bought in most supermarkets. This manipulation has not been achieved by drugs or additives but by reducing the rate of growth. Scientists are now also trying to develop special lean breeds of meat animals.

Intensive production can also alter the composition of carcass fat in a beneficial way. In all animals body fat is of two types: invisible fat, which is found in apparently lean meat, and visible fat, or depot fat, which is found in adipose tissue. Even apparently lean meat contains invisible fat because the cells out of which all living creatures are made are basically bags of protein surrounded by a thin membrane of fat. This fat is predominantly of a type called phospholipid (see page 15), which is rich in essential polyunsaturated fatty acids. Depot fat, on the other hand, is of the type called triglyceride, which tends to be more saturated. If the diet is low in fat, most of the fatty acids in depot fat will be made by the animal from carbohydrate or protein and will be saturated or monounsaturated. If the level of fat in the diet rises, so the composition of the fatty acids in the depot fat will alter accordingly.

High fat diets, therefore, not only promote rapid growth and fattening in non-ruminant animals like pigs and birds but the meat fat from these animals, besides being more plentiful, reflects the diet that they have been fed. There is no general rule for such diets but at present fishmeal forms an important component, so the carcass meat can have quite high levels of the very polyunsaturated fish-type fatty acids (the omega-three fatty acids), which many nutritionists now regard as beneficial. These fatty acids are more likely to occur in fowl than in pig because the incorporation of too high a level of these fatty acids in pig fat makes the back fat of the pig softer and reduces its acceptability to the consumer. The nature of intensive farming thus makes it possible to manipulate the fatty acid composition of non-ruminant meat in any way that is desired, and current practices make the fat less saturated.

Ruminant animals – cows, sheep and goats – cannot tolerate more than traces of fat in their diet because dietary fat upsets the fermentation in the rumen. So the ruminant always eats a low fat diet and makes the fatty acids of its depot fat itself. These are therefore saturated.

However some scientists have argued that grass is not the ruminant's original diet since fields of cropped grass are man made. The truly wild ruminant, they argue, browses on a vegetation that has *seeds* as well as *leaves*. These seeds float through the rumen safe from the fermentation and are digested only in the true gut. Seeds contain lipid, which is

> *The nature of intensive farming thus makes it possible to manipulate the fatty acid composition of non-ruminant meat in any way that is desired, and current practices make the fat less saturated.*

rich in polyunsaturated fatty acids and which would be absorbed intact and then incorporated into the tissue fats of the wild ruminant. Thus, while the fat of a free-range ruminant on a farm is relatively saturated, the fat of the wild animal is much more unsaturated which, of course, nutritionists now believe to be desirable for the consumer.

This, of course, is food technology at its worst, changing the composition of our meat. Or is it? For all the scientists are doing is seeking to produce healthier meat than we have had for many centuries.

Australian scientists have recently tried to imitate this effect that seeds have. They fed ruminants on a diet containing droplets of polyunsaturated fat coated in specially treated protein. The protein shell was not affected by the rumen, and, like a seed, the whole package floated through it and was subsequently digested, including its lipid. In this way the Australians have found that they can get meat and milk that are rich in polyunsaturated fatty acids, like the tissues of wild ruminants.

This, of course, is food technology at its worst, changing the composition of our meat. Or is it? For all the scientists are doing is seeking to produce healthier meat than we have had for many centuries. And which, of course, is no longer available to anybody except the rich and the few hunter-gatherers on our planet.

DOES FACTORY-FARMED FOOD HAVE LESS FLAVOUR?

A loss of flavour is one by-product of factory farming that is often complained about, particularly with high-yielding strains of fruit. But scientifically conducted tests have not, on the whole, supported these complaints. It is, of course, vital that these tests should be carefully conducted. After all, if I say to you "does this organically grown tomato taste different from this artificially fertilized one?", I am almost inviting you to imagine a difference. Even if both tomatoes were the same, many people in such a situation would answer "yes" because they would genuinely imagine a difference. If I give you two eggs and say "identify which is free range by the taste", I should expect you to be right half the time, just by chance. But in properly conducted experiments most people who believe that they prefer organic or free-range produce cannot distinguish them from intensive foods, or if asked which food they prefer, choose the intensively produced one as often as the organic/free-range alternative.

It is also possible that people who believe food used to taste better are affected by nostalgia. Just as the summers of remembered childhood always seemed hotter and sunnier (and longer) than those of today, so the food tasted better long ago.

The results of taste studies on different kinds of meat have not yet been published, but here it is possible that a real difference in taste does exist in meat products. It is easy to see why this might be so. It is possible that the type of feed can affect the flavour of meat (page 112), and perhaps this and the accumulation of other ingredients from the diet in the body fat of any animal may do so too. The stress on rapid growth and fattening means that the animals go to slaughter when they are younger. Since, broadly speaking, the taste of meat develops with the age of the animal, young meat tastes less strong than older meat.

There has also been a tendency to eat meat sooner after slaughter and to keep it chilled or frozen instead of hanging it, which used to tenderize it. Tenderizing is a by-product of *post mortem* chemical changes in the meat and also of enzymic action, which also imparted flavours. Those who eat game still usually insist on its being hung; if it is eaten earlier it is tough and tasteless. So is any freshly slaughtered meat (see also page 275).

IS FACTORY-FARMED FOOD DANGEROUS?

The answer to this question must be that we don't yet know. Certain techniques used in modern farming, such as growth promoters, antibiotics and hormones, may have undesirable effects, and these are discussed in Chapter 7. Some of the fears – for instance that factory-farmed food causes cancer – are just nonsense. Apart from the problems of factory farming already outlined, there is no evidence that it somehow produces food that is unfit to eat. If there are any yet undetected effects on health to be laid at the door of factory farming, they have to be very subtle, precisely because they have not yet been discovered. But exactly the same risk exists for "organic", "traditional" or "natural" farming, whose techniques are not God-given and safe but merely methods of producing food developed by fallible humans who know only that the food produced isn't instantly toxic. Generations of people ate traditionally produced food, and all of them are dead. We have no idea what role that food could have played in their demise. Scientists suspect that although some traditional techniques did kill some people, traditionally produced food wasn't responsible for many deaths. The same scientists also claim that factory farming is not causing most of today's problems. There is no reason to believe only some of their claims are correct.

——*FISH IN OUR DIET*——

So far, we have discussed the changes that have occurred in farming, the most significant method of food production, but a second method, hunting, is still important since it provides us with fish. Fish is currently a minor component of the British diet. National statistics suggest that we use on average about 1¾oz (50g) a person a day (40lb/18kg a head a year). The Japanese by comparison, the world's major fish-eating nation, buy nearly four times as much (150lb/69kg a person a year). Whereas most of the fish consumed in Japan is eaten by humans, much of ours is used as animal feed, mostly for chickens, pigs and the petfood industry, and fish contributes only 8 per cent of the total animal protein in the UK diet. The average consumer, it is estimated, eats fish once every five days, compared with once a day for the average consumer in Japan.

Although consumption of fish in the UK is increasing only slowly, the present level is about 50 per cent higher than in the 1950s and 1960s. The rise is largely attributable to the increased consumption of prepared fish products, especially frozen fish. The consumption of fresh fish had declined to very low levels, at least until recently when the new awareness of the health-giving properties of

> ❛
> *Generations of people ate traditionally produced food, and all of them are dead. We have no idea what role that food could have played in their demise.*
> ❜

fish boosted its popularity. Canned fish, once a regular item in the diet, particularly in "Sunday teas", has declined dramatically in popularity since the 1960s.

Until recently the low level of fish consumption in the UK did not worry nutritionists. Fish was regarded only as a source of good-quality protein, so its displacement by meat as the central savoury portion of the diet caused no change in the total protein content of the diet. Nutritionists therefore felt that there was no change in the nutritional quality of the diet and no cause for concern.

As has been explained, in Chapter 3, many nutritionists now, however, are concerned that the high level of animal fat in meat may be undesirable, and in particular may increase the risk of coronary heart disease. White fish (such as cod or plaice) has a very low fat content, and its substitution for meat reduces fat consumption. Even oily fish, such as herring, is probably better than meat as fish oil contains certain highly specialized polyunsaturated fatty acids (w3 fatty acid), which some nutritionists think may in some way be protective against coronary heart disease. This new enthusiasm for fish has led to a renewed popularity of cod liver oil, much promoted in wartime Britain as a source of vitamins A and D for children. It is now being promoted in a chemically refined form, without these vitamins, as a source of polyunsaturated fatty acids. The long underrated fishing industry is, of course, benefiting from this new endorsement of its products.

Even though it may have been of less importance in our diet, the fishing, or more precisely the fish-producing, industry has not been moribund and has undergone immense changes. The development of intensive farming of fish like trout, turbot and prawns, all important products for the consumer market, is probably the most obvious.

But the most profound impact on our diet has come from a revolution in fishing techniques and consequent changes in the areas fished. These have led to a marked change in the amount and type of fish that are available. The figures for landings of mackerel illustrate this change well: landings in the UK rocketed from under 5,000 tons a year in 1960 to over 300,000 by 1980. (Consumption did not show a similar rise since most of the catch was exported.)

Ever since the "Cod War" of the 1960s when Britain and Iceland quarrelled about British trawlers fishing in the waters around Iceland, there have been periodic disputes between fishing nations about who may fish where. The latest move is the unilateral decision by Britain in 1986 to declare the waters for 150 miles around the Falklands a fishing conservation zone, insisting on licensing all vessels that fish there and on inspecting their catch and equipment. Such restrictions and subsequent arguments occur because the advances in trawler technology now make it possible for any nation's fishing fleet to fish far from home waters, thus making over-fishing a constant danger. In the case of the Falkland waters the over-fishing came from Russian, Taiwanese and Polish ships, which between them were scooping up almost half a million tons of fish a year around the Falklands, inevitably depleting the fishing grounds of certain species such as squid. Countries such as Japan and Russia, the world's two leading fishing nations, which produce more than a quarter of the total world fish catch between them, have massive fishing fleets trawling grounds from the South Atlantic to the North Sea. What makes this possible is the use of onboard freezing to preserve fish and the introduction of factory ships sailing with the fleet so that fish stocks can be effectively preserved, and to some degree processed, during the days, or even weeks, it takes to get the fish home. Consequently trawlers now fish deeper waters further from shore and trawl a different mix of species.

Like the development of intensive farming, the development of the fishing industry is not a recent phenomenon but has been happening for many years. The origins of the modern industry may be traced back to the 18th century when the centuries-old tax on salt was removed. Before this, in all except port areas, most fish consumed was freshwater fish. The basic limitation on the consumption of sea fish was the speed with which it went off, both on the journey to port and the subsequent journey to market. The only practical methods of preserving fish were smoking or salting. Salting, although the more widely used, was prohibitively expensive because of the tax on salt, and throughout the 18th century there were complaints about the impact of this tax on the poor. The difficulties of keeping the fish from spoiling on the ship also meant the boats could not venture far from shore or indeed from the markets, because transport to market was also largely by water, for example up the Thames to Billingsgate. The main sea fish caught at this time were therefore shallow-water species, notably herrings and pilchards.

By the end of the 18th century the fishing industry, spurred on by the demand from the developing industrial centres, was beginning to develop. The trawlers began to fish further from home, discovering new fishing grounds. The problem of getting the fish back to port was tackled in several ways, but all involved bringing back the catches live, either by dragging them in nets behind the boat or by putting them in specially constructed tanks on board. Both systems limited the size of the catch a single boat could handle.

During the 19th century there were great advances in fish preservation. Collecting ice during the winter became a major activity. It was kept in large underground storehouses to give an almost all-the-year-round supply of ice for preserving fresh fish on its journey to market. And, of course, improvements in roads, and more importantly, the development of railways meant that fish could be transported from ports to great conurbations without serious spoilage.

The 19th century, therefore, saw a great expansion in the amount and type of fish in the British diet. The amounts of some fish eaten were prodigious. For example, at Billingsgate market in London in the mid-19th century something like 100,000 tons of fish were sold each year. Virtually all of this was consumed by Londoners themselves, and since the population of the conurbation was at that time only two and a half million, average consumption was of the order of 100lb (45kg) a person a year – two and a half times the amount eaten today.

This pattern of consumption was dominated by some very unusual fish by today's standards. Most notable was herring of which 400 million lb (181 million kg) were sold: 16lb (7kg) for every Londoner. Surprising as it may seem today, oysters were another major item. Nearly 500 million were sold: a figure equal to 4 oysters each week for every man, woman and child in the capital. These were not consumed by the rich gourmets but were predominantly the food of the poor, being sold by costermongers in the street to the cry of "Oysters a penny a lot". In fact, oysters were rather despised by the wealthy, much as winkles or whelks are today.

The cheapness and abundance of oysters may seem strange, but they thrived near the estuaries of the effluent-rich rivers, like the Thames and the Medway, which conducted the sewage of London to the sea. Oysters were just one of the shellfish that the Londoner loved, whelks were another. Unfortunately the sewage on which they thrived, besides providing food, provided many bacteria, which attacked the oyster and eventually led to its virtual disappearance. As stocks became depleted the humble oyster disappeared from the cockney menu, and an expensive import from France found its way onto the menu of the Savoy.

The firm of John Rouse in Oldham, which is still a fish and chip shop, claims to be the one that first produced fish and chips together, soon after 1880.

The abundance of fish in the 19th century and the difficulty in keeping them fresh gave rise to another British tradition: fish and chips. The large-scale frying of fish goes back to the Middle Ages, its advantages being that, as well as cooking the fish, it arrests and to a large degree masks, the development of off-flavours and putrefaction. Fish and chips became big business as stocks of fish arrived in towns in the early 19th century, being regarded as a method of "fish-saving", particularly popular among itinerant street sellers who fried cheap end-of-day stocks purchased at Billingsgate. The quality of these can be judged from the costermonger who told the social investigator and journalist Henry Mayhew in 1851 that it was an especially good food in a gin-drinking area "for people hasn't their smell so correct there". In Dickens's *Oliver Twist* (1838) a fried fish warehouse is mentioned as part of the normal scenery around Fagin's quarter of the East End. But this fried fish was sold on its own and often eaten cold.

Deep-fried fish and chips, as we know them today, are almost certainly a Northern rather than a London invention. It has been suggested that the primary reason was that Lancashire mill girls without the time to cook food for the family needed a ready-made snack. The early fryers seem to have been made in Lancashire and installed in shops that produced and sold traditional tripe and onions. The firm of John Rouse in Oldham, which is still a fish and chip shop, claims to be the one that first produced fish and chips together, soon after 1880.

No one knows what the overall nutritional effects of the changing pattern of fish consumption in the UK have been but some can be surmised. The demise of the oyster undoubtedly led to a decline in food poisoning, since the English oyster beds were heavily polluted and the oyster, being eaten raw, is always risky unless carefully grown. The progressive displacement of shallow-water fish like herring and sprat, by deep-sea fish like cod has meant that the amount of fish oil in our diet has declined much faster than even the fall in total fish consumption since the 19th century suggests. For herrings, sprats, trout, mackerel and eels belong to the class of fish known as oily fish and have much higher levels of fat, between 10 and 20 per cent in their bodies. By contrast, white fish, the deep-sea fish of the North Sea like cod, haddock, plaice and whiting, have relatively low levels of body fat (1-2 per cent).

Fatty fish play such a small role in the modern diet that the average person obtains little more than 2 per cent of his fat intake from fish. To judge from fish sales in Billingsgate the Victorians' pattern of fish consumption provided on average about seven times as much fish oil per unit weight of fish. Oily fish would have been particularly important as a source of both vitamin A (retinol) and vitamin D (cholecalciferol), which were generally at poor levels in the Victorian diet. White fish is not itself lacking in these vitamins – both cod and halibut livers are packed with them – but the livers are not usually eaten. The flesh of white fish provides only moderate levels, comparable to lean meat. Vitamin D deficiency or rickets was a particular problem in Victorian England and up until World War II. Although lack of sunlight caused by air pollution was largely to blame for this, as Chapter 3 explained, a diet rich in vitamin D would have offered some protection. It is interesting, therefore, that contemporary observers found rickets to be rare among the children of Jewish immigrant families from Eastern Europe for whom the herring in various forms was a delicacy. The indigenous British palate, unfortunately, ran to white fish if it got the chance and rickets was common. Of course, the reduction in atmospheric pollution over the years has meant that rickets has, by and large, disappeared (except among the new Asian immigrants, see pages 38-9), and so the vitamin D content of fish has become less important.

But probably the main reason to be concerned about the low level of fish consumption is that people are not benefiting from the possible ability of fish, and particularly fish-oil, to protect against coronary heart disease. If our present consumption of fish were to revert to the Victorian pattern, with a high consumption of oily fish, our fish-oil intakes would increase markedly, and some nutritionists believe this, like an increase in total fish consumption, to be desirable. But others argue that increased levels of fish oil consumption, whatever its benefits for the heart, may also carry risks. These arise for the same reasons that caused the spoilage of fish in Victorian markets: the ease with which fish oil goes rancid. This is due to the instability of the highly polyunsaturated omega-three fatty acids and to their vulnerability to oxidizing agents like the oxygen in the air. This could be an important area where advances in food preservation may remove the risk of rancidity.

Increased levels of fish-oil consumption would lead to a build up of these highly polyunsaturated fatty acids in the body fat where they would also be vulnerable to oxidative attack in this way. This is normally prevented by the protective effects of vitamin E so eating a lot of fish increases the vitamin E requirement. Some nutritionists think that complete protection can never be obtained and that if levels of consumption are too high (i.e., if oily fish is eaten much more than twice a week) the consumer is vulnerable to what scientists call peroxidation of body fat. The effects of this are not yet understood but may include an increased risk of cancer.

These are only speculations, as indeed are the purported benefits of eating more fish, and it would be wrong to jump to any conclusions about the desirability of consuming more fish oil. What can be said, however, is that fish meets with the approval of most nutritionists and has fewer detractors than almost anything else in our diet. Above all, fish provides, as it has done for centuries, a food that is completely acceptable to most people, around which delicious meals can be built. Unfortunately, the decline in fish consumption has meant that many consumers do not know how to cook fish. We have also grown so used to fillets that fish bones are even less acceptable than they were in the past. Increasing the consumption of fish is another area that might be encouraged by the food industry – for example, if more ready-prepared fish dishes were produced or if the take-away food sector diversified its menus more.

CHAPTER 6

FROM COSTERMARKET TO HYPERMARKET

THE GROWTH OF THE FOOD INDUSTRY

*L*ike generations of our long distant ancestors, we still obtain our food chiefly by farming and, to a lesser extent, by hunting (with perhaps just a little bit of scavenging in summer hedgerows). But the most dramatic change that has occurred over the last few centuries is that so few of us now produce our own food. Although the day is long gone when the cockney child could be astounded to learn that milk came from cows, not from bottles, most of us obtain most of our energy from the farm at one step removed – through the massive, much feared and greatly reviled food industry.

The food industry has three branches or levels: manufacturing, wholesaling and retailing. It is widely believed that these branches were originally quite separate and were only recently, as the individual companies increased in size, pulled together, so that the same conglomerate controls all three levels. Like many stories in nutrition, this is a half-truth. Certainly the food industry has become a megalith, dominated by a handful of companies with interests in everything from farming to selling. But equally this process does not represent a recent fall from grace. Integration and amalgamation have been inherent in the industry from the start. Even a superficial view of its history will show that there never was an idyllic past from which the industry has recently strayed but rather that it has grown in a consistent and continuous way to what we have today.

Clearly the food industry is an urban phenomenon that is of only minimal importance in largely self-sufficient farming communities. So, just as two centuries ago Britain was an essentially rural country, it was also a country with only a rudimentary food industry. This industry, like so much else, developed in the 19th century and grew rapidly. Even by 1841, a quarter of a million people were involved in it, 10 per 1,000 of the total population. Almost three-quarters of these were butchers, bakers or grocers. By the 1911 census the food industry employed four times as many people, as many as 23 per 1,000 of the population. The number of grocers and bakers had risen, and together accounted for more than half of the

> *Food processing has become even more important if measured in financial terms, and currently one-quarter of the cost of the food we buy is attributable to processing.*

employees in the industry, while butchery had declined in relative importance. To set these figures in context, in the 1981 census 25 per thousand of the total population were employed in the food industry.

Illuminating though they are, these figures do not show the full growth of the industry during this century, for two reasons. First, the industry has produced more per employee and second the nature of employment within the industry has changed. In 1841 nearly all those employed in the food industry had direct contact with the customer. Even those whose work could be described as processing usually sold the food too. Today, in contrast, food retailing accounts for less than 50 per cent of the employment. This, of course, reflects the growth of a separate food manufacturing or processing industry, which now provides nearly 40 per cent of total employment, and of a separate wholesale sector, which accounts for another 15 per cent. Both these sectors were of minimal importance in the 1840s. Food processing has become even more important if measured in financial terms, and currently one-quarter of the cost of the food we buy is attributable to processing. It is the growth of this processing sector that is at the root of so much current concern.

Townsfolk, of course, have always needed to buy food, so food retailing is as old as the towns themselves. But until the 19th century much of the food that the town dwellers consumed was bought in city markets. There it was sold by the producers themselves, and most of it was fresh and unprocessed in any way: live animals and fresh vegetables were brought to market by the farmer and fish catches were sold at dockside markets by fishermen. One of the few processed items was cheese, the manufacture of which was largely a cottage industry taking place on farms with dairy animals.

Insofar as a separate food industry existed in the early 19th century it was an urban retail industry, with costermongers and shopkeepers buying from such markets and selling to those who, for one reason or another, did not go to market themselves. These retailers did a very limited amount of food processing – for example, salting or curing meat, frying fish or stewing eels.

In the early 19th century the most significant retail specialist was the butcher. An ordinary household was, of course, unable to slaughter its own meat, and since the large meat animals provided too much for a single household to consume before it putrefied, the butcher jointed and dressed the carcass into different portions for sale. Butchers met the perennial problem of preserving meat with a traditional range of processes: salting, curing and producing ham, bacon and sausages. The manufacture of sausages is extremely ancient: the word comes from the Latin *salsus*, meaning salted, but sausages were known before the Romans. The traditional sausage was prepared in a way that helped to preserve the meat. Like Greek or Italian sausages today, it was usually dried or cured and frequently highly spiced, all of which prevent decay (with spices having the added advantage of disguising a degree of putrefaction).

At the beginning of the 19th century bakery was far less important. Although the baker had existed in many cities for hundreds of years, in all except the larger towns most bread was baked in the home. But as towns grew, bakers rapidly became more important and bakers' shops multiplied at an enormous rate. In 1800, for example, the town of Manchester already had a population of 70,000 people yet it had no commercial bakers; by 1835 the population of 200,000 had 650 bakers.

> *Ironically, although the neighbourhood baker is seen today as a bastion of traditional values and food advertisements try to evoke the picture of the traditional baker baking traditional bread, in the 1830s he was greeted by many social reformers as an agent of the devil.*

The reasons behind this rapid rise were complex. As we saw in Chapter 5, when the Corn Laws were repealed and the price of grain fell, wheat bread increasingly replaced barley and rye bread in the diet. Since grain was cheaper, the money saved on the flour could now be spent on processing (i.e., baking) without the price of bread rising and sales falling.

There was another reason behind the bakery boom too: bread didn't keep and so baking was a daily job. But the new factories were employing women who no longer had the time to bake every few days and were therefore willing to use the bakers' shops. The builders of the new slums capitalized on this by building cheap houses in which living and sleeping rooms replaced kitchens and which had no bread ovens in the fireplace, thus forcing everyone, except those who could afford a kitchen range, to buy their bread from shops. Ironically, although the neighbourhood baker is seen today as a bastion of traditional values and food advertisements try to evoke the picture of the traditional baker baking traditional bread, in the 1830s he was greeted by many social reformers as an agent of the devil. Shop-baked bread, this new processed food, was deplored both for being bad for health and because it encouraged laziness and moral decay in the women who bought it!

Besides the butcher and baker, the other major retailer to emerge in the 19th-century town was the grocer. As we shall see, the development of our modern food industry was largely spearheaded by the changes that occurred in the grocery trade. The term grocer had entered the language in the Middle Ages to describe a spicer, a merchant who dealt in the lucrative business of bringing spices from the East. But only towards the middle of the 19th century did the retail grocer's shop come to exist. The Victorian retail grocer dealt in relatively non-perishable foodstuffs – items like sugar, tea, coffee, dried beans and peas, cheese, cured meat, butter and fat. Because such goods were non-perishable, the grocer was not tied to local production and so with grocery began the wholesale and distribution side of the food business. Indeed, in one sense the grocer developed because of the importance in our diet of the main imported components – tea, coffee and sugar. These commodities were imported over vast distances by sea, which required considerable outlay in the cost of ships and crew, quite apart from the costs of setting up plantations. But the prices obtained at auctions when the cargoes arrived

> *The development of our modern food industry was largely spearheaded by the changes that occurred in the grocery trade.*

showed that money could be made in food wholesaling both by the grocers who bought to resell and by the individuals or syndicates who financed the voyage.

Our modern food industry has also been shaped by the strange and corrupt nature of Victorian grocery. As the towns grew and the new suburbs developed, so the grocer in the town centre was cut off from a larger and larger proportion of the urban population and was confronted by itinerant grocers who hawked tea and other groceries from door to door. Larger dealers working in town centres met this challenge by advertising their goods and offering to deliver them, usually as ready-made-up parcels, under a proprietary name. This was the origin of both the multiple grocer and the idea of a brand of goods.

In selling under a specific name the grocer was seeking to offer the consumer a guarantee of quality. Quality was important because retailers were often accused of adulterating food and the itinerant hawker could certainly do this with impunity. Tea, being both expensive and popular, was particularly prone to adulteration and the sale of tea in packets was originally a response to the problem of illegal but profitable adulteration. One practice was to dry used tea leaves and sell them again. (In the 1840s eight factories reprocessing tea from hotels existed in London alone!) The addition of other leaves to teas was more harmful, since the adulterant was often toxic, as were the chemicals that were often added as well to get an inferior mix looking and behaving in an acceptable way. Victorian tea was often contaminated with lead salts and copper carbonate, both of which are toxic.

Since the retailer bought loose tea leaves from the wholesaler and only packaged it upon sale to the customer, a guarantee against adulteration depended not only on the retailer's honesty but also on his acumen in selecting a source of supply. In 1826 a Quaker grocer, Joseph Horniman, attempted to provide a guarantee of quality to his customers by selling his specially chosen tea in sealed lead-lined packets, which could not be tampered with. Although we might now express concern at his unfortunate choice of a potentially toxic packaging material, Horniman's tea clearly met a national need because by 1870 sales had reached 5 million packets a year.

The mechanized mass production of packet tea followed in 1884 with Mazawattee tea. Then, in 1889, a young Scots grocer, Thomas Lipton, introduced his own brand of tea, not merely guaranteeing the quality but also the price, which he set at 1s 7d (9p) a pound to undercut the prevailing retail price of 2s 6d (12½p). The success of this venture encouraged him to produce other branded goods and to guarantee his supplies by purchasing everything from tea estates in Ceylon to hog packaging facilities in Chicago. Lipton was the first modern multiple grocer, and by 1914, thirty-eight years after he opened his first shop, he had 500 retail outlets.

More importantly, Lipton soon had dozens of imitators and rivals; the modern retail grocer had arrived. The competition was, of course, intense and both the retailing and processing sides of the industry were constantly involved in bankruptcies and takeovers.

Just as the growth of grocery wholesaling was stimulated by grocers importing food, so butchers, too, were affected by the rise in imported meat. Even before this, the retail butcher had sometimes

❛—————————————————

Lipton was the first modern multiple grocer, and by 1914, thirty-eight years after he opened his first shop, his empire had 500 retail outlets.

—————————————————❜

found it difficult to find the capital to buy carcasses at his local market, while the scale of the investment now needed to import boatloads of canned or refrigerated meat from Australia or the Americas was far beyond him. The importation of meat from overseas became the preserve of large combines from which the retail

The millers also became bakers and factory baking produced cheaper bread and bigger profits. The soggy cut white loaf became our heritage.

butcher had to purchase his supplies. Such meat had, of course, been chosen, slaughtered and dressed in its place of origin, so the retail butcher's contribution to processing became limited to jointing meat.

Towards the end of the century advances in milling had likewise limited the crafts involved in the baking industry. The independent miller had all but disappeared as the roller mills took over. The new large milling combines began to control the baking of bread both by buying bakers and by controlling bread prices through their monopoly of flour supplies. The rapid staling of bread, however, meant that baking had to remain a local process until after World War II. Then plastic wrapping and new additives to preserve bread enabled the shelf-life of the loaf to be extended from a day to a matter of weeks. The consequence was almost inevitable. The millers also became bakers and factory baking produced cheaper bread and bigger profits. The soggy cut white loaf became our heritage.

It will be clear that in the evolution of the modern food industry two different changes have occurred simultaneously: an increase in the size of companies involved and a concentration of skills. By the early 20th century, after a series of takeovers, effective control for whole areas of food production was approaching a monopoly. Already by the 1930s, for example, 40 per cent of the bacon cured in the UK was produced by one company, Marsh and Baxter. Virtually all imported sugar was in the control of Tate and Lyle, and nearly all London's milk supplies were controlled, directly or indirectly, by the United Dairies. Likewise meat imports, milling and tea supplies were all in the hands of oligopolies.

In the 1930s there were still many independent retail outlets: for example, there were 80,000 grocers, of which less than 20 per cent were part of chains, and 40,000 butchers, while greengrocers' and bakers' shops each numbered 30,000. But we have seen how the development of the food industry had changed them, stripping away many of their independent skills and converting them from craftsmen to tradesmen. As always, the grocery business led the way. The grocers' skills had been reduced by the turn of the century to cutting cheese and wrapping butter.

New priorities therefore developed in retailing, particularly retail grocery, with more attention being paid to the art of selling, to shop design, advertising and the provision of a good service. It may seem strange to us now when we hanker after old-fashioned service, but it was this change in emphasis that rang the death knell for the independent grocer. He now had nothing useful to do except sell, and

It may seem strange to us now when we hanker after old-fashioned service, but it was this change in emphasis that rang the death knell for the independent grocer. He now had nothing useful to do except sell.

success would depend on how well that was done. Literacy was becoming more widespread by the end of the 19th century and the level of sales was mainly influenced not by the quality of service, or even of the goods, but by newspaper advertising, particularly in the new popular press. With advertising, as with so much else, the advantage is with the conglomerate, and the independent grocer could not survive for very long. Even by the beginning of World War II chain-store grocers were responsible for over half of all grocery sales.

As the food industry has grown it has aggregated into larger and larger units. Consider Unilever, the large manufacturing combine whose founder was William Lever (later Lord Leverhulme). His original company, Lever Brothers, was founded in 1885 to manufacture soaps by a new process. William Lever had dreams of revitalizing the moribund Scottish fishing industry, and as a step in this direction he bought a retail fish shop in 1919. By 1921 he had a chain of 360 such shops, which he named Macfisheries. The shops were taken over by his company, which also purchased trawling companies and a wholesale fish business at Billingsgate. At that time sausages were an indispensable part of the fish shop stock, so the company of Walls was acquired, too, to provide them. This was the beginning of Unilever, now the ninth largest company in the world. In 1986 its total worldwide sales from a total of 75 countries amounted to over £17 billion, a large proportion of which came from food and the remainder from such diverse activities as toiletries, packaging and plastics. Many apparently independent UK manufacturers are, in fact, part of the Unilever conglomerate, including Batchelors, Birds Eye, Brooke Bond, van den Burghs, Liptons, Macfisheries, Mattessons, Walls and John West.

The history of Macfisheries demonstrates that one by-product of the growth of the food conglomerates is the disappearance of the independent food wholesaler. As both retailing and manufacture have increased in size, so manufacturers now sell their own produce directly to retail chains. The food wholesaler had a role only when the retail chain was both independent and small-scale.

Inevitably the power of food manufacturing has increased as it has grown in size. Birds Eye, for example, foremost among our packers of frozen vegetables, has contracts with over a hundred East Anglian farmers. In such a situation they can virtually dictate farming policy for a whole region.

—FOOD PROCESSING: CURSE OR BLESSING?—

In the 20th century the food industry has grown from being a supplier of food to being a supplier of meals. That is to say, it has become a distributor of processed food. Processed food is a subject guaranteed to provoke an argument. Quite apart from the question of whether the processing of food somehow makes it less healthy (which is dealt with in Chapter 7), processed food attracts a lot of criticism because much of food processing is devoted to the production of convenience foods.

Some of the criticism of convenience foods is not very different from the 19th-century reaction to bakers. A good cook can undoubtedly produce food with a taste and flavour that convenience foods can rarely, if ever, mimic. However home cooking, at least in British cuisine, is extremely time-consuming. If fruit and salad play a major role in the diet, home cooking may be compatible with the fast preparation of food (although the preparation of a good salad is fairly time-consuming). Many people in Britain today are no longer willing to spend much time on food preparation. There are those who deplore such an attitude, feeling that home cooking is somehow virtuous, especially for women. But those who stress the traditional virtues of cooking are often ignorant of its history

Cooking, as we have now come to understand it, hardly existed until the late 19th century, when the first step in the

> *Cooking, as we have now come to understand it, hardly existed until the late 19th century, when the first step in the convenience food revolution made it available to all. This was the development of the controllable stove.*

convenience food revolution made it available to all. This was the development of the controllable stove. Cooking is an extremely complicated process in which we seek to alter the chemistry and physics of food by the application of a limited range of agents, foremost among them heat. Until the 19th century, cooking was limited by the fact that there was no controllable source of heat. Most people cooked over an open fire or used brick ovens, either built into the main fireplace or set in the scullery. Temperature control was non-existent so that even relatively simple cooking operations required constant supervision because foods needed to be removed from the heat frequently to regulate the rate at which they were cooked. In the grand houses of Victorian times this could be achieved by an army of kitchen-maids, each one supervising different components of the meal. But most people, of course, could afford no such army, and so the meal was limited in scope by the need for simple cooking techniques. Broiling, roasting, boiling or frying were the limit of the culinary horizons and ordinary people seem to have eaten hot meals only two or three times a week.

The first controllable stove was the closed kitchen range, invented by the famous eccentric scientist Sir William Thompson (later Count Rumford) at the very end of the 18th century. It did not come into general use, even in middle-class homes, until the 1850s. Although a great advance on the open fire, it had relatively crude temperature control, and the first truly adjustable stove was the gas stove, which provided an oven in which temperature could be reliably and precisely adjusted. The great French chef, Alexis Soyer, had used such an oven in the Reform Club in London in the 1830s, but the domestic gas oven really dates from 1855 when one was put on sale at the price of £25. Since this was about three or four months' wages even for a well-paid working man, it is not surprising that the gas stove remained confined to affluent households and did not come into general use until the 1890s.

The gas stove was a transforming influence, enabling the development of some kind of basic cuisine in ordinary homes and a more complex cuisine than ever before in the homes of the rich. It is no coincidence that the great French chefs L'Escoffier and Montagne, who created modern *cordon bleu* cooking, lived at this time. But as cooking became more complex it took up more of women's time. There are no figures available, but it is easy to see that as the gastronomic horizons of ordinary people were extended so the time that had to be spent preparing food increased. In a period when servants were common and even the lower middle classes could usually afford a cook, this might have been tolerable to the housewife. But by the end of World War II, when the cook had almost disappeared from all but the richest

> *Whatever reservations may be expressed about the quality, or even the safety, of processed food, no one denies that food processing contributes to the liberation of the housewife.*

homes in Britain, cooking had become a major occupation for many housewives just at the point when they were demanding more freedom from the stove and the sink, not least because the war had made the phenomenon of the working wife common and acceptable. At the same time the reaction against the restrictions imposed by wartime shortages was leading to a demand for a change from the plain food that dominated cooking in Britain. The food-processing industry is the way that *impasse* has been resolved. Whatever reservations may be expressed about the quality, or even the safety, of processed food, no one denies that food processing contributes to the liberation of the housewife.

The food industry does not, of course, produce processed foods with the liberation of women in mind. It exists to make profits or, as is the nature of most industries, to make continually larger profits. In its early days the food industry went on increasing its sales because there were progressively more people to feed. Otherwise, as long as it sold predominantly unprocessed food, its chances of increasing its profits were restricted. As poor people get richer they consume more food but this process does not continue indefinitely; few humans consistently eat much more than 3,000 kilocalories each day. Thus the market is not infinite. Of course, as people get richer they eat more expensive food – for example eating less bread and more meat – but again there is a limit to any growth in consumption. If profits are to continue to increase once these natural plateaux were reached, the food industry has to sell us the same foodstuffs at higher cost. It achieves this by processing that food. Thus, instead of buying fresh vegetables, we buy them frozen or processed in some other way. Instead of buying raw meat, we buy meat dishes that are ready to reheat.

Many people view this change as reprehensible. Undoubtedly some skills are lost and a generation of women has now grown up who are far less skilled at cooking than their mothers were. But is this necessarily so bad? As long as someone knows how to produce ready prepared food and provided that producer does not produce foods with health risks, there is no need for us all to know how to cook any more than we should all know how to be farmers or tailors. Nor is cooking really a long-established tradition. Indeed, for generations before the late 19th century women

> *As long as someone knows how to produce ready prepared food and provided that producer does not produce foods with health risks, there is no need for us all to know how to cook any more than we should all know how to be farmers or tailors.*

of "breeding" (and almost all men) couldn't cook at all. Cooking was a menial job, not a task for men or ladies but for servants. Probably very few of the 19th-century moralizers who condemned the working woman for her inability to cook knew any more about cooking themselves than ringing for cook. Then the skills of a lady of leisure were to know how to judge quality. Just as they might know a good tailor, these women would

126

pride themselves on knowing how to recognize a good cook. Today's consumer needs to know how to recognize a responsible and reliable food manufacturer – which is perhaps not always easy, given the rapid advances in food technology and the obscure terminology on food labels.

A more valid argument against convenience foods is the frequently voiced criticism that they don't taste as good. Of course, taste is subjective, and there is no objective measure of what tastes good and what doesn't. Some people probably prefer home-made to convenience foods because they were brought up on them and have acquired a palate for their particular balance of tastes. The basic mistake is to compare the taste of the convenience food with the real food that it claims to be like. Canned cream of tomato soup, for example, is a poor imitation of real (i.e., home-made) tomato soup, even though the food industry sells it under that guise. It is rather itself, for there is no natural, home-made tomato soup to match its taste. There is, of course, a sameness about canned tomato soup because the process by which it is produced is more constant and more finely controlled than even the most excellent chef can achieve. But most people have experienced the sensation of meeting a particular processed food for the first time and finding it an exquisite new experience. Then after they have eaten it a few times, the taste begins to pall.

Having thus defended processed convenience food, it must be admitted that there is also much wrong with it. Perhaps the worst aspect is the way in which it has come to be associated with low-quality ingredients and with a wide range of additives. This has happened because the processor has seized the opportunity to use the skills of food chemistry to trick our palates.

The most famous example of this is the English sausage, a processed convenience food that predates the modern food industry. But the modern sausage is a very different object from its ancestors. Although regarded as meat by most consumers, the sausage is at best a meat sandwich, for it contains up to 40 per cent cereal and the meat it does contain is largely the by-products that we otherwise reject: excess carcass fat (the product of our intensive agriculture), offal, skin and other undesirable bits of lean meat. There is perhaps some ecological justification for this practice, for it is better to consume such animal by-products than to throw them away. There is also the economic argument that the more of these by-products that are used, the more money is got for the carcass and so the price of muscle meat is lower. But many people find these by-products unacceptable. So, by the use of additives and other tricks, the food industry packages them as though they were something different. The same is true, although to a lesser extent, of many of the immensely popular burgers, and in a similar way of many ice creams, which are a mixture of sugar and of fat that has never been near a dairy.

Because items like sugar and fat are incorporated into convenience food in disguise, they can make it extraordinarily difficult to eat a sensible diet. A hamburger that looks like lean meat can provide up to 50 per cent of its energy as fat and, unlike a fatty pork chop, you can't cut off the fat if you want to. Fat and sugar are, of course, added to produce convenience food at prices that will compete with, or undercut, unprocessed food. But neither low quality nor additives are the inevitable consequence of processed or convenience food. The revolution in eating habits that has occurred in the last few years has led to the production of a whole new series of convenience foods in which the number of additives have been reduced, while items like low fat sausages made with lean meat can now be purchased in the high street supermarket. Rising incomes among the middle classes, accompanied by an increasing disposition to spend money on food, has also led to the development of a range of delicatessen processed foods such as ice cream that contains real cream and beefburgers that are really made with ground lean beef.

Such foods inevitably cost more, and this is the nub of the problem, for surveys suggest that the average British consumer still rates cheapness as a major reason for choosing a given food, even though most consumers spend a much smaller proportion of their income on food than ever before. The choice is in effect ours: if we recognize that the labour we would otherwise put into the food has a cost, that our time is worth money, convenience foods may provide as much value for money as high grade ones.

But before we get too complacent it is also worth remembering that for many people in our society no such choice exists. Many people cannot afford to eat a diet of new healthy processed foods. For a single parent family, for example, where pressures on time make it necessary to use processed foods, only the cheap ones can be afforded. And the cheap ones are the traditional high fat or high sugar concoctions.

CHAPTER 7

THE MULTIPLE STORE AND THE RISE OF THE SUPERMARKET

The current passion for nostalgia has given a certain vogue to old photographs, and in almost every branch library it is possible to find sepia photographs showing what your local high street used to be like. Almost anywhere the comparison between such a photo and the modern high street will reveal three related changes.

First, in almost every high street there are now fewer food shops, even though there will be more people living and shopping in the area. Second, there is a reduced diversity of shops; that is, there are fewer specialist shops, like butchers and bakers, and instead more and more types of food are now being sold in the grocers' shops. Third, if different high streets are compared, there is now a certain repetitiveness in the names that those shops bear. In the sepia photographs the shops usually have the names of local traders. Now, all over the country, certain names – like the Co-op, Sainsbury's, Tesco, Safeways, Dewhursts and Broomfields – tend to recur. These three changes are the easily visible signs of the food retailing revolution that has involved the progressive coalescing of small independent specialist shops into large multiple retailers, almost all of which now are supermarkets.

The biggest of the multiple chains is the oldest, the Co-op, which has over 3,000 separate retail outlets. The "high profile" stores that run the big high street supermarkets are a long way behind in the number of stores, although individual stores tend to be larger than the Co-op ones. Sainsbury's, for example, has nearly 300 stores, Presto, over 500, Tesco, 300 while Asda has 100. The extent of the concentration of power in a few firms is now so great that almost half of the grocery sales in this country occur through the shops of the six major multiples.

But the multiple store is not a new phenomenon. It has been with us on an increasing scale for more than a hundred years, ever since the beginning of the Cooperative movement. Nevertheless the extent of its domination is surprising. Multiples and Co-ops could already claim over 40 per cent of grocery sales before World War II; by 1960 the figure had risen to 50 per cent; by the early 1970s to 60 per cent; and it is now well over 70 per cent.

The multiple chain has always had an advantage over the private shop since the volume of stock that it orders enables it to get cheaper prices from the manufacturer. Originally individual companies would bargain for the best terms. Today there is a system of discriminatory discounting whereby manufacturers offer different wholesale prices to different sectors of the retailing industry. In other words the multiples can buy branded foods at wholesale prices below – often far below – those offered to the independent retailer. This whole arrangement was investigated by the Monopolies and Mergers Commission in 1985 after complaints about its being against the public interest. But the Commission found this was not so.

——THE ARRIVAL OF THE SUPERMARKET——

The supermarket began to make a major impact on the retailing scene from the 1950s onwards (although the first UK supermarket, a Co-op store in London, was opened as early as 1942), and it was the multiples that pioneered their introduction. Although the word is used very loosely, what is generally meant by the word supermarket is a large self-service store, typically stocking between 3,000 and 5,000 separate items of grocery. This, of course, represents a large increase in the scale of high street food shopping even over the large multiple store. The superstore, or the even larger hypermarket, represents a scaling up of the whole supermarket idea, with perhaps 25,000 lines being stocked by hypermarkets, although many of these, of course, are not food items. The hypermarket is a European idea. The first one opened in Belgium in 1961, and most of Europe's thousand hypermarkets today are sited in France and Germany. In the UK the idea is still a fairly controversial one. The sheer size and impact of hypermarkets frequently make any plans for new ones the target for objections from established traders, consumer groups and environmentalists.

The supermarket philosophy has always been concerned with maximizing profits from a high volume of sales, rather than with achieving a high profit from limited sales. The multiples, with their ability to buy cheaply, were bound to succeed in this. Self-service shopping was also an essential part of low prices since it cuts staff costs. But although this may have been the initial attraction, self-service in supermarkets quickly evolved into something much more.

> *The supermarket philosophy has always been concerned with maximizing profits from a high volume of sales, rather than with achieving a high profit from limited sales.*

SELF-SERVICE PSYCHOLOGY

It was soon realized by the major supermarket chains that self-service shopping brings to the fore a whole new psychology of selling, quite unlike that involved in the efforts of a sales force to persuade us what to buy and much more effective because it functions at a level we do not usually perceive. Its importance has been revealed by American surveys that suggest that more than two-thirds of purchases in supermarkets are made on impulse – i.e., they are goods that the consumer didn't intend to buy when he entered the store. Some psychologists have suggested that this remarkable phenomenon occurs because shoppers are in a trance-like state as they walk round the store, which is packed with items that not long ago were unobtainable or luxury goods.

> *American surveys suggest that more than two-thirds of purchases in supermarkets are made on impulse – i.e., they are goods that the consumer didn't intend to buy when he entered the store.*

There are many ways in which supermarket customers can be influenced to buy goods. The placing of items is one key consideration. It was quickly realized that it was a good idea to display sweets on shelves near to the check-out queue because so many shoppers were accompanied by young children who would ask for sweets while they queued or be promised sweets to keep them under control, or who would simply add them to the basket and embarrass their parents into buying. The shelf upon which food is placed also affects its chances of selling. Items placed at eye level tend to be selected more frequently, so these shelves are used for the items on which profit tends to be highest. Keeping the shelves full is also important because people are reluctant to be the last to take a particular item. One study showed that shoppers tend to buy 22 per cent more from full shelves. It is also beneficial to position items in the store so that the average shopper has to pass as many shelves as possible, thus maximizing the chances of impulse buying. This is why aisles of shelves tend to run longitudinally down the supermarket, encouraging the shopper to visit as much of the store as possible.

In such ways the supermarket soon became not merely a discount system but a much more efficient selling machine. Prices could be held down by large-scale purchasing, by cheaper selling methods and by large turnovers, but at the same time profits were increased.

THE EXPANDING SUPERMARKET

In their early days the supermarkets were virtually confined to groceries and dry goods, that is, packaged and processed foods that could be kept on open shelves for a reasonable time. While the supermarket therefore rapidly displaced the high street grocer, the specialist stores like the greengrocer, baker, dairy and butcher who sold fresh foods were less affected.

The arrival of commercially viable fast-freezing techniques, which made it possible to preserve foods without much change in their flavour, transformed this. Frozen foods began to appear in the 1950s – the now ubiquitous fish finger arrived in 1955 – and supermarkets began to stock a progressively wider range of frozen foods: meat, fruit and vegetables as well as processed foods like ice cream. This brought them into competition with the specialist shops, although only in some areas. The advantage of frozen

> *The supermarket soon became not merely a discount system but a much more efficient selling machine.*

In 1965 less than 2 per cent of households had freezers; by 1971 this figure had risen to only 4 per cent. But since then the increase has been startling: by 1975 25 per cent of UK households had a domestic freezer and today the figure is over 70 per cent.

foods for supermarkets was not merely that such items could be stored with minimal spoilage, but also that they could be stocked all year round. Thus instead of, say, the pea harvest being associated with a glut of peas and very low prices, the excess production could be frozen for sale later. Frozen peas are thus always available at a price that does not fluctuate seasonally.

But until the late 1960s frozen foods were bought by the consumer in small amounts for consumption within a few days of purchase because home freezers were too expensive for all but a small minority. Most vegetables and much meat continued, therefore, to be purchased fresh from specialist shops. This pattern has begun to change only recently. In 1965 less than 2 per cent of households had freezers; by 1971 this figure had risen to only 4 per cent. But since then the increase has been startling: by 1975 25 per cent of UK households had a domestic freezer and today the figure is over 70 per cent. The change paralleled the rise in freezer centres, shops, usually supermarkets, dedicated to selling frozen foods. None existed in Britain in the mid-1960s. By 1970 there were 150 and by 1975, 900. Today there are 60,000.

The supermarket has now made significant inroads into the butchers' and greengrocers' share of the market but still has a long way to go. Thus, while only 30 per cent of grocery sales in 1981 were through independent shops, 75 per cent of butchers' sales and 90 per cent of greengrocers' sales were still made through independents. But butchers, dairies and bakers, even when overtly independent, are in fact restricted by the fact that so few wholesalers or processors control each trade. But whether overtly or truly independent, the individual retailers are rapidly losing their share of the specialist trades as the supermarkets take up the marketing of fresh food. The rate of turnover for supermarkets has risen to a point where the short storage times of perishable foods are no longer a problem. The increased use of chiller cabinets also extends the keeping time, while still allowing the food to be displayed.

So, as the years have passed, the supermarkets have enlarged the range of non-grocery items they stock and have increased the effectiveness with which they sell them. Thus it is now a common phenomenon to find that supermarkets stock fresh, unwrapped bread, chilled fresh as well as frozen meats and unpackaged vegetables.

In effect the major supermarket chains have become their own middle men, often concluding long-term contracts with producers, like fruit farmers, or with wholesale butchers or bakers.

As supermarkets have moved into the retailing of fresh or minimally processed foods like meat, so they have accelerated the process of vertical integration referred to in Chapter 5. In effect the major supermarket chains have become their own middle men, often concluding long-term contracts with producers, like fruit farmers, or with wholesale butchers or bakers.

Even before supermarkets sold much fresh food, they were gaining control over the wholesale and manufacturing sectors of the food industry. With the production of "own name" brands of processed and packaged food items, the supermarket was not only selling the food but manufacturing it as well. In the case of canned and packaged foods this was (and still is) usually achieved by making a deal with a company that already manufactured an item to produce more of it but to the supermarket's specifications and under the supermarket's own brand name. It may seem strange that manufacturers should help supermarkets to produce own brands that in the long run would effectively undercut the manufacturer's own products. But in the short term this process is mutually beneficial, for while the supermarket is able to sell the "own name" food at a cheaper cost and/or higher profit, producing it enables the manufacturer to increase turnover, using his machinery and plant to a higher capacity. But even if the manufacturer is worried about the long-term consequences, ultimately he has no choice but to co-operate. As the multiples grow, their power to boycott a specific product becomes more of a threat. Thus it becomes progressively less feasible for nominally independent manufacturers to argue with them.

Even nominally independent manufacturers have found that supermarket chains and all multiples have considerable control over them simply by virtue of the volume of foods they purchase. This does not just mean that supermarkets negotiate the best profit margin for themselves. Massive purchasers can actually affect the composition of what they buy. One example comes from New York City, where the moguls who affected food composition were not a retail company but the city school system. New York City has 10 million pupils, most of whom eat at school, and since the school meal system uses a single planning and purchasing department, it has a lot of clout. Recently this department decided to switch to a healthier diet, and it found it very easy to bring pressure to bear on major manufacturers to modify the composition of their products by removing sugar or additives.

Supermarkets have the same clout. They don't necessarily refuse to stock a product that the manufacturers do not make to their specifications, but if they feel there is a consumer preference for a modified alternative, they get it produced as their own brand and stock it alongside the original item, perhaps even preferentially positioned. One example of this has been the way in which the supermarket chains, notably Sainsbury's and Tesco, have spearheaded the recent more health-conscious changes in much processed food. Once Tesco made nutritional merit a selling point, the manufacturers had to fall in line with the production of low fat/high fibre and sugar- or additive-free products on a truly massive scale.

In all this, the key to the supermarkets' success has been the volume of their sales, which enable them to negotiate from a position of strength and to dictate the quality and cost of what they want. This volume of sales is maintained on the one hand by having outlets in as many places as possible and on the other by ensuring that as much as possible of the household shopping is done within the

> The key to the supermarkets' success has been the volume of their sales, which enable them to negotiate from a position of strength and to dictate the quality and cost of what they want.

supermarket. Getting the customers to enter the supermarket has always been recognized as vital because once they are in they can be enticed to buy other things. Since supermarkets often involve lengthy delays at the check-out, they are particularly unattractive to someone who believes he wants only a few items. One way round this has always been to sell "loss leaders" – that is, staple foods offered at prices involving little or no profit, or even a loss – so as to undercut the high street specialist stores and attract the customer into the supermarket. Sliced bread has been a regular loss leader for years together with a constant stream of bargain offers for other regularly purchased items such as tea, canned soup, breakfast cereals, baked beans and biscuits, which figure in most households' shopping lists.

The other way to entice the shopper to enter the store is to make it possible to purchase a very wide range of goods. The more that can be loaded into the trolley, the less important seems the delay at the check-out. As well as stocking traditional grocery items like soap powders, most supermarkets stock non-food items like alcohol and cigarettes that would not have been found at a traditional grocer's. The larger supermarkets have now proceeded far beyond household consumables into selling clothes, toys, DIY and gardening items, and even books, which makes it possible to do almost all the shopping in one go.

The hypermarket takes this philosophy to its extreme in stores so massive and extensive in their range of stocks that no other retail outlet need be visited. This expansion of the supermarkets' range of goods is viable only because of the high proportion of shoppers who now own cars. It is obviously inefficient to ply your shopper with a wide range of goods if the purchases are going to be limited to what can be carried home in a couple of plastic bags. From the late 1960s onwards, the supermarket has therefore placed a great stress on providing integrated parking space to enable the shopper to wheel a loaded trolley out to the car. The hypermarket takes this one step further. Rather than site the shop in a centre of population close to the shoppers but with limitations on parking space, the hypermarkets tend to be built on the outskirts of towns or on old factory sites, requiring the shoppers to drive some distance to the store, but compensating them by the range of goods and the ease with which they can park and load up their cars.

THE FUTURE OF THE SUPERMARKET

The very combination of a self-service system and a high throughput of customers that has been the key to the supermarkets' success has also been the chief source of their special problem – the check-out queue. Supermarket shopping fluctuates, with peak shopping times being Friday and Saturday. If staff numbers are set at the levels needed to deal with these crowds, the supermarket would be overstaffed for the rest of the week. Supermarkets are, of course, major employers of schoolchildren at weekends and part-time staff provide one solution to this problem.

But the long-term solution seems likely to come from technology. Already supermarkets are beginning to automate checking-out by using laser scanning of the bar codes that goods now have on their labels. This will become standard practice within a few years. Sainsbury's, for example, hopes to have laser scanning in all its stores by 1990. As well as speeding up the check-out, this will incidentally provide the customer with a detailed printout of what was purchased, and will also mean that a supermarket can keep more precise details of what is being sold. This will facilitate stock control and will make it easier to assess the effectiveness of different sales strategies: what, for example, is the effect of a price reduction on different days of the week? Is it necessary at weekends?

Paying too is soon likely to be automated. Although some supermarkets, like Sainsbury's, still refuse to accept credit cards, they will probably gain ground as more people use them. Automatic reading and debiting of credit cards is already technically possible, as is the cheque printer which fills in your cheque so that all you need do is sign it. Such changes will make supermarket shopping more attractive and will reduce the viability of the independent store even more.

Even the one advantage that the neighbourhood store does still possess – accessibility – is being eroded by an even newer development. This is the phone-in supermarket, where orders are given over the phone and goods are delivered the same day. Two such systems already exist in London and the idea seems likely to spread elsewhere in the country. Although the phone-in supermarket is in its early days, it already has a likely successor with details of goods available being displayed on the television screen and a linked home computer transmitting orders down the telephone line. Progress towards this system is systematic if unsung; a system of standardized code numbers for different products, the UK Article Number Bank, has been set up, and it is thought that it will be accepted generally within the next ten years. In America, where progress has been more rapid, the computer shopping market is already estimated to be about £90 million. So, it seems likely that the system will flourish here and eventually provide a challenge to the conventional supermarket as well as to the local shop.

In terms of giving the customers what they want, supermarkets have been a mixed blessing. On the one hand they have responded with alacrity to the new views about healthy eating and have been quick to stock vegetarian dishes, wholemeal cereal products, leaner joints of meat, a wide range of fish and so on. They have, too, been quick to satisfy the public demands for more esoteric health foods and for more exotic foods to tempt the palate. It seems likely that the health food stores and the delicatessens are going to feel the squeeze from the supermarket chains as surely as the butcher and the baker did before them.

But the supermarkets have shown curious blind spots – perhaps, a cynic might argue, where not enough profit was involved. Thus supermarkets will not cater for minority tastes or demands. For example, with the exception of Asda, no supermarket chain until recently would stock cling-film made without plasticizers because they felt there was no demand for it. Consumer activists argued cogently that since the product was not stocked, the supermarkets had no way of estimating that demand. It took a report from the Ministry of Agriculture, Fisher-

> *Even the one advantage that the neighbourhood store does still possess – accessibility – is being eroded by an even newer development. This is the phone-in supermarket.*

> *But the supermarkets have shown curious blind spots – perhaps, a cynic might argue, where not enough profit was involved.*

Traditional shops became important only in the 19th century. They represent a passing phase, not an inextricable part of our tradition. In fact the market stall is the nearest thing to a traditional shop.

ies and Food arguing that ordinary cling-film was not suitable for use in micro-waves to get the plasticizer-free product on the shelves in most stores where it now sells well.

It is not unreasonable to suggest that an increasing concentration of our food purchasing into the supermarkets might be at the expense of such minority demands simply because, when people find it too difficult to get precisely what they want, they accept second best. Against this must be set the fact that supermarkets have realized that our palates can be tempted in all sorts of ways besides the traditional duo of sweet or creamy and are now encouraging more variety in our diet.

It is difficult to predict what the continued displacement of the independent specialist shop by the supermarket will lead to in the long term. So far it has meant cheaper food, and although the owners of specialist shops complain that super-markets cannot provide the advice the customer wants, the British consumer is apparently willing to forgo the advice to get a lower price. The corner shop that is open at unsocial hours will probably have a role in the foreseeable future since consistent very late night or Sunday opening is not economic for large supermarkets. The consumer seems prepared to accept that "Open All Hours" shops will charge higher prices. Similarly nearness and the convenience of being able to buy 1 or 2 items easily will probably preserve the village shop, while in the towns the independent specialist shops may reappear under a system of franchise as independent points of sale within the supermarket. Or the door-to-door delivery van might get a new lease of life, perhaps linked to computer ordering or (as has already happened to some degree) appended to the doorstep milk delivery. But the shops as the sepia photographs portray them are going to disappear. But before you get upset about this and bemoan the passing of another tradition, just look back at Chapter 6 and remember that such shops weren't, in general, much older than the sepia photographs. Traditional shops became important only in the 19th century. They represent a passing phase, not an inextricable part of our tradition. In fact the market stall is the nearest thing to a traditional shop.

THE ROLE OF ADVERTISING

It would, of course, be a mistake to assume that our shopping habits have been entirely dictated by changes in production and in retailing. The other great influence is advertising.

Advertising has been a growth industry throughout the 20th century. The most reliable figure for total expenditure on food advertising in the UK now puts it close to half a billion pounds (£500,000,000). The three confectionery giants – Cadburys, Mars and Rowntrees – between them spend £70 million each year advertising sweets alone. Anyone can judge the importance of advertising expenditure by the food industry by looking at the commercial television channels for a few hours. Up to 50 per cent of the advertisements shown will be for food.

Advertising by the food industry is principally aimed at three intertwined objectives: to encourage the consumer to eat new types of food (almost totally, of course, processed food); to increase the demand for a given type of food; and to persuade the consumer to switch brands. There can, after all, hardly be a citizen in the country who doesn't know about baked beans, but advertising by Heinz, the market leader, shows no sign of abating. What Heinz is trying to do is to sustain the image of the baked bean (it is presented variously as fun, appetizing, nutritious and liked by children), and to preserve the idea that the only real baked beans are Heinz ones, fighting off competition from retailers' own brands as well as other manufacturers.

> *Fresh foods receive very little advertising, particularly those that would now be regarded as important in our diet.*

There are two objections to food advertising. The first is to the huge amount that is spent and the foods that it is spent on. Fresh foods receive very little advertising, particularly those that would now be regarded as important in our diet. The advertising expenditure on fruit and vegetables, for example, is minuscule. The total expenditure on advertising food is at least twenty times as great as the total expenditure on advertising healthy eating.

The second objection to food advertising is one that applies to advertising in general; that it does not seek to inform the consumer, helping him to a more balanced choice, but it aims to manipulate him, leading him to choose the object advertised for reasons of which he is not aware. American journalist and author, Vance Packard first brought this to general attention in his book *The Hidden Persuaders* as long ago as 1957. Packard argued that much advertising and research into advertising was aimed at getting across a message of which we were not aware, at speaking directly to our unconscious. This is what advertisers do when they create an image for a food. It is difficult to believe, for example, that Rowntree's After Eight Mints would have been as popular if marketed simply as peppermint creams. Instead, they were endowed with a chic image, as something to be served on its own silver tray, to be eaten at dinner parties where the guests glitter in conversation and in style. It was an attempt to make the consumer associate the food with a lifestyle that for most people is desirable but unattained. Other chocolates aim at different images: the image of Black Magic, for example, is that it is a romantic gift from a man to a woman.

Nor does advertising just involve what one might normally regard as advertisements; it is part of all aspects of packaging goods. Mr Kipling's Cakes, for instance, are promoted as traditional and possessing all the virtues associated with home-baking at its best. The packaging aims to strengthen that image, from the old-fashioned typeface used on the label to the way in which the packet illustration is photographed to suggest the cakes are not all regular in shape and are therefore more like home-made ones.

Of course, food advertising makes specific claims too: about price, nutritional value and value for money. But such factual claims have not been a major component of the advertising message in the past. They are now increasing and are often phrased in such a way that they can be a minefield for the unwary. Claims that a

> *It has been proved that hitherto both gastronomic appeal and nutritional value are far less important determinants of consumption than price and image. Although health criteria are becoming increasingly important to the consumer, they are not yet a major determinant of the nation's food habits.*

food contains "no artificial ingredients" begs the question of how nutritionally desirable are the natural ingredients it does contain, while statements that a food contains no artificial preservatives say nothing about other additives such as colourants (see Chapter 8).

Food advertising, like all advertising, is often the cause of unease among consumer activists, and many questions are asked about it. Why are advertisers not restricted to making specific claims, rather than working by innuendo and implication? Why should unlimited advertising be allowed? Should it not be restricted by law? And, above all, why is it not regulated to prevent false claims being made?

Any legislation would have to cover all advertising, not just food, and no government will introduce such legislation until there is an overwhelming case that it would be beneficial. Even then, it would probably not act until consumer lobbies forced it to. Any ban would probably be only partial and would be circumvented in various ways, as the tobacco industry has demonstrated since the ban was placed on cigarette advertising on television.

Legislation already exists to regulate the factual claims made in any advertisement. Offending television and radio advertisements, which are those judged to mislead the average consumer, can be removed by the Independent Broadcasting Authority and the Advertising Standards Authority deals with printed matter in a similar way. Unfortunately, these bodies are relatively toothless and act only after an advertisement has appeared at least once. They rarely complain about the food industry's advertisements because straightforward factual claims are fairly rare. The food industry can point out that nutritional value of food is only a minor consideration among the reasons why most people choose food. Surveys show the British public claims to eat the more nutritious food far more often than it actually does. It has been proved that hitherto both gastronomic appeal and nutritional value are far less important determinants of consumption than price and image. Although health criteria are becoming increasingly important to the consumer, they are not yet a major determinant of the nation's food habits. Unless we change our reasons for buying, advertising is hardly likely to change its style.

——*PRESSURE AND CONSUMER GROUPS*——

It must be clear to everyone that there has been a great revival not only in public interest about food but also in the groups that write, lobby and argue for dietary change. The most vociferous of these are the "food reformers" who are arguing for a variety of sweeping changes in our diet. But they are not alone, nor even the most powerful lobby. To understand what is going on it is necessary to begin with NACNE (the National Advisory Committee on Nutrition Education).

The revival of interest in the health value of what we eat began less than ten years ago; it dates from the activities of NACNE, which started in 1979. This body was a working group of scientists convened to provide a set of guidelines on healthy eating for the Health Education Council and the British Nutrition Foundation. NACNE did not discover anything new; there was already a growing body of scientific evidence on the link between diet and the degenerative diseases. But there was no overwhelming consensus among scientists on what was a good diet, apart from a few vague generalizations like "eat less fat" and "eat less sugar" – such as those published in a DHSS booklet *Eating for Health*, which appeared in 1978.

What NACNE did in 1981 – which led to the subsequent storm when it was made public two years later – was to put figures to the amounts of fat, sugar, salt, alcohol and fibre that it thought were acceptable or advisable in a healthy diet.

NACNE's job was to distil from the scientific literature on diet and degenerative disease the most probably correct view and to recommend a diet that could improve the national health. Even in this NACNE was not unique. Groups of doctors and scientists periodically issue such reports, and the DHSS has a standing committee of scientists and physicians called the Committee on Medical Aspects of Food Policy (known generally as COMA) to advise on such matters, although in the past its reports have either been so bland as to amount to nothing at all or have concentrated on the relationship between diet and individual disease rather than between diet and health as a whole.

In order to give health educators something positive to work on, NACNE tried to tackle two needs that health educators felt had not, up to then, been adequately met by the standard government advisory bodies. The first was to decide whether, in diseases like dental caries or coronary heart disease, efforts should be made to improve the eating habits of the population as a whole, or whether advice should be targeted only at those individuals known to be at particularly high risk. The second was to tackle the conflict between health educators, who needed detailed guidance about how much less fat, salt, etc. should be eaten, and research scientists, who have not yet been able to devise the sorts of experiments that can provide such information with certainty. Although a number of expert committees in other countries, such as Sweden, Canada, Norway and New Zealand, had made recommendations, at least, for acceptable amounts of fat in the diet, the British government had fought shy of this approach. What NACNE did in 1981 – which led to the subsequent storm when it was made public two years later – was to put figures to the amounts of fat, sugar, salt, alcohol and fibre that it thought were acceptable or advisable in a healthy diet. These figures were essentially judgements by a working group of the committee based on the evidence available at the time, judgements which might well be expected to change as a result of future evidence or in response to changes in public health or eating habits.

What made NACNE famous was its failure to produce a report. Various drafts were produced by a sub-committee of scientists but were scotched in the main meeting by objections from representatives of the DHSS, certain sections of the food industry and from sincere, but perhaps ivory-towered, academics who had little experience or understanding of public health education. While this wrangling was going on stories were leaked to the press suggesting that the food industry was trying to strangle the truth because it feared for its profits. This created a sensation and focused attention on the politics of food and health to an extent that had not occurred since World War II.

Eventually, in 1983, a somewhat modified NACNE report did appear. Its recommendations were widely publicized and were accepted by many consumers as definitive. Since then a loose coalition of food reformers has developed, who might be defined as non-industry, non-government lobbyists interested in changing our diet. Long-standing groups, like the Vegetarian Society, find themselves in broad agreement with much newer groups like the London Food Commission. All are criticizing current diets and arguing for broadly comparable changes. What might still be called the "NACNE view" (less fat, less salt, more fibre) commands almost general agreement, although some groups press in addition for more specific changes, like fewer additives or no irradiation. These lobbies have gained much support in the media, and all adopt a broadly anti-food-industry posture.

The food industry, of course, has its own lobby groups to promote its interests in the public and political arena. There are general bodies like the Food and Drink Manufacturers Association, and sectoral interests like the Milk Marketing Board, the Butter Information Council and the Sugar Bureau. Although these seem to be listened to attentively within Whitehall, they are less successful in the media, where cries of "sectional interests" almost invariably ensure that they are vanquished.

Since the publication of NACNE's findings, the nature of government reports on diet has shown a change. In 1984, COMA (the Committee on Medical Aspects of Food Policy) published a report on coronary heart disease that, for the first time for that committee, gave a figure to the maximum amount of fat acceptable in the diet.

Opinions on diet also emanate from a bewildering number of bodies. These range from distinguished institutions like the Royal College of Physicians to more fringe groups like the Society for Nutritional Medicine. Two particularly grand-sounding bodies are currently active. One is the British Nutrition Foundation, which is funded by the food industry, but nonetheless claims to be unbiased in its pronouncements. The other is the Parliamentary Food and Health Forum, which is a meeting point for parliamentarians and all interested bodies in the food and health debate but has no governmental standing. Finally there is government advice, from committees like COMA and from quangos like the Health Education Council. This continues to be more moderate than the extreme pronouncements of the food radicals but is now more "reformist" than it was before NACNE.

Faced with such a surfeit, the consumer might wonder who to believe. The answer is no one – experts can give general advice for the average person but it is only the individual who can decide how relevant or how practicable such advice is to him or her. The object of this book is to help you to make up your own mind.

—— *TECHNOLOGY IN THE KITCHEN*——

In Chapter 6 we saw how the arrival of technology in the Victorian kitchen altered people's diet. The same is true of today's technological advances, which have been important not only for their direct impact on our pattern of consumption but because they have done so much to facilitate the supermarket revolution.

Foremost among these new technological wizards of the kitchen are the refrigerator and the freezer, which have both relatively quickly moved from being the prerogative of the affluent to indispensable items of household equipment. The growth of freezer ownership was mentioned earlier (see page 132); refrigerator ownership is now virtually universal, with over 95 per cent of UK households having one.

Both the refrigerator and the freezer extend the life of foods by reducing their temperature. The principle on which they work is simple. Foods go bad in two ways. First, spontaneous chemical reactions can lead to undesirable changes in texture, smell or flavour. Second, bacteria or moulds can grow on the food, either spoiling its flavour or threatening the consumer with food poisoning. Almost all chemical reactions vary in speed with temperature, almost always going faster at higher temperatures and slower at lower temperatures. This applies to bacterial growth as much as to any other chemical reaction. So, reducing the temperature reduces the rate at which foods spoil, and the more the temperature is reduced the greater is this slowing up, which is why a freezer at −20° Centigrade (−4° Fahrenheit) keeps food so much longer than a fridge, which has a temperature of about +4° Centigrade (39° Fahrenheit). Although reducing the temperature slows up the growth of all food spoilage organisms, there are a few exceptions to this rule about the effect of temperature change on chemical reactions in food. Bananas, for example, blacken faster if kept in the cold. But these exceptions are rare, and the overwhelming effect of refrigeration and freezing is to reduce food spoilage and bacterial food poisoning.

Although it is less effective in slowing up food spoilage, the fridge has certain advantages over the freezer. The process of defrosting can take hours, and frozen foods are not therefore always easily available for use. A more important problem that initially spoilt all early attempts at freezing food was caused by the effect that ice had on the structure of most foods. It is well known that when water turns to ice it expands (this is why frozen pipes burst). All living creatures are made up of cells, which are, in effect, microscopic balloons filled with a mixture of proteins and water. In early attempts at freezing foods, ice crystals formed and pierced the skin of the cells, so that when the food thawed the cells leaked and the food became inedible. This process can be seen spectacularly in the effect that snow, or freezing, has on green leafy vegetables, which become limp and unpalatable upon thawing. Foods that do not have a cellular structure, like cheese or ice creams, are not open to this form of damage and prove relatively easy to freeze, although milk has been less easy because the fat and protein separate out. Therefore +4°C (39°F), safely above the temperature at which water freezes, seemed for a long while the lowest temperature at which most food could be stored.

The problem was partially solved when it was realized that if water was frozen rapidly enough, very small ice crystals did not form so that little or no damage was done to the cells and the food was still palatable on thawing. The secret of the freezer revolution has not been the ability to maintain low temperatures but the ability to reduce food to those temperatures very quickly. Commercial freezing can achieve this fastest of all, but even home freezers now have a fast freeze switch.

Because the fridge and the freezer have extended the time that food can be kept at home they have removed the need for frequent shopping and have thus aided the supermarket revolution. Shopping need no longer be a daily chore; intermittent trips to the supermarket can keep the family well provided. The final implications of this have yet to be felt because we still have not abandoned all our pre-refrigeration shopping habits. The daily doorstep delivery of milk, for example, was an innovation of the 1930s, encouraged by a government determined to get people to drink more milk. The refrigerator made this unnecessary since milk no longer goes off in a single day, and increasingly people buy their milk on trips to the supermarket every two or three days. The dairies are fighting both a public relations campaign, which, with some justification, portrays the milkman as a social service, keeping an eye on the old and infirm, as well as desperately diversifying and delivering other foods besides milk in order to defend their market.

The extension of food-keeping time is, of course, quite different for the two pieces of equipment, the refrigerator keeping most foods a few days while the freezer keeps them for months on end. During that keeping time all chemical processes are slowed up but not prevented completely, and foods do slowly change their composition. Even before these changes manifest themselves as spoilage, there will be some loss of nutrient content and many people fear that this means our diet is less nutritious.

Such fears are based on exaggeration and misconceptions. While some nutrients are lost in deep freezing, many others are not vulnerable. The nutrient that is most vulnerable to deep freezing is vitamin C. But this does not mean that our vitamin C intake is reduced. Most of the vitamin C eaten by most people comes from potatoes, and here the method of storage hasn't changed. Even for foods that are frozen the vitamin C intake can be higher after freezing, despite the losses that occur. For it must be remembered that losses of nutrients occur if the foods are kept at room temperature, although they don't become as important because spoilage usually intervenes. If the introduction of the freezer meant we ate the same amount of fruit and vegetables but ate them frozen instead of fresh, there might be a case for alarm. In fact its impact has been to increase intakes of fruit and vegetables, particularly in the winter months when formerly there were few very fresh sources of vitamin C.

The effect of the fridge on the diet is extensive. There is less waste of vegetables and left-overs need not be eaten at the next meal, so the diet can be more varied. Milk kept cold and in the dark (for the light does go out when the fridge door is shut!) doesn't lose its riboflavin content and doesn't go off before it is all consumed. Nor, of course, does butter. Soft margarine is more palatable from the fridge, keeps better and, since it is easier to spread than cold butter, tends to be eaten in preference, and this also pushes up the intake of polyunsaturates. The effect of the freezer is even more profound. Stored packages of out-of-season foods can be used a little at a time. Thus

If the introduction of the freezer meant we ate the same amount of fruit and vegetables but ate them frozen instead of fresh, there might be a case for alarm. In fact its impact has been to increase intakes of fruit and vegetables, particularly in the winter months when formerly there were few very fresh vitamin C sources.

sea-food risotto is now easily made with frozen shellfish of all kinds from the freezer. Snack meals prepared in a rush are often nutritious, for although the frozen peas or white cabbage may have less vitamin C than the fresh ones, consumption is also higher since they are so easy to add to a meal or snack.

> *Charming though the mythology is, the nutrient content of soups and stews, no matter how home-made, is no higher (and often less) than that of the ingredients that went into them.*

Before the introduction of the fridge the main way of extending the life of perishable food like meat was to cook it in a soup or stew. One direct result of the fridge has been a reduction in the importance of home-made soups and stews in the UK diet. It has been suggested that this has led to a decline in nutritional quality but this is a fallacy. Home-made soups have long been endowed with special (but completely spurious) magical properties as regards their nutritional value. Hot soup is somehow thought to be especially nourishing because it is hot, but although it may seem thoroughly warming on a cold day, it has no physiological advantage over a cup of tea, or even hot water. Soup does not acquire any special nutritional properties from its heat (see page 10). Specific kinds of soup have their own special fanclubs. Beef broths have been popular at least since the early 19th century when the German expert Professor Liebig lent his reputation to their nourishing powers and a belief in the nutritional value of chicken soup is part of the folklore of European Jews. The traditional Yiddish mother always kept a pot simmering on the stove and greeted any catastrophe with, "Never mind, have a bowl of chicken soup and you'll feel better." With characteristic self-mockery, Jews today call chicken soup "Jewish penicillin", and tell such stories as the one about the old lady who had two chickens. One got ill so she killed the other to make a nice bowl of chicken soup to help the sick one get better!

Charming though the mythology is, the nutrient content of soups and stews, no matter how home-made, is no higher (and often less) than that of the ingredients that went into them. Their only special nutritional value was derived from the continual boiling up, which stops the ingredients from going bad. Now that we can achieve the same end by using the fridge or freezer the soup is redundant as a method of keeping food.

One advantage of traditional meat soups – and the one loss that can be laid at the refrigerator door – is that soups rendered edible the otherwise inedible parts of the animal carcass. They did this in two ways. First, a considerable part of the protein in the animal carcass is a substance called collagen, which is important in the skin, blood vessels, tendons and ligaments and which comprises what generations of schoolchildren have disdainfully called the "gristle" on the meat. Collagen is a poorly digested protein in its intact state (for which reason it is sometimes called animal fibre), but when it is boiled it yields gelatin, which is much better digested. This same gelatin is a major component of jelly – indeed it is what makes a jelly gel. Its effects in a meat stew are to cause it to become thick and jelly-like, the properties that make us regard the stew as nourishing. As it happens, gelatin is about as poor a quality protein as it is possible to get, but with other likely proteins in soup, such as split peas, the value of gelatin is improved a bit, by what is called protein complementation (see pages 13-14). This, therefore, made soup a little bit better than plain cooked meat.

The second way that soups render the inedible edible is by using bits of the carcass that otherwise we would not eat. Here the advantage is economic rather than nutritional: it is thrifty not to waste and in straitened times it might be necessary. Europeans gave up cracking bones to get at the marrow a long time ago since traditional home-made soup provided an easier way to the same end as the marrow is extracted into the soup by boiling. The importance of this should not be exaggerated: although it is nourishing enough, there are no special nutritional properties in bone marrow, and if you never eat it you won't suffer. Other parts of the carcass that we usually reject include the feet, the skin, offcuts of muscle and entrail meat, all of which can be made into a palatable soup.

Before the demise of the soup becomes a cause for too much regret, it should be remembered that it is precisely these unwanted parts of the carcass and digestible gristle that find their way into sausages and burgers, where their presence is now regarded by many food activists as extremely undesirable.

THE MICROWAVE COOKER

The microwave oven became valuable once the freezer became the standard way of storing food. With a microwave as an adjunct, one obvious use of the freezer is not merely to freeze foodstuffs to be used later in meal preparation, but to store pre-prepared dishes or even whole meals. The microwave has accelerated the spread of convenience frozen foods because the standard household microwave oven can cook such dishes in about one-third of the time taken by the conventional oven and without changes in flavour associated with conventional cooking. This makes it possible to eat when you feel like it and takes away the planning needed for preparing meals.

The microwave and the freezer have together contributed to two major changes in our pattern of eating. The first is the decline in importance of the family meal. With the microwave and a stock of convenience foods it has become possible for individuals in the household to prepare their own meals when they want them. The second change has been an increase in what is called 'grazing', the eating of a large number of small meals, rather than a small number of large ones. At present no one knows what the effect of this is likely to be, although in animal experiments there are detectable differences in physiological function and the pattern of disease between meal eaters and nibblers. Meal eaters, for instance, tend to put on more weight if they over-eat.

The microwave oven's contribution to labour-saving should also enable the housewife to spend more time away from the kitchen. It should also make it possible for people living on their own to prepare food easily and if it becomes more widespread it may even help the solitary house-dweller who can't be bothered to cook.

The microwave oven is basically a very simple idea. It is a metal box with a magnetron that generates microwaves. The metal walls of the oven reflect the microwaves back so that they bounce around all parts of the oven. There is nothing special about microwaves: they are one type of what scientists call electromagnetic waves, one example of which are light waves, another are the radio waves used in radio and TV broadcasting, to which microwaves are closely related. Like radio waves or light waves, microwaves are not hot but can heat up substances that absorb them. Microwaves are readily absorbed by water, which all foods contain. As they strike the molecules of water in the food, and to a certain degree the sugar and fat as well, they cause these molecules to vibrate very fast, and this raises the temperature of the food. The microwaves penetrate the food only to a depth of about 2in (5cm) from whichever side they strike, and the heat of their absorption is generated in this outer layer. If the food is deeper than about 4in (10cm) the centre gets heated not directly by microwaves but by conduction of heat from the outer layer. The oven and the air it contains remain cool because they do not absorb microwaves. The dish that the food is contained in does not absorb them either and so heats up much more slowly than the food inside, becoming hot only because it is in contact with the hot food.

Much concern has been expressed about the possible adverse effects of microwaves, but there is little to fear. In the domestic microwave oven microwaves are generated only while the oven door is closed and the British standard for microwave ovens requires that only a minute amount of microwave energy leaks out while the oven is operating or when the door is opened. The microwaves that are absorbed by the food do not stay there, contaminating it, but cease to exist once the energy they contain is converted to heat.

The prohibition on putting metal in microwave ovens has nothing sinister about it. Microwaves pass through materials like plastic or china – just as light passes through glass – and so, as they bounce from the sides of the oven, they heat the food from all sides, from underneath as well as from the top. Since metals reflect microwaves, food heated in a metal or foil dish would not get heated properly because the microwaves would not penetrate the sides or base of the metal container. Because metal reflects them back if a metal container is used, there are more microwaves bouncing around inside the oven and if there is enough metal the magnetron can get overheated or small sparks can be generated, which pit the oven walls. But nothing untoward happens to the food itself.

The other common fear is that microwave cookery somehow reduces the goodness in the food. This is another myth. The chemical changes in microwaved food are different from those that occur in a conventional oven. A simple microwave, for example, does not brown meat or cause the skins of baked potatoes to harden. But these differences arise because the microwave is doing less damage to the food being cooked, not more. Scare stories that extraordinary losses of vitamins are occurring are simply not true. Indeed, to some extent there are more vitamins in microwaved food. The microwave oven also enables the delicate flavour of foods like fish to be preserved, enhancing their palatability and hence increasing our intake of the nutrients they contain.

Anxiety about microwave cooking is another instance of fear of the unknown. It is different from the ordinary oven, just as the oven was different from the roasting spit. These differences are most notable in the impossibility of browning or crisping in a microwave. For this reason it is unlikely that the microwave will ever therefore completely displace the traditional oven, but it is likely that hybrid microwave/ conventional ovens will become standard equipment.

CHAPTER 8

HOW HEALTHY IS OUR FOOD?

THE RISKS OF EATING

*I*s eating bad for you? Many people today are convinced that the answer to this very silly question is "yes", and it is fair to say that the apparent risks of eating have increased dramatically in the last twenty-five years. However the crucial word in that sentence is "apparent". It is not necessarily that food has become any more harmful but we NOW see food as dangerous in all sorts of ways that were hardly thought of twenty-five years ago.

Before that time diets were assessed for their health value purely in terms of their adequacy: did they provide all the nutrients that were needed to prevent deficiency? Then came concern about excess: was there too much sugar? Too much fat? Too much cholesterol? Now attention is focused on the possibility that diets contain toxic substances such as additives and pollutants, which are sapping our health and disturbing our behaviour. These effects are often referred to loosely as food allergies, but allergies and toxic effects are quite different. As is explained below, allergic responses to food are not due to the toxicity of what is consumed but to a failure of the consumer's own physiology. The difference is clear if you consider hay fever. Some people find pollen induces an allergic reaction, but most of us do not. What is a miserable time for the hay fever sufferer is glorious summer for the rest of us. Returning to food, there is concern on two points: first, that some components of our diet may be associated with an allergic response in some people, and second, that for all of us our diet is toxic. The special focus of concern is that these allergic and toxic responses are produced by food additives or by accidental pollutants.

Before discussing these it is worth making some general observations about what we mean by toxic substances and how far they are found in our diet. The word toxic is often defined in dictionaries as poisonous, but when scientists talk of toxins and toxic effects they mean something more general and often less fatal than Agatha Christie does. To a scientist, a toxin is anything that causes an unwanted change in the normal running of the body

> *It is not necessarily that food has become any more harmful but we now see food as dangerous in all sorts of ways that were hardly thought of twenty-five years ago.*

146

that is regarded as adverse – i.e., not beneficial. This does not mean that a toxin kills. Thus one of the adverse effects associated with various additives is that in excess they can lead to flatulence. By this measure pickled onions, cabbage, baked beans and curries are all toxic. And indeed, if you look them up in one of the standard scientific texts on food toxins you will find them listed as such. But such toxins have never figured as important in a detective story!

——*NATURALLY TOXIC FOOD*——

Nutritionists have long been aware that enormous numbers of toxins occur quite naturally in our diet. Indeed, so many are present that it is difficult to conceive of a food that does not contain toxic components. This should not engender any alarm; there are very few cases of illness – let alone death – attributable to toxic substances in our diet, except, of course, to alcohol, which is probably the most dangerous single additive but which almost 90 per cent of the adult population consume.

Alcohol illustrates one of the paradoxes about food toxins, for not only is it an extremely toxic compound but we consume it precisely because of its toxic effects. The mortality from alcohol consumption is incredible: deaths from drink-driving currently run at over 1,000 a year. There are no reliable estimates of deaths in the UK due to the direct effects of alcohol poisoning or from the indirect effects of its over-consumption, but they run into thousands each year. Undoubtedly this represents a greater sum of human tragedy than all the other deaths and misery that can be attributed to other toxins in the diet. Yet we are not only unlikely to ban alcohol consumption; we will take few serious steps to reduce it. Any government even tempted in this direction knows it would face a huge public outcry. Alcohol is exceptional for the amount of damage it causes, but it is not the only product that is desired because of its toxicity.

The other outstanding example is the group of chemicals that we call methyl xanthines and that are found in tea, coffee and chocolate. Of these the best known is caffeine, which is contained in particularly high levels in coffee, although it is also present in tea and chocolate. Tea contains about 60 per cent of the caffeine of coffee, as well as high levels of another methyl xanthine called theophylline. Cocoa contains about the same level of caffeine as tea, as well as high levels of yet another methyl xanthine called theobromine. Chocolate, of course, is made from the cocoa bean and so also contains the same methyl xanthines, while manufacturers of cola drinks and some other drinks add caffeine to these too.

The effect of all these methyl xanthines is the same, although caffeine is by far the most potent. They stimulate the brain, helping to keep the consumer awake and thinking clearly; they are also diuretics, that is they make people urinate. It is the effect of these compounds on the brain that accounts for the popularity of the drinks that contain them, although most consumers are unaware of this or the extent to which they are dependent on their "cuppa". People seem to differ quite widely in their response to caffeine:

> *Alcohol illustrates one of the paradoxes about food toxins, for not only is it an extremely toxic compound but we consume it precisely because of its toxic effects.*

> *The toxic side effects of these compounds become visible at quite low levels of consumption – eight to ten cups of coffee a day. These effects include irregular heartbeats, confusion, ringing in the ears, stomach upsets and convulsions.*

some, for example, are unable to sleep if they drink coffee in the evening, while others have it as a bedtime drink. However there may be a degree of self-delusion in all this. Many of those who avoid coffee will happily drink a bedtime cup of tea, while cocoa has come to be widely regarded as a bedtime drink, not a stimulant. Any soporific effect is probably due to the fact that it is usually drunk warm and made with milk and lots of sugar.

The toxic side effects of these compounds become visible at quite low levels of consumption – eight to ten cups of coffee a day. These effects include irregular heartbeats, confusion, ringing in the ears, stomach upsets and convulsions. In animal experiments they also include damage to the foetus. Less than ten times this toxic level can be fatal.

But mankind also seems to like the consumption of toxic flavours whose effect is to burn or sting. Peppers of various kinds are prized in many cultures, and what we perceive as the heat of a curry is in fact a misinterpretation of a message from the pain receptors in our mouth. The attraction of foods as diverse as radishes, onions, leeks and cabbage is their pungency, although the adverse effects of the compounds that cause this can be testified to by any cook who has had to cook onions, as well as by anyone who likes fried onions. All of these are examples of what might be called socially acceptable toxins, foods whose powerful toxic activity is an essential part of their attraction. The fact that, quite rightly, we don't become neurotic about this provides a perspective within which to evaluate concern about the effects of additives and contaminants in our diet.

It could be argued that the effects of these socially acceptable toxins are very different from the adverse effects of some other foods. But the foods in our diet are by no means either acceptably toxic or harmless. Obviously we try to avoid toxic foods in which the toxic effect is not desired. But we do consume some of them, particularly if they are only intermittently toxic, or only toxic at high intakes, or only toxic to some people. Among the intermittently toxic foods are potatoes, which are toxic when green, which they become if stored in the light; quail, which can be toxic if the birds have eaten hemlock berries before they are killed; and mussels, which can be contaminated by food-poisoning bacteria. We have, of course, developed well-established procedures for dealing with such problems: we don't store potatoes in the light to prevent them from turning green; quail are fasted for some days before shooting; and freshly harvested mussels are traditionally kept for some days in a pail of water containing oatflakes as food while they clean themselves.

> *Many foods can be toxic at high levels of consumption but not at the levels at which usually consumed.*

Many foods can be toxic at high levels of consumption but not at the levels at which usually consumed. Nevertheless unwanted effects do occur, even with unlikely foods such as cabbage and sprouts, which can adversely effect the thyroid gland. But to have a measurable effect, a diet would have to consist of little else but these compounds, preferably eaten raw. That is a fairly improbable recipe, although some people have managed it.

Of the foods that are toxic only to some people, the most famous examples are probably cheeses, which can cause migraine attacks or other unpleasant symptoms. Although often loosely described as an allergy by the sufferer, what is happening is that a substance found in cheese, called tyramine, stimulates the blood vessels in a way that can cause a variety of symptoms, ranging from giddiness and nausea to headache and even in some rare cases a stroke. Tyramine is made by bacteria from the amino acid tyrosine, and it is found in cheeses whose production involves a bacterial fermentation. Other fermented foods like wine, sauerkraut or pickled fish can also contain tyramine, or similar compounds like histamine, and can therefore precipitate symptoms in vulnerable people. In addition, mackerel and fish of the same family can produce increased levels of histamine if stored at too high a level, while certain other foods like bananas, chocolate and avocado pears also contain similar substances.

Most of us can eat all these foods with impunity since our body chemistry is quite capable of dealing with these compounds as rapidly as we consume them. But a few people are less able to defend themselves. Any of us can become sensitive if our normal defence system is disabled. Tyramine and histamine belong to a class of compounds called vasoactive amines, and we dispose of them in our body by the action of an enzyme called monoamine oxidase (MAO). Unfortunately, the most powerful anti-depressants that are commonly prescribed, called MAO inhibitors, work by switching off that enzyme. People taking these anti-depressants can therefore become very sensitive to the effects of vasoactive amines and have to avoid foods like cheese and wine. (Fans of *Rumpole of the Bailey* may recall the story of "Rumpole and the Expert Witness", in which this interaction of food and medicine was used to commit murder.)

This list by no means exhausts the possible adverse effects of food. It merely serves to set out the nature of the problems that exist even without additives. The list is not intended to cause panic. After all, how many people die from eating avocados or have had their life cut short by a cup of cocoa? There are probably many more who feel they are dying from all the artificial additives and pollutants in their diet. The next time one comes to visit you, give him mackerel with potatoes and cabbage and a nice cup of tea to calm him down, and then read him the next section of this book.

FOOD ALLERGIES

It was noted on page 146 that the toxic effects of food are quite distinct from allergic ones, but an allergy to a particular food or food additive is another reason why the consumer can experience adverse effects from eating. Much publicity has been given to this possibility, and this has led to a marked increase in the number of people who claim to be allergic to some components of their diet. Where such claims have been investigated the overwhelming majority have been shown to be unfounded. One recent study, for example, showed that 75 per cent of a group of people claiming to have an allergy to some component of their diet did not show a response when tested under scientific conditions.

Allergic reactions are responses of the body's immune system to a foreign sub-

> **Food allergies are not confined to additives or to "junk foods". Allergic responses can occur to any of a wide range of foodstuffs, just as they can to other chemicals in the environment, and there is no evidence that additives are particularly likely to induce an allergic response.**

stance to which the body has become sensitized. The potential to react to foreign substances that invade the body is our defence against bacteria and other germs and is clearly vital. The disease AIDS is fatal primarily because it paralyses the immune system, making the body unable to defend itself against normally minor infections.

The body's immune system works on a principle of overkill. Because it is difficult to decide whether or not an invader is potentially harmful almost any foreign substance can cause a reaction. The reason that most substances do not induce an allergic response is that they do not penetrate the body. People who are allergic somehow respond more easily to normal chemicals in their environment. The reasons why this is so are complicated, but the problem lies with the body not with the substance to which it is reacting. Now, undoubtedly, some of the adverse reactions to food additives are allergic in nature and people who have developed such an allergy have little choice but to avoid the additive that causes the trouble. But food allergies are not confined to additives or to "junk foods". Allergic responses can occur to any of a wide range of foodstuffs, just as they can to other chemicals in the environment, and there is no evidence that additives are particularly likely to induce an allergic response.

The most common food allergies are an allergy to wheat or similar cereals (or any food containing wheat products) and an allergy to cow's milk. But allergies can exist to almost any food. There are some people who are allergic to fruit and fruit juices and others who are allergic to shellfish, so an additive-free or wholefood diet is not a guaranteed way of avoiding food allergies. Nor are they caused by junk foods. Indeed, one of the few foods to which allergies do not occur is white sugar, that supreme ingredient of "junk" food. It is worth remembering that many more people have an allergy to the protein of cow's milk than have ever been found to have an allergy to any additive. Moreover, allergic responses are very specific. Just as hay fever sufferers often find that while they will react excessively to pollen from one plant another will have no effect, so someone who is allergic to one food or even one additive may be able to consume the others with impunity. So consuming an additive-free diet is not the solution to the problems of food allergies.

Allergic responses to food or food additives can involve very variable symptoms ranging from digestive disturbances (anything from stomach cramps or flatulence to diarrhoea and vomiting) to symptoms like urticaria (nettle rash), rhinitis (a runny nose) or asthma, all of which are easily identified as allergic responses. Of course,

> **One of the few foods to which allergies do not occur is white sugar, that supreme ingredient of "junk" food.**

the presence of these signs does not always indicate an allergy: there are obviously many more causes of a runny nose. Moreover, allergies can cause other less definable symptoms. Not surprisingly, therefore, allergies can be difficult to identify, and foolproof diagnosis can be made only by a doctor. Allergies to a food item can start at any time, so the fact that something never used to affect you is no guarantee that it won't now. Nevertheless, unless you always react after eating a particular food, you are unlikely to be allergic to it. (See also pages 90-4.)

——FOOD ADDITIVES——

In the last two years food additives have become the subject of much public concern. It has now reached the stage where manufacturers and retailers use "additive-free" as a selling point. This concern has mostly been generated by the implementation of EEC rules requiring virtually all additives in a food or food product to be identified.

Public concern has been fuelled, not merely by the length of the list of additives, but also by the system of E numbers used by the EEC to identify permitted food additives. The aim of this system was to identify additives unequivocally, even within the multilingual Common Market, and to make it clear that any additives present were permitted ones. Although the system was intended to control the use of additives and to provide more information about food composition, the anonymity and extent of the E classification system has probably generated more anxiety than it has dispelled.

Not all additives in food have E numbers. Some that are still being considered by the EEC are nevertheless permitted in the UK where they have been allocated a number but no E prefix, and this is not shown on the label. Thus the dye used in the UK to colour kippers, which food chemists call Brown FK (the initials stand for "for kippers") is called 154. If it is approved by the EEC it will become known as E154. Meanwhile it is shown on food labels just as Brown FK.

Maurice Hanssen, a consumer activist, responded to the arrival of E numbers on the retailing scene with his now famous directory *E For Additives*, which provides a complete guide to which chemical each E number describes and to the possible risks that might be associated with consuming it. The book has been a run-away success and went through seventeen editions within two years of publication. The publicity that publishers put on the jackets of books should always be taken with a pinch of salt, but when Hanssen's publishers described his book as "the bestseller that started a food buying revolution" they were being, if anything, rather coy.

Hanssen lists nearly 400 additives, for three-quarters of which he admits there are no known harmful effects. But he claims that eighty additives have produced harmful effects. The regulations covering food additives require, not surprisingly, that where the balance of the evidence shows that a specific additive is harmful it must be withdrawn. Is it fair to conclude, therefore, that for most of those eighty additives for which Hanssen suggests that there is some evidence of adverse effects, this evidence would be still regarded by most scientists as controversial?

> *The publicity that publishers put on the jackets of books should always be taken with a pinch of salt, but when Hanssen's publishers described his book as "the bestseller that started a food buying revolution" they were being, if anything, rather coy.*

> *For an additive to be approved, the committee must be convinced it is safe. This does not mean that, were the evidence made public, the majority of nutritional scientists would be convinced by it. The very fact that committees in different countries make different decisions about additives shows how expert opinion can be divided.*

The answer to that question must be "only sometimes". The great problem with evaluating additives is the secrecy with which they are tested. Most testing is done by the food industry – it is, after all, only fair that the people who will make a profit out of additives should pay the costs necessary for their introduction. But the results of those tests, like the results of much industrial research, are rarely published or made available to anyone else. The government-appointed committee of experts which judges whether an additive is to be permitted has access to the results of such tests, although it guarantees that it will treat this information as confidential. For an additive to be approved, the committee must be convinced it is safe. This does not mean that, were the evidence made public, the majority of nutritional scientists would be convinced by it. The very fact that committees in different countries make different decisions about additives shows how expert opinion can be divided.

It is frequently suggested that such committees contain a disproportionate number of scientists connected with the food industry. This is hardly surprising since it is the food industry that does most of the testing and therefore has the most expert scientists in this field. The objection to their presence has some justification, but it is difficult to resolve without reducing the level of skill in the committees. Most scientists regard cheating in their scientific work as an unpardonable sin, so flagrant distortion of results is unlikely. But scientists are as prone as anyone else to being subconsciously biased by their loyalties.

While the more outspoken charges that there is a food industry/government conspiracy to cover up the damage caused by additives can be dismissed, it is necessary to consider carefully the evidence that activists say is ignored and to evaluate its importance. The evidence of harm that Hanssen and others quote but that the government committees have not accepted is of three types: unconfirmed reports; evidence of sensitivity occurring infrequently; and evidence of toxic effects at very high levels of consumption.

Unconfirmed reports of adverse effects are not uncommon. When a scientist thinks he has discovered something he is not always correct. In all sciences isolated reports tend to be treated cautiously until they have been confirmed by another group of scientists. This is the case with E450(b), sodium tripolyphosphate, which is an emulsifying salt added to some foods. As Hanssen notes, some French scientists have suggested it could cause digestive disturbances. This claim has not been confirmed by other scientists and is not, on balance, regarded as correct.

The second type of evidence on toxic effects consists of reports that some individuals have shown allergic or hypersensitive reactions to certain additives. Much publicity has been given to this, but the existence of sporadic allergies to additives is no more a reason for restricting their use than comparable evidence relating to cow's milk is a reason for declaring it to be dangerous. There are also claims, much publicized recently, that certain additives cause behavioural changes, particularly hyperactivity in children and, according to some experts, criminal behaviour.

Undoubtedly some individuals do have allergic or other adverse reactions to certain food additives. But most people show no reaction at all to the permitted additives. Those people who do have adverse reactions have them only to relatively few additives. The extent to which people react to additives has sometimes been claimed to be extraordinarily high, but most of these reports cannot be substantiated. So far the best survey data that have been collected come from Denmark where scientists have shown that for two much criticized additives, tartarazine (E102) and benzoic acid (E210), true sensitivity is somewhere between one person in every thousand and one in every ten thousand.

Scientists have shown that for two much criticized additives, tartarazine (E102) and benzoic acid (E210), true sensitivity is somewhere between one person in every thousand and one in every ten thousand.

The final and more problematical type of evidence cited by consumer groups shows that a toxic effect exists for a specific additive but only at very high levels of consumption – much higher than could be achieved if the only source of the additive were the amounts contained in a food. This is the case with E412, guar gum, a compound commonly used as an emulsifier. Very high levels of guar gum cause flatulence and abdominal cramps, but there are no reports of any adverse effects at the low levels at which it is used as a dietary additive. However the existence of toxicity at high levels raises the problem of how to deal with the risks this poses.

With any compound that causes an adverse effect, the problem is to define a safe level of intake. This applies not only to food additives but to many kinds of environmental hazard. If an additive is toxic at high levels, is there a level of intake that we may regard as safe? It is tempting to say that anything that has a toxic effect at any level should be banned. But this is not really sensible. After all most vitamins have adverse effects at high enough intake levels (see pages 32-41). What is needed is to determine an acceptable level of risk and this is something we all do every day, since almost every human activity carries a risk, yet we regard most of them, to all intents and purposes, as safe.

The rule that has been instigated to deal with additives that can be toxic at high levels is to take as an "acceptable daily intake" (ADI) one-hundredth of the level at which no adverse effect has been demonstrated experimentally. Whether the ADI is truly safe is a moot point. There are three aspects that must be considered. First, there is the problem that experiments on toxicity are almost all conducted on animals, not people, and it is always possible that effects differ between species. This does not mean that everything will be more toxic to humans. For example, an intake of chocolate that is acceptable to us will cause dogs to become seriously ill. Many experiments now use more than one animal species for tests, but we can still never be quite sure that humans are not going to be different.

But even if the animal tested is representative of the way humans will respond, there is a second problem, that of variability. In experiments with toxic substances it is found that animals differ from one another in their sensitivity to the toxin. Indeed it is usual to express toxicity as an LD50, the dose that is toxic to 50 per cent of the

> *While one molecule of cyanide can be dealt with, one molecule of a carcinogen may set off the train of events that will eventually lead to cancer.*

animals. This is because the level that is toxic can vary quite widely between one person and another. In the case of vitamin A ten times the dose that produces adverse effects in one person may have no effects at all in another.

For what might be called "traditional" poisons, such as cyanide and arsenic or the fat soluble vitamins, there are probably levels that can be safely consumed at which no one has a chance of being killed. Vitamins A and D, for example, do not cause any toxic effects at the levels needed to meet our vitamin requirements. Low levels of arsenic can probably also be consumed without harm. However many scientists believe that certain other types of poisons, notably carcinogens, cannot be treated in the same way. Although the risk of cancer diminishes the lower the dose and may be so remote that it could never be demonstrated in any experiment, it never quite vanishes. While one molecule of cyanide can be dealt with, one molecule of a carcinogen may set off the train of events that will eventually lead to cancer.

Imagine, for example, a compound that was so weak a carcinogen that the chances of an individual getting cancer after consuming it for a year were a million to one against. Thus an individual could consume it for a million years before he was certain of getting cancer. Most of us would regard that as no real risk. But in the view of most scientists, in a population of 50 million people all consuming that compound, fifty cancer deaths would result each year. Do we still regard that as an acceptable risk? Although in the past many scientists have tried, rather arbitrarily, to claim they should decide when a risk is unacceptable (some American scientists have supported the idea of a million to one chance as safe), clearly such problems cannot be solved by scientists alone. Only the consumer can say what he or she regards as an unacceptable risk. But risks must, of course, be weighed against any benefits.

Some consumer activists have argued for a no-risk policy. They maintain that if there is the remotest chance of something being harmful, it must be banned. Fear of cancer is so great that this view easily commands support when carcinogens are involved, without any attempt to quantify the risk. At one point the no-risk philosophy became enshrined in American law in the infamous Delaney amendment of 1958, which required that any substance shown to cause cancer at any level of consumption in any species should be banned from the diet. Scientists pointed out this often meant the banning of substances that undoubtedly reduced the risk of other diseases. One example was the nitrates that were used in curing meat to prevent microbial growth. Other substances falling within the scope of the ban like cyclamate, were extremely unlikely to cause cancer in humans, and were replaced in the diet by far less desirable substances such as sugar.

In the debate about additives and food components we are still in a position where, for many additives that carry a possible risk, we lack clear evidence about their benefits. For some (such as nitrates) we can show a clear gain in health terms. But for most others, benefits are more nebulous and difficult to define. Reducing additives might, in many cases, reduce the range of convenience foods available.

The cost of food might rise and employment in the food industry might fall. We cannot assess all the implications of banning additives, nor do we have any consensus as to how the undesirable effects of such a ban should be weighed against risks. How many people should be made unemployed to save one life? The development of a consumer consensus on such matters is still a long way off.

Meanwhile concern must be kept within reason. It is illogical to accept the real, if remote, increase in the risk of cancer that results from central heating and home insulation (which give the natural radioactive gas called radon more chance to build up) while panicking about equally remote risks from plasticizers in cling-film.

Toxic effects and allergic responses caused by additives are probably much less significant than is often supposed. We have seen that the question of whether they should therefore be banned is a difficult one. We do not consider banning any natural food (such a potatoes, cow's milk and wheat products) because it has some toxic effects or is associated with allergic responses in some consumers. We could not survive without food. The additive issue must be dealt with in the same way, by balancing the risks against the benefits. To elucidate these we must now consider exactly what additives are.

WHAT ARE FOOD ADDITIVES?

For many people the phrase 'food additives' inevitably evokes the word 'artificial'. This is a misconception as there are a variety of natural food additives. Indeed the bulk of food additives are probably natural. A natural food additive is a biological product that has not been manipulated or extracted by modern chemical processes. An artificial additive is either something that has been synthesized by a chemist or a natural product that has been chemically modified in some way. Only artificial additives are given E numbers. So garlic, rosemary or thyme or sugar or salt, which are all natural food additives, are not given E numbers. Most natural additives do not induce the same mistrust as artificial ones. Indeed the presence of herbs or spices in food is likely to be a selling point, even though, as will be realized from the discussion of natural toxins in food, there is no special reason why a natural additive should be any better than an artificial one. Indeed when the tartrazine came under suspicion it was replaced in the USA by the natural colourant croescin, which in turn had to be withdrawn because of inadequate information on its safety.

Many of the "natural food" enthusiasts who, nevertheless, divide additives into natural and artificial, thereby create a good deal of confusion. For a given chemical compound, for example L-ascorbic acid (vitamin C), it does not matter at all whether it comes from a natural biological source, or whether it is chemically synthesized. It will have the same properties regardless of its origins.

Of course, it is sometimes possible to distinguish between artificial and natural vitamins chemically. Many vitamins are not single chemical compounds and exist in a variety of chemically distinct, although closely allied, forms. For example, a variety of compounds share the same vitamin E activity known as α-β- and γ-tocopherols. Natural vitamin E

For many people the phrase "food additives" inevitably evokes the word "artificial". This is a misconception as there are a variety of natural food additives.

155

tends to be a mixture of all tocopherols in varying proportions, depending upon the source, whereas synthetic vitamin E is usually one particular type, DL-α-tocopherol. A chemical analysis can in this case distinguish natural from synthetic vitamin E so they must be regarded as different. But even here there is no scientific evidence that one kind has any advantages or disadvantages, and the division of natural from artificial remains, nutritionally, meaningless.

There are various categories of food additive of which three attract most criticism: colours, preservatives and flavourings. This division leads to some interesting advertising claims. For example, a manufacturer might proudly declare a jam free of artificial preservatives and not only omit to point out that it contains natural preservatives in the form of sugar but also to fail to declare that it contains colourants. Since most of the concern that is expressed about food additives actually relates to colourants, preservative-free food may still not be what the consumer requires.

COLOURANTS

Colourants are compounds added to food to provide or enhance its colour. They can be identified easily because they have E numbers in the range 100-180. There are also two groups of permitted colourants in foods that do not have an E number. One group comprises natural vegetable extracts, which are often a complex and variable mixture of chemicals and include paprika, sandalwood, saffron and turmeric root. The second group is composed of colourants that are permitted for use in the UK but that have not yet received an E number because not all EEC governments regard them as safe. These include Brown FK (see page 151) and similar compounds.

These official disagreements make colourants in many ways the most controversial group of additives. The differences between nations in the colourants that are permitted are astonishing. At one extreme the UK government allows eighteen, five more than the EEC standard. In the USA, on the other hand, there are only five colourants in general use, while Norwegians manage to get by with no colourants at all. In the UK colourants can be added only to processed foods. Thus fresh fruit and vegetables, meat and fish cannot be coloured, although in certain circumstances coloured dyes can be used to mark such foods. (For instance, fresh citrus fruit can be marked with methyl violet.) However, colourants may be added to canned fruit and vegetables.

> *The differences between nations in the colourants that are permitted are astonishing. At one extreme the UK government allows eighteen, five more than the EEC standard. In the USA, on the other hand, there are only five colourants in general use, while Norwegians manage to get by with no colourants at all.*

Criticism of colourants is of two types. First, critics point out that colours are not necessary and that often their function is not to benefit the consumer but the food industry by enabling the nature of processed food to be disguised. One example of this has already been mentioned on page 127 where we saw that much of the "meat" contained in meat products like pies and sausages is made up largely of waste from the carcass that has been treated to make it edible. Many critics argue that the addition of colourants to such products to make them look like cooked meat deceives consumers who would reject the product if they realized what it consisted of. Now that nutritionists recommend a reduction in dietary fat, this argument has gained strength because it is undeniable that attempts to make high fat products look as if they were made from lean meat runs

> *The azo-dyes became famous when the American physician Dr Ben Feingold suggested that sensitivity to food colours, and particularly to these dyes, caused behavioural problems, most notably hyperactivity in children.*

counter to this advice. Another example of misleading the consumer are carbonated soft drinks which contain the much criticized colourant tartrazine (E102), added to impart an orange colour to a drink that usually has little or no connection with real oranges.

The second criticism is aimed at the addition of colours to jams or canned peas, which lose their natural colouring during processing. This is justified by the food industry on the grounds that the consumer does not want foods that lack colour, as was demonstrated some years ago when Marks and Spencer briefly introduced canned peas that had no added colour. Their dull grey peas found few buyers. Consumer activists point out that this demand for coloured products is only habit and that consumer attitudes have changed so much recently that were Marks and Spencer to repeat the experiment it would now produce the opposite effect. Norwegian consumers, after all, manage quite well without any added colours in their food. The popularity of the new products to which no colours are added seems to support this view.

The reason much of the criticism of additives is aimed at colourants is that they include the azo-dyes or coal tar dyes. The two terms are sometimes used interchangeably, but they do not quite mean the same thing. There are sixteen colourants which are coal tar dyes – that is, dyes were originally extracted from coal tar, although now they are all chemically synthesized. Of these, eleven are azo-dyes.

The azo-dyes became famous when the American physician Dr Ben Feingold suggested that sensitivity to food colours, and particularly to these dyes, caused behavioural problems, most notably hyperactivity in children. These claims remain highly controversial and they are not yet widely accepted among scientists and clinicians. Some clinicians do regard them as correct and base their treatment accordingly, while at the other extreme some scientists claim that the whole syndrome of hyperactivity does not exist at all and is the medicalization of an extreme form of normal behaviour. Recent British studies showed that behavioural responses to tartarazine did occur, but were always associated with physical signs (e.g., eczema). They underlined the fact that wheat and cow's milk were more important triggers than tartrazine or chocolate. Certainly, diagnosing hyperactivity or assessing changes in its severity is a difficult matter, largely dependent on the subjective judgement of the observer. Feingold's claim is likely to remain controversial for some time yet.

Many parents of supposedly hyperactive children are convinced that, while scientists dither, the Feingold treatment of eliminating certain additives has worked on their child, and some have set up their own organization to publicize the treatment. The "Hyperactive Children's Support Group" regards food sensitivity as a major cause of behavioural and learning problems in children. Of the 23 additives that they recommend should be avoided by children with these problems, 16 are colourants and include 10 azo-dyes and 14 coal tar dyes.

However, these parents do not carry the majority of interested scientists and clinicians with them in their views. The situation is like a Scottish court of law, where there is not enough valid evidence to convict and the verdict has to be one of "not proven". Nevertheless, parents at the end of their tether with an extremely trying child cannot be discouraged from trying to give the child a diet free from colourants. If they believe that this does their child good, the lack of scientific proof need not be a reason for discontinuing the diet. But equally parents who feel unable to feed their child a Feingold-type diet should not torture themselves with guilt, since current scientific opinion is that they are unlikely to be doing any damage thereby. A recent controlled survey showed that about 3 people in 10,000 reacted to an additive, so it is a rare problem.

Nevertheless, in the long term it seems likely that, with or without good reason, pressure will mount for the removal of colourants, or at least artificial colourants, from the diet. Whether this will result in any measurable improvement in health remains an open question, but it certainly will not do any direct harm. Once we have become accustomed to a loss of colours in some processed foods, it is likely that no one will miss colourants greatly. And since this will reduce the opportunities for food to be presented as something it is not, we may even find that the changes are beneficial.

PRESERVATIVES

It is impossible for most people to eat a diet completely composed of fresh foods and so some method of food preservation is necessary. Preserving food is one of mankind's oldest skills, and many of the methods still used long predate the E classification system and do not come within its scope. These include the adding of salt, sugar, alcohol and certain herbs and spices, as well as processes like drying and smoking.

Indeed, so old are many of these processes that we hardly think of them as preservation techniques. Instead the preserved version of the food has become valued in itself. We regard jam as a foodstuff in its own right, not merely as fruit preserved with sugar, and few people think of a kipper merely as a herring that had to be smoked to preserve it, or treat pickled onions as preserved onions. The currying of food also acts as a preservative, and its origins may stem from that. But curries are now regarded as a gastronomic treat, not as processed foods.

Preserving food is one of mankind's oldest skills, and many of the methods still used long predate the E classification system and do not come within its scope.

In the main, the preservatives that are covered by the E number legislation are newer ones that have enabled us to extend the range and type of preserved foods. The consequences of removing these preservatives from the diet would be adverse. For unless we are willing to restrict the type of foods that we eat, at least some of the 47 common preservatives (whose E numbers are in the range E200-299) are vital. This is eloquently illustrated by the controversy that has raged for some years now about the use of nitrites and nitrates (E249-252) as preservatives in cured meats such as bacon. Both sides in the food additive controversy agree that these additives do have some untoward effects, notably that they can cause illness in young babies (and for this reason they are not allowed to be added to babyfoods). There is agreement, too, that in the gut of the normal adult some are converted to a class of chemicals called nitrosamines, which in large doses are carcinogenic. But both sides also concur that this is no reason for removing them from cured meats, for without them such products are vulnerable to the growth of a food-poisoning micro-organism called *Clostridium botulinum*, which has the unenviable reputation of producing the most toxic poison known, a poison that is particularly dangerous because it cannot be destroyed by cooking.

> *Any slight risk of cancer that may result from the use of nitrates and nitrites as preservatives is more than outweighed by the virtual certainty of a continuing mortality from botulinism that would follow their removal.*

Overall, it seems that any slight risk of cancer that may result from the use of nitrates and nitrites as preservatives is more than outweighed by the virtual certainty of a continuing mortality from botulinism that would follow their removal. Of course, both risks could be avoided if all cured meat products – bacon, hams, salamis – as well as pressed meats, canned meats and sausages were eliminated from the diet. But such a diet is impracticable except for vegetarians (and very strict ones because these additives have also to be included in many cheeses). A few people are obliged to avoid nitrates and nitrites because they cause a type of asthma, but we do not, as with colourants, have the option of continuing with the same foods that we eat at present but with preservative-free versions. But, in general, there is a health risk from dispensing with additives – something reflected in the more than 50 per cent rise in salmonella poisoning in the last five years.

There are some preservatives that could be dispensed with without any know direct health risk, although this would lead to increased food wastage. Notable among these are the anti-fungal compounds that can be applied to the skins of citrus fruit to inhibit fungal growth. Without the addition of these compounds there would be much more spoilage of fruit in storage and during transport which would mean that such fruit would be available for shorter periods and would be more expensive. It is difficult to predict what the health implications of a prohibition of fungicides would be. Nutritionists now believe the consumption of fruit to be important for its fruit fibre (pectin) content, as well as for the vitamin C it provides. Whether the fall in fruit consumption that might well result from a prohibition would have adverse effects that would outweigh any benefits is at the heart of the problem. At the moment the risks of these compounds to our health are seen as sufficiently slight, and the potential disruption of their removal sufficiently great, for them to be kept in our diet.

ANTIOXIDANTS
Antioxidants can be identified by the E numbers from E300 to E321. They have a

Antioxidants can be identified by the E numbers from E300 to E321. They have a similar effect to preservatives in preventing food from going bad but they protect against chemical deterioration caused by oxygen in the air rather than microbial attack.

similar effect to preservatives in preventing food from going bad but they protect against chemical deterioration caused by oxygen in the air rather than microbial attack. The combination of oxygen with certain components of food causes the development of flavours that we regard as "off". Only certain foods, including those containing polyunsaturated (essential) fatty acids, are susceptible to this form of chemical attack. After attack by oxygen these fatty acids form compounds that have a characteristic smell that we recognize as rancid. Fish is an obvious example of a food susceptible to this type of chemical damage, and the smell of rancid fish is one almost everyone has met at some time. Cooking oils are another obvious victim, although they are now routinely sold with antioxidants so detectable deterioration is rare. Oxidative damage is not confined to fatty foods, however. The browning of cut apple or the blackening of cut potato are other examples of changes that result from attack by oxygen. And "scald", the browning of apples and pears that can result from slight contact damage, is also a form of oxidative damage. Another is the deterioration of wine on contact with the air, which is why an opened bottle of wine cannot be kept for long.

Antioxidants are a class of chemicals that mop up any oxygen that comes into contact with food, thus preventing oxidative damage. Rather than oxidizing the food, the molecule of oxygen oxidizes the antioxidant molecule and is thereby chemically neutralized. Preventing this sort of attack is important to all living creatures who have their own antioxidants to protect their tissues. Two of these are vitamins: vitamin E – the tocopherols (E307-309), which protect fatty substances – and vitamin C – ascorbic acid and its variants (E300-304), which protects water-soluble substances. It is no coincidence that these two vitamins are antioxidants. Their importance is largely due to their ability to prevent oxygen damage in the body. Neither of these vitamins pose any risk when used as food additives.

Concern about the antioxidant additives centres around two groups, the gallates (E310-312), and the closely related pair, Beta-hydroxy-anisole, or BHA (E320), and Beta-hydroxy-toluene, or BHT (E321). There has been some concern that the gallates could be dangerous to asthmatics and to people who are sensitive to aspirin. They are also among the additives that are forbidden in babyfoods, although they are added to a wide variety of other processed foods, including oils and fats (as well as margarines), breakfast cereals and snack foods. BHA and BHT also have only restricted use in babyfoods, but they are used in a wide range of processed convenience foods. They have been the subject of several criticisms. The Hyperactive Children's Support Group identifies them among the additives that it believes can trigger hyperactivity in some children. On the basis of animal experiments, they have also been suspected of being carcinogenic.

While there may be a case for withdrawing gallates, it is not a strong one. The charges levelled against BHA and BHT are even more difficult to deal with and show how difficult it can be to balance risks and benefits in this area. Although some experimenters claim that BHT might cause cancer in laboratory animals, others have claimed that BHA might prevent it. On the basis of other animal experiments it has even been suggested that BHT might actually extend the human lifespan beyond its normal limits!

Despite the contradictory nature of the evidence, it may seem strange that the

According to one estimate in 1985, the UK food industry spent £55 million on a total of about 1,000 tons of 3,500 flavouring compounds that were added to the diet.

Acceptable Daily Intake (ADI) of BHT has recently been reduced. This action illustrates another aspect of the decision-making process. The fact that BHT appears to extend the life of laboratory animals is also evidence that it is not biologically inert to the animal that consumes it. This evidence, even of good effects, calls for considerable caution because ideally the additive should have no effect on the consumer at all.

Although the ADI of BHT has been reduced, there is no suggestion from the regulatory bodies that BHT or the other antioxidants should be banned altogether. On balance, it seems likely that the disadvantages of consuming oxidized fat (which besides causing rancidity can cause real damage to health if eaten in too great an amount) make the retention of BHA and BHT desirable. But clearly there is much more scientific work to be done before the current confusion can be resolved.

FLAVOURINGS

Flavourings make up the largest group of additives used, but few are included on the E numbers list. According to one estimate in 1985, the UK food industry spent £55 million on a total of about 1,000 tons of 3,500 flavouring compounds that were added to the diet. Consumer activists have not yet displayed much concern about flavourings, and most scientists would argue that the majority are unlikely to be harmful to health. Natural flavours are made out of combinations of quite simple chemicals, and to a large degree the flavour chemist seeks to recreate the natural flavour by blending those same chemicals together. Since one natural flavour may be the result of more than a hundred chemicals in varying proportions, the art of flavour chemistry lies in blending them in the right proportions to obtain the most pleasing and realistic flavour. It is exactly like the perfumery business where a blender's most precise instrument is his nose, and because blending is so individual, flavour combinations are closely guarded secrets. As you might expect, there is a thriving business of trying to crack other companies' flavour mixtures. The secrecy is such that flavours are not individually declared. All that is required is a declaration that all flavourings used are on the permitted list.

Most of these flavourings are as harmless as food whose flavour they mimic since the flavour chemist does not create new chemicals that mimic a particular natural flavour but seeks to analyse natural flavour and rebuild it. The artificiality of some of the results, for example the crudity of artificial apple or other fruit flavours that are often found in sweets or drinks, does not indicate that a new chemical has been used. The problem is just that the balance between the hundreds of compounds that make up the natural flavour has not yet been found. Indeed, often only the crudest imitation of the real flavour is made deliberately. In pear drops, for

> *Any lack of subtlety is disguised by making the flavour very strong, in much the same way that the loudness of music can be used to disguise its banality.*

example, only one or two compounds are used to give an approximation to pear flavour. The manufacturer does not find it worthwhile to add small amounts of other compounds that would give a closer resemblance to the real thing. Instead any lack of subtlety is disguised by making the flavour very strong, in much the same way that the loudness of music can be used to disguise its banality. The main risk from using such artificial flavours is that we have our palates blunted by them, the gustatory equivalent of deafness from listening to loud music.

However, the flavourings that generate most anxiety on health grounds are not these true flavourings but the artificial sweeteners that are used to make food taste sweet without the addition of sugar. These are treated differently in law from other flavour compounds (probably because no one is so secretive about them). They are declared individually on foodstuffs and are entitled to have E numbers. In fact only two do: sorbitol and mannitol (E420 and E421). Both of these are natural sugars, different from ordinary sugar but still providing calories. Their main use is in food for diabetics. But hypersensitivity has been reported to high intakes of both – even though both are natural!

More fear is expressed about the chemical sweeteners that are hundreds of times sweeter than sugar and provide few or no calories. These are included in slimming foods. The oldest, discovered a hundred years ago, is saccharin, which has often given rise to concern but has still not been proved to be harmful. Another is cyclamate, which was removed from the UK permitted list in 1970 because of evidence of its possible carcinogenicity at high concentrations. The recently introduced aspartame also has its critics. It is made of two amino acids joined together, and one of them, phenylalanine, is an amino acid that people with the genetic disease phenylketonuria cannot metabolize. Such people must avoid aspartame, but since almost all cases of the disease are diagnosed in early infancy, sufferers know they are at risk. It has been suggested that other people may also be unable to metabolize large amounts of aspartame, but the evidence is inconclusive. However, the point has been made that, considering all the known and suspected disadvantages of ordinary table sugar (sucrose), none of the artificial sweeteners are anywhere near as harmful, even considering their possible disadvantages.

Another group of additives related to the flavours includes the flavour enhancers or modifiers. Here the major criticism centres around monosodium glutamate or MSG (E621), which is used to enhance meaty or savoury flavours. Some people are particularly sensitive to large quantities of MSG. At its mildest it causes headaches, and at its worst a mixture of giddiness, nausea, muscle pains and heart palpitations. This response is sometimes called "Chinese Restaurant Syndrome" since it was first identified in people who became ill after eating Chinese food, which makes extensive use of MSG as it is found in large amounts in soy sauce.

OTHER ADDITIVES

Additives with E numbers between 322 and 999 are a mixed bag, which have had fewer accusations levelled at them than those discussed so far. Only the more famous – or infamous – are relevant here.

Emulsifiers are a common additive. They enable oil and water to be mixed into a stable emulsion as, for example, in mayonnaise, salad cream and other dressings. Old-fashioned cooks use egg yolk to achieve this. The active component within egg yolk comes from a group of compounds called lecithin. Lecithins differ slightly according to their source, but all are classed under the same E number, 322. Because it is cheap, the major lecithin used in commercial food processing today comes from soya bean; neither this nor egg lecithin have been accused of having any harmful effects. Indeed lecithin supplements have been promoted as "health foods".

Polyphosphates used in this way therefore enable the industry to cheat the customer out of 10 per cent of the meat that he is charged for. Indeed, they were advertised in the Meat Trades Journal *under the revealing caption "Why sell meat if you can sell water?".*

A different kind of criticism can be levelled against the polyphosphate additives listed as E450(a) to E450(d). Although these can be used as emulsifying salts in meat and meat products to prevent the loss of fat and meat juices during cooking, they have perhaps an even more important use to the food manufacturer because water can be injected into the meat, so increasing the weight by more than 10 per cent without any visible sign. Polyphosphates used in this way therefore enable the industry to cheat the customer out of 10 per cent of the meat that he is charged for. Indeed, they were advertised in the *Meat Trades Journal* under the revealing caption "Why sell meat if you can sell water?" New labelling regulations will require the processor to say how much extra water has been added in this way, but will not outlaw the practice.

As is the case with many other kinds of additive, it is now becoming common to promote products, such as frozen chicken, with labels declaring them to be free from polyphosphates. Although this guarantees that the product will not be diluted with massive amounts of water, it does not mean that no excess water has been added. Manufacturers now often "glaze" such products with a surface layer of ice that ensures that the consumer is still spending money on added water. This process occurs most excessively with frozen prawns, which can have more than 20 per cent of their weight as added water – even though no polyphosphates have been added to them.

THE ECONOMICS OF ADDITIVES

It is impossible to assess the cost of additives. One recent estimate was that, in 1985, £225 million were spent on additives to food, of which 88 per cent was on "cosmetic" additives (i.e., mostly colourants and flavourings). It is difficult to see why this vast expenditure should not be cut simply by reducing the number of additives used. The food industry always claims that such reductions would lead to increases in costs, but this is true of only some additives in some cases. Additive-free versions of some foods are available but only the most optimistic would expect these to be cheaper. Rather, these foods would be more expensive, since processing would be more complex, or would require more expensive ingredients.

——*POLLUTANTS AND CONTAMINANTS*——

Besides fears about food additives, there is anxiety, too, about the potential risk from environmental pollution and compounds like agricultural chemicals. There is a widespread fear that these might leave potentially toxic residues in the food we eat. Such contaminants do, undoubtedly, find their way into our diet, and the subsequent outbreaks of poisoning receive justified publicity. What is less certain is whether there is a risk to our health from serious and continuous contamination from the residues of intensive farming or from environmental pollutants such as lead and mercury.

CONTAMINANTS FROM AGRICULTURE

Pesticides and weedkillers are an inevitable part of modern intensive agriculture, and they have caused outbreaks of poisoning. One such case, for example, happened in Sri Lanka when young Tamil girls working on tea estates suffered partial paralysis after consuming oil that had been accidentally contaminated with an insecticide. Such spectacular outbreaks usually arise from confusion or negligence, in this case from storing cooking oil in metal drums that had been contaminated with the insecticide.

Even with perfect procedures, however, small amounts of the hundred or so pesticides and weedkillers used in the UK do find their way into our diet. The pesticides represent a more serious threat because they are generally fat soluble and therefore become concentrated in body tissues unlike water-soluble compounds which are usually excreted in the urine. The levels found in human tissues are low and their effect is completely unknown. The best-known effect is the way in which DDT damages carnivorous birds, in particular causing the production of eggs with thin shells and increased mortality of the young. Apart from accidents leading to direct spraying of the animals, there are probably two reasons why carnivorous birds are particularly at risk. First, they often have a physiology that is less able to deal with poisonous substances than that of herbivorous or omnivorous animals. The second reason is related to the concentration of the toxin in "the food chain", a matter of great importance to the problem of contaminants in human diets.

Everything that lives is food for something else. Thus, if a small amount of the DDT sprayed on crops gets eaten by herbivorous animals, the DDT will slowly build up in the tissues of these animals. If such animals are themselves then eaten by a carnivore, the carnivore will receive a much higher dose of DDT with its food than the herbivores received originally. If this carnivore is then preyed upon by another carnivore, the effect will be magnified yet again. So the animal at the top of this pyramid of consumption can receive quite toxic doses of DDT from this process of biological concentration.

By and large we do not eat carnivorous animals so we are spared the worst consequences of this phenomenon and there is no suggestion that levels of pesticides in other animals are sufficient to present a problem to human consumers. We do eat carnivorous fish, for example turbot, but levels of DDT in the marine food chain are

> ❛
> *Everything that lives is food for*
> *something else.*
> ❜

not toxic. Currently the UK is almost alone within the European Community in not having statutory residue limits on pesticides, which might seem worrying were it not for the fact that we do have an elaborate system for licensing pesticides and monitoring the residue levels in foods, which not all other countries in the Community have. The situation in Britain is regularly reviewed by a government working party. In its latest report (1986) it noted that levels of pesticide residues in the diet have gone down in the last 20 years or so. Also, home-grown foods and animal products have been found to have reassuringly low levels of pesticide residues, as do human body fat and breast milk. On the other hand, some food imports from China have been shown to have higher levels which need to be watched. The monitoring of residues is probably necessary, not so much because they represent a real risk as because we need to assure ourselves that they are neither a problem nor will they be allowed to become one.

ANTIBIOTICS AND GROWTH PROMOTERS

Antibiotics have no direct effects in our diet, but the widespread use and abuse of antibiotics in animal production has contributed to the development of antibiotic-resistant bacteria, which are therefore more difficult to treat when they infect us. But antibiotic resistance in bacteria is not entirely due to the use of antibiotics in agriculture; the profligate use of antibiotics in medicine has also contributed. The problem is a serious one, and the use of antibiotics in agriculture has been restrained. Greater use is being made of antibiotics not used in human medicine, and the addition of antibiotics to animal feeds as growth promoters is now illegal.

The steroid sex hormones are also used as growth promoters and fattening agents. Growing unease about these during the 1970s has led to their total banning within the EEC since 1986, and between 1968 and 1981 Italy, among some other countries, banned the used of all anabolic steroids. This followed evidence that pregnant women who were treated with very high levels of a particular synthetic steroid called di-ethyl stilboestrol (DES) had children who were more likely in later life to develop a normally very rare form of cancer. DES was present in intensively produced meat, particularly beef, although at relatively low levels compared with those used in medical practice. Unfortunately the ban simply meant that the use of anabolic agents was driven underground. The illegal use of anabolic agents has no in-built safety measures and, in the belief that "if some is good, more must be better", some farmers are not only likely to inject large doses of whatever is cheapest but will not feel obliged to inject only into the ear – the part which is normally thrown away. In 1981 it was shown that Italian children who ate veal-based baby-foods containing DES developed enlarged genitalia and breasts.

Although there was undoubtedly a good case for banning DES, other steroids that were used as growth promoters or fattening agents, particularly those chemically identical to the animal's own steroid hormones, probably did not represent a risk to human health. Provided they were not injected immediately

> *The widespread use and abuse of antibiotics in animal production has contributed to the development of antibiotic-resistant bacteria, which are therefore more difficult to treat when they infect us.*

165

Such a total ban on steroids might seem prudent, but the ironical consequence has been the development in Europe of an illegal trade in steroids for use in animal husbandry by unscrupulous farmers. The dangerous steroid DES, is the cheapest and most available on the black market.

before slaughter, levels in the tissues were the same as those found in normal animals. The balance of the scientific advice was that these other steroids should continue to be used, under strict regulations.

However the EEC parliament worked itself into a frenzy about the subject and banned the use of all steroids as growth promoters. The German government was particularly keen on this ban for reasons that quite possibly have more to do with placating the politically powerful "Greens" in German politics than with producing safe meat for German consumers to purchase.

Notwithstanding the politicians' motives, such a total ban on steroids might seem prudent, but the ironical consequence has been the development in Europe of an illegal trade in steroids for use in animal husbandry by unscrupulous farmers. The dangerous steroid DES, is the cheapest and most freely available on the black market. The ban has probably been self-defeating for unless the illegal trade can be stamped out, there will be no improvement and possibly even a deterioration in the safety of meat. A limited ban, allowing only natural steroids under veterinary supervision, would have presented no risk to humans and would have stamped out this unregulated trade.

INDUSTRIAL CONTAMINANTS

Industrial waste intermittently finds its way into the food that we eat, usually as a result of accidents or of improper disposal of waste. As the scale of industry gets larger, the potential consequences of something going wrong increase. However, the sheer scale of such pollution makes its detection more likely, and although foodstuffs, animals and crops may have to be destroyed, the chances of the contaminants finding their way into our diet are small.

Continual low levels of contamination present a much more real risk. One outstanding example of this is the heavy metals, of which mercury and lead are probably the most important contaminants of our diet. (The next most important is cadmium.) Mercury and lead are both important in a variety of industrial processes and both are highly toxic. They are excreted from the body extremely slowly, so continuous small doses can lead to a build-up in tissues that will eventually reach toxic levels. The major route for such contamination of our diet, particularly mercury, is fish because the heavy metals tend to be discharged with industrial effluent into rivers and seas and are therefore found in inland and coastal waters. By a process of biological concentration along the aquatic food chain, the mercury becomes concentrated in certain fish at levels that are many times higher than those in the water. However the levels of mercury cannot rise too high in the fish without killing them and levels of mercury that are high, but not fatal, for the fish are unlikely to deliver enough mercury to damage humans unless the level of fish consumption is very high, although this can occur. One case of mercury poisoning was recently reported from New York where the patient was a lady who regularly ate 1lb (0.5kg) of swordfish every day. On a far more extensive scale, before this pheno- menon of biological concentration was appreciated, there were severe problems with mercury poisoning in fish-eating communities in areas that were indus- trially polluted, the case of the Minimata Bay epidemic in Japan being the best-known instance of this.

> *One case of mercury poisoning was recently reported from New York where the patient was a lady who regularly ate 1lb (0.5kg) of swordfish every day.*

RADIOACTIVE CONTAMINATION
Radioactive fallout has become detectable in our food as a by-product of the atomic age, and radioactive contamination of food received much publicity during 1986 following the Chernobyl accident. Before the nuclear test ban treaty of 1963, some foods from a number of countries had levels of radioactive contaminants that caused much concern and in some localities levels were sufficiently high that live- stock were unfit for consumption. Overall, though, the UK diet was not much affected and, even after Chernobyl, the levels are now generally much lower than they were in 1963, and they will continue to fall as long as governments do not renew their programmes of nuclear testing.

DELIBERATE ADULTERATION
Finally, our food can be contaminated by criminal acts of deliberate adulteration, a topic that has a long history, having been of great concern in the early 19th century, as we saw in Chapter 7. Two recent cases deserve mention, if only because the scale completely dwarfs all risks of accidental contamination. In 1981 cooking oil sold fraudulently by doorstep traders as pure olive oil proved to contain rapeseed oil, which had been denatured with the poison aniline for industrial purposes. A total of 13,000 people were admitted to hospital with symptoms of poisoning and over 100 died. Another example, from 1985 this time, is the sale of low-grade Austrian wine contaminated with the toxic compound ethylene glycol, which is normally used as the major component of antifreeze. It was added to the wine deliberately and illegally to improve its flavour.

REAL RISKS OF CONTAMINANTS IN FOOD
Although the list of contaminants in food is a long one, this should be thought of as a good, rather than a bad, thing. For the contaminants that we are aware of are un- likely to be a real problem. Their levels in food are monitored, and scientific work on the maximum safe level can provide guidelines of safety. It is the unknown poison that presents the problem. If, as is sometimes claimed, there is conspiracy of scientists, food industry and government to disguise contaminants in the diet, there is little, if any, reasonable evidence for it. There is sometimes complacency, but monitoring and continual debate on risks are probably the best safeguard. The risks are unavoidable. They are not avoided even by eating wholefood. Really major risks have come from foods that a "wholefooder" would regard as completely acceptable. The aflatoxins and other toxins produced by fungi that can flourish on

nuts and grain can cause anything from insanity and cancer to immediate death. These fungi thrive on products that are badly stored or packaged (particularly if kept in hot, humid conditions). It is, of course, the small wholefood concerns, not the big companies, that are particularly prone to this risk because they have neither the clout nor the expertise to provide safety checks against potential contaminants.

IRRADIATED FOOD: IS IT SAFE?

The irradiation of food involves no additives nor contaminants, and although it makes use of radioactive sources, it does not cause the radioactive contamination of the food itself.

It is well known that, in high doses, radioactivity kills, and it is precisely this knowledge that is put to use in the irradiation of food. Ionizing radiation, like X-rays, is directed at a food to kill any micro-organisms that happen to be present. The food can be already sealed in a container, through which these ionizing rays will pass. This means that food can be packed before it is sterilized. The net result is the same as heat sterilization but irradiation has a number of advantages. The first is that the food is not cooked in any way, and so irradiation is suitable for raw foods, such as fresh fruit and vegetables. Irradiation does not leave the food completely unaffected, the changes that occur being progressively greater with increasing doses. However, even quite low doses will inhibit the natural biochemistry of the food. Irradiation can therefore be used to slow, or inhibit, ripening and to extend the life of fresh food.

The aim of irradiation is to cause no detectable changes in the texture or flavour of food, but, as is discussed below, this is not always achieved. In addition, because the food remains cold during this process, the packaging need not be heat stable. Packaged foods that are to be heat-treated need to be bottled or canned, whereas foods that are to be irradiated need to be packaged in cardboard or plastic containers. Irradiation is not without some disadvantages, as it can cause unwanted changes in the texture and flavour of some foods.

Concern about irradiation focuses on three issues. The first is whether it makes food radioactive. The answer is that it does but only slightly and only briefly. When the ionizing radiation passes through the food, some atoms absorb it and become radioactive. But they rapidly revert to their non-radioactive state by the process known as radioactive decay, which is the tendency for the radioactivity of any substance to decline with time. All food has some degree of radiation in it, anyway, and the increase due to irradiation is small compared with this. Indeed, irradiation may make the food less radioactive by the time we consume it. Since it enables the food to be kept for longer, decay of natural radioactivity will have proceeded further than in a non-irradiated food.

The second cause for public concern is that irradiation can cause changes in taste or texture. Irradiation results in a wide variety of chemical changes (although far fewer than cooking does), and although these changes do not make

> *Irradiation may make the food less radioactive by the time we consume it. Since it enables the food to be kept for longer, decay of natural radioactivity will have proceeded further than in a non-irradiated food.*

the food harmful in any way, they can make it unpalatable. Certain foods are parti-cularly prone to these changes. Meat, for example, develops an unpleasant flavour variously described as "scorched", "goaty" or "wet dog". The flavour of eggs and dairy products is also easily damaged. The chemical changes responsible for this are not yet understood and limit the use of irradiation on these foods. Other, better understood changes may also occur such as changes in colour: meat goes dark red and then brown, while lobsters and shrimps turn black. There are alterations in texture too: meat may become over-tender while tomatoes may become squashy. Food scientists are trying to find ways of minimizing these changes and have already discovered that the alterations in meat are much slighter if air is excluded during irradiation.

But the major source of public concern about irradiation, and the reason why it is still restricted in the UK, concerns not the changes that it induces but the absence of changes. For since many foods do not show any obvious changes on irradiation, there is no reliable test for detecting it. It is therefore possible for irradiation to be used to allow old items of food to be sold as fresh. For the time being, until this problem of detecting irradiated food is solved, the process looks like remaining an attractive technical advance but of no practical use.

——HEALTH FOODS——

All the risks associated with modern food technology, whether real or imaginary, have done much to encourage the consumption of health foods. Although nutri-tionists find it hard, if not impossible, to say what health foods are, the health food industry seems to be thriving by making and selling them. In the UK there are approximately 1,500 health food shops, 500 wholefood shops, and 3,500 of the 10,000 chemists shops stock and sell some sorts of health food products. In addi-tion, in the last year or two most high street supermarkets have begun to stock, and to some degree stress, foods that most health food adherents would find highly acceptable. However, there is still room for expansion, for, relative to the popu-lation, the UK still has only half the number of health food shops that there are in West Germany.

It may seem silly to say that there are no simple definitions of what health food, organic food or wholefood are, since most people believe they have a clear under-standing of them, but it is difficult to arrive at a definition that is legally leak-proof. Indeed, the US Federal Trade Commission in Washington has proposed that the expression "health food" be banned, a proposal supported by both the American and British Consumers Associations. Neither "health food" nor "wholefood" can be defined in any legally binding way, simply because neither term has any real meaning. An attempt by the Canadian government to define the word natural runs to several pages of legal prose. Health food definitely excludes certain foods, for example commercial confec-tionery, yet acceptable health food pro-ducts include snack bars containing raw sugar, honey and dried fruit that do just

> *Neither "health food" nor "wholefood" can be defined in any legally binding way, simply because neither term has any real meaning.*

169

as much damage to teeth as traditional sweets. Professor Arnold Bender, formerly a professor of Nutrition in London University, has savagely criticized both, pointing out, for example, that if whole wheat is wholefood whereas white flour is not, then logically unpeeled potatoes or oranges are wholefood while peeled potatoes or orange segments are not!

Some definitions have been advanced, although none of them is legally satisfactory. For example *The Health Food Guide* by Michael Balfour (published by Pan Books, 1981) offers one definition. Health food is food "produced from or reared on soil that is unpolluted by chemical fertilizers, is free of chemical sprays, artificial stimulants to growth and additives, has not had the goodness refined out of it, and is prepared for the table with the least possible delay and loss of nutrients". The UK Health Food Manufacturers Association, together with the European Federation of Associations of Health Food Manufacturers, spent three years coming up with their agreed description of health foods. According to this, health food is as naturally based as possible, and includes both foods with their full nutritional content and also food supplements intended to prevent deficiency on a normal diet. Health foods, the description maintains, should be prepared with the specific intention of maintaining and/or improving health. They should, therefore, be accompanied by consumer information regarding their health benefits and preferably be sold in specialist stores by trained staff. The fact that, on the products that health food shops sell, such information as is given is often quite simply untrue, while the verbal claims made by staff are sometimes preposterous, would seem to reduce the usefulness of these fine sentiments.

Wholefood does not have even the benefit of a manufacturer's definition, but the term is increasingly used as an alternative description to health food. It appears to be used to imply that the food in question has not been intensively produced, or refined so as to reduce its nutritional value. This, at least, has the advantage over health food in that it is not claiming that such food will improve health. The wholefood bandwagon is rapidly gathering speed in two interesting ways. First, wholefood seems to be the term that has been taken up by the orthodox retailing sector when it sells such products. Secondly, there is a new generation of shops that call themselves wholefood shops. The name is not copyright and anybody can describe their shop as anything they like, but the tendency is for wholefood shops to sell foods rather than the ancillary products such as dietary supplements, which are so important in health food shops since they are the really profitable items. Wholefood shops, moreover, often sell items like nuts or dried legumes to the consumer in bulk at discount rates.

The only really objective definition of health food or wholefood is that they are items that health food or wholefood shops sell. Such shops, like most specialist shops in the high street, charge more for their goods than the equivalent in the supermarket. One published survey showed that items cost from 7 to 225 per cent more in a health food shop. Sometimes this was because the shop had a different type of product. For example, sea salt in the health food shop cost 225 per

> **The only really objective definition of health food or wholefood is that they are items that health food or wholefood shops sell.**

cent more than the cost of ordinary salt in a grocer's. But often there was no justification for the differential. Lemons cost 100 per cent more in health food shops and six branded foods 10 to 28 per cent more.

A *Which?* magazine survey in 1978 showed that health food stores charged 5 to 20 per cent more than supermarkets for the same brand goods. Equivalent quality items like dried apricots, wholemeal flour, brown rice and clover honey could be bought from wholefood warehouses somewhat cheaper than ordinary prices, but health food shops charged on average 40 per cent more than the ordinary price.

Whether health food shops are worth patronizing must depend on whether the health claims they make for their foods are valid, for this is implicit in the Health Food Manufacturers Association's definition of health foods. It must be said at the outset that there is no reason why they should be. The proprietors, and more crucially the counter staff, of a health food shop need have no specific qualifications or specialist knowledge on which to base their advice. Many health food shops belong to the Holland and Barrett chain, a company that is part of the giant Booker group. Booker has no special commitment to producing only health foods – it is, after all, one of the major sugar producers in the world. Presumably it can ensure a standard level of knowledge among its health food outlet staff, but it is not clear how, or if, it does this. Many other health food shops are independent, but the sources of the sales staff skills are equally unknown.

Of course, the staff are probably all readers of the specialist trade magazines. But these pose a problem. For while the law restricts the advertising claims that a manufacturer or retailer can make about the health effects of a product, there is no restriction on what a journalist may say in an article. It would appear that sales staff in a health food shop will make claims exceeding the stated claims on a product by quoting articles that they appear to believe. Thus the manufacturer makes no specific claims but the second arm of the health food movement, the publications that it produces, will make it on his behalf. Professor Arnold Bender quotes an example of this occurring:

> Holland and Barrett (Natural Choice No 14) correctly and honestly stated that because of the lack of full scientific evidence neither they nor advertisers could claim good effects for this practice (of people taking large doses of vitamin E every day). They did, however, suggest that the potential customer read a book on vitamin E which makes the usual extravagant claims.

Of course, it is undeniable that the health food movement was the leading apostle of dietary fibre during the long period when the medical profession and scientists ignored its possible health benefits, and full credit should be given for this. However it would be illogical to claim that this single success justifies all its other claims.

Once modern nutritional science could be persuaded to turn its attention to fibre it was able to prove a large number of advantages from consuming it. However nutritionists are unable to demonstrate any advantage of brown rather than white sugar, arguing that both are equally undesirable. Nor is there any

> *Nutritionists are unable to demonstrate any advantage of brown rather than white sugar, arguing that both are equally undesirable.*

evidence to support the health claims made for honey, molasses, kelp, buckwheat, royal jelly and nearly all the host of other items sold by health food shops.

The claims that are made for health foods are so many and various that it is impossible to consider them all in detail. Vitamin E supplements seem to be taken for a variety of reasons including high blood pressure, complications of diabetes mellitus, heart disease, aiding wound healing, increasing fertility and delaying senility. It can, however, be confidently said that so far there is little evidence for any of these claims. Vitamin E has been very thoroughly researched in the past as medical researchers and nutritionists have wanted to find out as much about it as the other vitamins (see also page 40).

The reader may wonder how such extravagant and unscientific claims come to be made and while it is, of course, not possible to show how they all arose, some examples will show the kind of thing that happens. First there are undoubtedly people who sincerely promote a nutritional theory that has not yet gained general scientific support. Scientists often think that something might be true but cannot prove it satisfactorily. Establishing scientific proof is a slow process and before it is completed there is a stage where acceptance of claims is based on faith, not evidence. Such claims are often supported by the health food industry. This, for example, is the basis of the current enthusiasm for gamma-linolenic acid (GLA) in health food products. There is some evidence that GLA does affect the human metabolism, but there is no sound evidence that it improves health in any way. Only real enthusiasts accept the claims that are currently made, while the scientific world remains uncertain about its purported effects.

In addition to these premature but perfectly sincere claims, there are many less pleasant reasons that account for some of the assertions made about health foods. Some statements are deliberately fraudulent (these are by no means restricted to the health food industry). It is claimed, for example, that various products will make the consumer lose weight without having to restrict his food intake – a claim that is attractive enough to promote sales but is quite simply false.

There is also the superstitious association of ideas. Ginseng, for example – which is considered a food supplement and so does not come under the strict supervision accorded to medicines – has for centuries been granted magic powers by the superstitious because the root looks a little like a human penis in shape. A surprising number of people today reject science and its approach and instead prefer to accept ancient or traditional beliefs. For such people the fact that ancient Chinese herbalists knew of ginseng is reason enough to believe in it, despite the fact that many modern scientists reject the claims made for it. Objectively, of course, the fact that something was first described 2,000 years ago does nothing to increase its chance of being true.

Then, of course, there is the attraction of the exotic. Ginseng comes from the mysterious East and such scientific enthusiasm for it as does exist comes from Tokyo and Russia (although interestingly, as Professor Bender points out, the Russians appear to be talking about a different plant from that which the Far Eastern traditional medicine is so enthusiastic about). Scepticism, on the other hand, seems to be home-grown and is found in Western scientific journals which lack the appeal of the exotic. But to those who want to believe in a substance like ginseng, the sceptical attitude of the orthodox scientist, when it is not backed up with convincing proof, is seen simply as narrow-mindedness if not "sour grapes" about claims that are not the product of Western technology. However, ginseng is an excellent example of just why it is so difficult to provide the much-wanted proof – one way or another. For a start, there are at least five different species of ginseng, each with different properties. Second, it is very difficult to get hold of reliable preparations on which reliable research can be performed. Third, ginseng is not patentable, so no pharmaceutical company is likely to be willing to put up the huge amount of money necessary to test any new type of medication. The money could come from government funding bodies, but they only fund research on well-defined research materials as this is the only way they can get meaningful results. Fourth, the government agencies are likely to be further discouraged from funding research into ginseng because of the growing number of adverse effects being reported in the medical journals, including high blood pressure, morning diarrhoea, skin problems, sleeplessness, depression and loss of menstrual periods. It may be that these side-effects arise only in those taking large doses, but until there is reason to believe that ginseng might prove a potential public health menace there is little reason for a government health department to do anything more than support orthodox scientists who try to discourage the public from using it.

But ginseng is by no means the only doubtful "health food" that has been imported from overseas or revived from some ancient form of the healing arts. A remarkable number of far-reaching claims for vitamins and mineral supplements come from remote Swiss clinics. The sceptic may find it incredible that such a small country could support so many brilliant scientists working outside the mainstream scientific system. Similarly, the supposedly beneficial effects of yoghurt first reached this country from Bulgarian peasants who claimed to live to be nearly two hundred years old, thanks to the effects of yoghurt. This story was later disproved, but the legend lingers on. Claims made for vitamin and mineral supplements are often justified by reference to ancient scientific papers, which are now thought by most scientists to be wrong. A particular brand of sea salt carried, until recently, a medical testimonial to its properties – but that medical opinion was first published one hundred years ago.

Above all, the growth of the health food industry is aided by the gullibility of most health food enthusiasts and their failure to appreciate scientific method. In a recent edition of the health food newspaper *Health Now*, Barbara Cartland recommended a particular vitamin and mineral mix to childless couples. The evidence that she presented to justify this was that soon after she had recommended it to one childless couple, the wife had conceived. (It is impossible to say why she recommended it to them in the first place but, since it was composed of various vitamins and minerals known to have an effect on reproduction, the reason may have been based on theory.) No scientist would accept that as evidence, any more than he would accept that, if you correctly guessed once on which side a tossed coin would fall, this showed you had second sight. Hithertho childless couples do sometimes eventually conceive, and Barbara Cartland's young friends might well be one such example. To investigate the effect of her dietary supplement properly, a scientist would need to have evidence of its effects on more than one childless couple, and also evidence on what happened to couples who did not take the supplement. This is what scientists call a controlled trial, and in medical research such an approach is fundamental. But it is singularly lacking from the health food literature.

An example can be found in two books, *Healing and the Vitamin Factor* and *Addiction and the Vitamin Factor*. Their author, Vic Ramsey, is an enthusiastic proponent of a mixture of evangelical Christianity and health foods as a cure for a variety of illnesses and social problems. (In much the same way as the evangelical Dr John Kellogg originally promoted his cornflakes at the end of the last century.) He claims that incipient hypoglycaemia (low blood sugar) due to the consumption of a diet lacking in vitamins and minerals, is at the basis of much disease and makes people prey to drug addiction. But nowhere in these books does he quote any scientifically acceptable evidence to support his theory. It is all done by anecdotes, false arguments and rhetoric. Overall Mr Ramsey comes across as a very reasonable, deeply religious, humane man but he does not emerge as a scientist, and his undoubted sincerity is no more reason for letting him tinker with your body's chemistry than for letting him tinker with your car.

This is not a false analogy. After all someone who works on your car without any knowledge of what he is doing could damage it or could misdiagnose the fault so that you fail to take it to the garage until too late. The same risks apply to health foods. Though by and large they are probably harmless, they can lead to the consumer failing to seek medical attention for a real ailment. And some are not harmless at all. One recommendation for a vitamin mixture to alleviate childlessness includes high levels of vitamin A to be taken throughout pregnancy. Vitamin A in excess is what scientists call a teratogen, something that can lead to the development of deformed babies. Until recently the common health food "solution" to premenstrual tension included high doses of vitamin B_6 (pyridoxine). Following a flurry of cases of damage to the nervous system in such women due to the toxic effect of vitamin B_6, enthusiasm for this solution has declined.

Some people ask why, if there are so many potential problems with health foods and so many false claims, scientists do not investigate them. There is a variety of answers to this. First, the nature of the claims that are made often makes them difficult to investigate. A claim that a health food fills us with energy is difficult to pin down. A claim that a compound or particular diet protects against cancer would take decades to investigate. No one is willing to do it: after all if the claim is made without good reason, it is unreasonable to expect someone else to pay for the research needed to disprove it.

A few claims can be directly and easily investigated. For example, Professor Bender has reported that some vitamin mixtures labelled as "natural" contain particular chemical forms of certain vitamins that do not occur in nature and must therefore have come from the laboratory. A *Which?* report studied 20 samples of dried fruit from health and wholefood shops and found that nearly half of them had been treated with sulphur dioxide to preserve them but, illegally, did not say so on the label. According to the public analyst, a civil servant responsible for investigating food standards, many of the descriptions on health food products are misleading and are therefore breaking the law.

Nutritionists should be forgiven for taking the view that it is a waste of time to disprove even the easily investigated claims. For the health food lobby seems to have stock answers to such investigations. It frequently claims that scientists are in the pay of the conventional food industry or that they are part of a government conspiracy. Another argument is that science cannot investigate the more extravagant claims made because they are beyond the area that science can study. There may be a case for saying that scientists should be more open-minded about unorthodox or "alternative" forms of treatment. However, unless such claims are based on sound, reasoned arguments there will be few respected researchers who will take them seriously.

—CONCLUSIONS—

This review of the possibilities of toxic effects of food and food additives, coupled with a brief review of the health food industry's claim to provide many of the solutions to the problems of our modern diet, underlines two messages. First, that though there are glaring problems with our diet, they are not overwhelming us to the extent that discussion of them in the media might suggest. Improvements can and are being made, but only as fast as our science allows us to make them. If we want faster change we must be prepared to fund the research for finding scientific solutions to unresolved problems, or accept the risks that apparent improvements might not be what they seem.

Secondly, there are no wholly good nor any unequivocally bad guys in the food safety business. While the government, the scientists and the food industry can be complacent and lethargic, in need of constant prodding if improvement is to occur, the now flourishing health food industry is not a new voice of unparalleled honesty and beneficence but is at least as prone to suspect practices as the conventional food industry it seeks to replace.

PART III

FOOD
AND THE
FAMILY

ANNE HEUGHAN

CHAPTER 9

CHOOSING FOOD

Besides individual reasons for choosing food, many external influences control the supply and affect choice. In Part II we saw how exterior forces such as government policy, EEC regulations and the structure of the food industry affect our choice. But there are many other factors involved, including tradition, advertising, income and even religious and moral considerations.

One of the earliest influences on children's choice of food is, of course, their parents. At home choice is determined to a greater extent by what parents provide, even though their own preferences will decide whether or not they like what they are offered. Taste is frequently subject to change. For instance, many young children will not eat spicy food, yet they learn to like the taste, and even to prefer it, as they get older.

Peer group pressure is also extremely important in determining what a child chooses to eat, and adolescents may use food as a means of expressing conformity (with their friends) or rebellion (against their parents and teachers). Teenagers may eat lots of sugary food partly because they know their parents disapprove of their eating it, but also because their friends eat lots of sweets.

Food can also be a sign of friendship. Inviting people to a party and giving them food and drink is one of the conventional ways of creating new relationships. In these situations we may feel impelled to eat something, whether we are hungry or not, because it would be considered impolite to refuse hospitality. This can put those trying to diet under immense pressure, unless they can choose low-calorie food and drinks.

Income may affect both what is purchased and also the total amount spent on food. As a nation becomes more affluent, people spend more on animal protein and fatty foods, such as meat and cheese, and less on starchy, fibrous food. Western households on restricted incomes usually spend more on sugary foods and less on fruit and vegetables.

Most religions have rules connected with the symbolic role that food plays in religion. The banning of certain foods for religious reasons obviously restricts choice; strict Hindus, for instance, must be vegetarians. Even if you don't follow a particular religion you probably have strong moral feelings about food. For example some people deliberately buy free-range eggs instead of those from battery hens, and most people feel strongly about not wasting food.

Many vegetarians decide not to eat meat or fish partly because of taste preferences but also because they object to the killing of animals. Some are also concerned about the long-term effects of farming and the resulting damage to the balance of nature.

Occasionally people will decide not to eat a food from a particular country for political reasons. For example, for a short time French farmers were unpopular within the EEC and British housewives boycotted French produce. Such actions are unlikely to limit the variety of foods we eat because food is now available from so many countries, but it can occasionally make a food more expensive for a time.

Cultural influences also affect what we eat. Most British people have an aversion to eating horsemeat; yet it is perfectly acceptable in France. In countries such as India and China food is considered in terms of "hot" and "cold". This is not the temperature of the food but the effect it is supposed to have on the body. "Hot" foods are supposed to excite the emotions while "cold" foods are supposed to soothe the body and mind. During certain times of the year you are supposed to eat more or less of these different types of food.

Food is used to celebrate events from weddings and christenings to harvest festivals. The very word, festival, stems from feast, a celebration of food and drink. Certain foods associated with these events may be used to symbolize some part of the happening. For example, a christening cake is used to symbolize a birth; in Italy rice is showered over the bride to symbolize health and prosperity. Families try to buy the food that is traditionally eaten at these festivals, and because our ideas of special occasion foods are firmly fixed, it can be particularly difficult to get used to the idea of serving a "healthier" food for such occasions. Old customs die hard, and so items such as cream may be accepted by visitors even though they may not eat it in their own homes.

Advertising may be the key to making the first purchase of a new product or as a reminder about a forgotten product, and the food industry spends millions of pounds advertising and marketing foods. A food manufacturer will usually gear the advertising (and marketing) of a product to one particular age group, and then emphasize qualities such as taste, nutrition, health or fun that are most likely to appeal. Today advertisers increasingly stress qualities that are beneficial to health, but this can often confuse the customer. Labels and advertisements will frequently draw attention to certain qualities of a product, but they will underplay or even not mention others. Until pressure from dentists and dietitians forced them to change, companies marketing "health" drinks high in vitamin C failed to mention that their drinks also had a high sugar content. Other manufacturers emphasize that their foods are free from additives but fail to point out their high fat content. Over the next few years food labels, particularly the nutrition information on the labels, will almost certainly play a large part in influencing what food we buy but the labels need to provide simple nutritional information that can be interpreted

> *Until pressure from dentists and dietitians forced them to change, companies marketing "health" drinks high in vitamin C failed to mention that their drinks also had a high sugar content.*

by the consumer at a glance.

Finally, the choice of food will be affected by the time available to cook, by the cost of the food and by the availability of the food. Today it is certainly possible to buy virtually anything. But the everyday availability of foods is what matters so it is important that foods we use frequently are not too expensive.

—LEARNING TO CHANGE—

As described in Part I, the quality of the diet depends not so much on individual nutrients as on the overall balance of the foods eaten. The various reports on diet agree that it is largely made up of "excesses". Most of us eat far too much refined food, which contains little fibre, too much fat (particularly saturated fat), too much sugar and too much salt.

So, in light of this new nutritional information, how should we set about improving our diet and that of our family? The first point is that changes are likely to be most successful if they take place gradually. Some people can manage suddenly to turn over a new leaf, but most of us have to familiarize ourselves more slowly to new ideas. There is no single way to change a diet, as much depends on previous dietary habits. There is, unfortunately, no instant recipe for successful change. It demands forethought and planning, especially at first; it may mean stocking a few different foods, adapting recipes and even learning some new recipes.

Improving the diet means putting more emphasis on some foods and less on others. Unless a health problem requires you to avoid certain foods, there is no reason to give up any food you like – although you may have to eat it less frequently. Giving up completely, or too soon, may well discourage you from sticking to your new eating plan.

If you enjoy cooking, making changes may well be simpler because it is often easier to adapt your own recipes than to find acceptable alternative manufactured foods. Making a few small changes to your old recipes will need only a little thought in both the planning and cooking; try adding baked beans to shepherd's pie or using skimmed milk and low fat cheese in a cheese sauce. Eventually you will be able to revise your menus considerably; some of the old regulars may disappear as you find new, healthier favourites to take their place.

It may be necessary to introduce completely new foods or to use familiar foods more often. It is important, therefore, to keep some of these in the store cupboard. Cartons of longlife skimmed milk, tins of tomatoes, cans of kidney beans and chick peas, herbs and spices are all useful and, if you buy lean cuts of meat, fish and chicken, that will make it easier to adapt old recipes or try out new ones.

Food manufacturers and retailers are beginning to respond to public interest in healthy eating. Manufacturers are developing new products or highlighting the nutritional merits of those already in existence. Unfortunately, some manufacturers are concerned with only one particular issue, like adding bran to everything or stressing that items are free from artificial colours, flavourings and

Most of us eat far too much refined food, which contains little fibre, too much fat (particularly saturated fat), too much sugar and too much salt.

preservatives. Many of the new processed foods avoid one pitfall only to fall into another; a low fat dish may be extremely high in salt or a high fibre product such as those that are bran-supplemented may be short on the extra vitamins and minerals a wholefood contains. So when buying processed food it is advisable to look out for those points the manufacturer does *not* draw attention to.

——*HEALTHY EATING IN EVERYDAY LIFE*——

The following eight rules for healthy eating are designed to help you to introduce beneficial changes into your diet and to cut down on foods that are least desirable on health grounds. But it is one thing to know what the basic rules for healthy eating are and quite another to follow them on a permanent basis. So we will also look at each rule in turn and discuss the best ways of both introducing it and sticking to it!

RULE 1: EAT A VARIETY OF FOODS

Everyone, whatever age, should eat a variety of foods. Living off the same items day after day would be both boring and nutritionally undesirable. This means eating fish as well as meat, salads as well as cooked vegetables and fresh fruit as well as fruit juice. Eating a variety of foods is not a problem for most people, and if you like trying out different fruit and vegetables or experimenting with new recipes, your diet is probably already full of variety.

However there may be certain times when particular care needs to be taken that our diet doesn't become monotonous. For example, students moving away from home could end up eating such a diet because they have few cooking skills or because they are uncertain how much of their budget should be spent on food.

CHECKLIST
* Make sure to include some food from each of the groups listed on p. 231 at each meal, but try not to choose the same foods all the time.
* Learn to experiment with new foods or to cook one new dish each month.

RULE 2: INCREASE FIBRE INTAKE

It has been recommended that an adult's average daily fibre intake should be just over 1oz (30g). The precise amount will vary in proportion to the calorie intake. For example, a child consuming 1,400 kilocalories a day is unlikely to eat the same amount of fibre as a man consuming 2,700 kilocalories. Although changing to high fibre products should not be difficult, fibre intake is still low in the UK.

CHECKLIST
* Make sure that your diet includes a variety of fibre-containing foods such as green and salad vegetables, root vegetables, fresh fruit, cereals, nuts, pulses and wholegrain foods.
* Include some raw fruit and vegetables as they will not only ensure that your diet includes some of the vitamins and minerals that are easily destroyed by cooking but will also add extra interest and texture to a meal.
* Choose wholegrain products such as brown rice, wholemeal pasta, wholemeal bread and rolls and wholemeal breakfast cereals as often as possible.

* If you don't like products made with all wholemeal flour, use half white and half wholemeal flour in baking.
* Use more dried fruit and nuts, both to eat on their own as snacks or to add to food such as salads and breakfast cereals.
* Include more beans and pulses in your diet. In many meals you can replace some of the meat with beans. This is not only healthier but cheaper too. There are not enough high-fibre, ready-made dishes available and people are only slowly incorporating beans and pulses into their dishes. Baked beans, chilli con carne, lentil soup and chick peas are all acceptable, but beyond this many people seem reluctant to add more or do not know how to.
* Eat potatoes baked in their jackets. These are not only a valuable source of fibre but are a good source of vitamin C. If filled with sweetcorn, peppers or chilli beans there will be additional fibre rather than just the extra fat if butter or margarine were used.
* Don't sprinkle food with bran. Bran should be thought of like a vitamin pill – a temporary boost for times of need. It doesn't contain all the other nutrients supplied by wholegrain products such as wholemeal bread and wholemeal breakfast cereals and so does not transform a refined diet into a "healthy", whole one.

Adults, unless specified by their doctor, should try to have ten portions a day from the fibre chart below. Try to include a variety of fruit, vegetables, pulses and cereals. If some of the portions are too large, have half a portion and make the rest up with another half portion. Use the chart to work out approximately how many fibre portions you are eating already.

FIBRE CHART

The quantities below give approximate 3g fibre portions. Ten portions will provide 30g of fibre. The average amount of fibre eaten each day is approximately 20g.

Vegetables
375g (13oz) asparagus, boiled
125g (4½oz) aubergine
100g (3½oz) French beans, boiled
100g (3½oz) runner beans, boiled
75g (2¾oz) broad beans, boiled
60g (2oz) butter beans, boiled
40g (1½oz) haricot beans, boiled
40g (1½oz) baked beans
125g (4½oz) red kidney beans, boiled
100g (3½oz) beetroot, boiled
75g (2¾oz) broccoli, boiled
100g (3½oz) brussel sprouts, boiled
100g (3½oz) red or white cabbage, raw
125g (4½oz) savoy cabbage, boiled
100g (3½oz) carrots, raw or boiled
150g (5¼oz) cauliflower, raw or boiled
150g (5¼oz) celery, raw
75g (2¾oz) leeks, boiled

75g (2¾oz) split lentils, cooked
1 whole large lettuce
½ large marrow
125g (4½oz) mushrooms, raw
75g (2¾oz) mushrooms, cooked
225g (8oz) onions, raw
125g (4½oz) parsnips, boiled
30g (1oz) frozen peas, boiled
60g (2oz) split peas, boiled
50g (1¾oz) chick peas, cooked
300g (10½oz) raw green or red pepper
50g (1¾oz) plaintain, boiled or fried
300g (10½oz) potatoes, boiled
150g (5¼oz) potato baked in skin
100g (3½oz) chips
50g (1¾oz) spinach, boiled
100g (3½oz) swede, boiled
60g (2oz) sweetcorn, boiled
125g (4½oz) sweet potatoes, boiled
200g (7oz) tomatoes, raw
150g (5¼oz) turnips, boiled
75g (2¾oz) yam, boiled
Other salad vegetables, like radish, water-

cress or cucumber, all contain fibre but you would have to eat a large portion to account for 3g fibre.

Cereals
1 slice wholemeal bread
2 slices brown bread
4 slices white bread
½ wholemeal roll
2 white rolls
15g (½oz) All Bran
30g (1oz) Cornflakes
70g (2½oz) Rice Krispies
40g (1½oz) muesli
20g (¾oz) Puffed Wheat
1 Shredded Wheat
1 Weetabix
40g (1½oz) oatmeal
125g (4½oz) white rice
75g (2¾oz) brown rice
3 digestive biscuits
50g (1¾oz) wholemeal pasta
175g (6oz) pasta

Fruit
2 small eating apples
1 large baking apple
150g (5¼oz) apricots, raw
15g (½oz) dried apricots
175g (6oz) stewed apricots
1 medium banana
40g (1½oz) blackberries, raw or cooked

200g (7oz) cherries
30g (1oz) blackcurrants, raw
50g (1¾oz) blackcurrants, stewed
75g (2¾oz) damsons or plums, raw
100g (3½oz) damsons or plums, stewed
30g (1oz) dates, no stones
15g (½oz) dried figs
100g (3½oz) gooseberries, raw or stewed
300g (10½oz) grapes
300g (10½oz) grapefruit (approximately 1 whole)
50g (1¾oz) loganberries or raspberries
500g (1lb 1oz) melon, weighed with skin
2 nectarines or tangerines
200g (7oz) oranges (approximately 2 small)
200g (7oz) peaches (approximately 2)
175g (6oz) pears (approximately 2)
250g (8½oz) fresh pineapple
30g (1oz) prunes, dried
40g (1½oz) raisins, sultanas
150g (5¼oz) rhubarb, stewed
150g (5¼oz) strawberries

Nuts
20g (¾oz) almonds, without shells
50g (1¼oz) Brazil nuts, without shells
50g (1¾oz) chestnuts, weighed with or without shell
50g (1¾oz) hazelnuts, without shells
30g (1oz) coconut
40g (1½oz) peanuts, without shells
60g (2oz) walnuts, without shells

RULE 3: INCREASE CONSUMPTION OF COMPLEX CARBOHYDRATES

Many countries that have a lower incidence of heart disease and bowel cancer than the UK have a higher intake of complex carbohydrates. In addition most of these countries have a lower fat, particularly saturated fat, intake.

At present, most of us plan our meals by choosing the meat or the equivalent part of the meal first, but the emphasis needs to be shifted away from the meat and fish components to building upon a base of starchy staples, preferably high fibre foods like jacket potatoes, brown rice or wholemeal pasta. You may find it useful to adopt a different philosophy: select the cereal or staple first, then vegetables and finally the meat or fish.

> ❛
> *The consumption of bread and cereals has been declining since the beginning of the century, and the tradition of serving bread with meals, so that those who are still hungry could fill up on bread, has been discontinued in many families.*
> ❜

The consumption of bread and cereals has been declining since the beginning of the century, and the tradition of serving bread with meals, so that those who are still hungry could fill up on bread, has been discontinued in many families. Perhaps this idea should be reinstated and we should eat the bread, as they do in many parts of the Continent, without butter or margarine.

> *It is the butter on the bread and the oil in the chips that provide the bulk of the calories and thus make such foods "fattening".*

CHECKLIST

* If you are eating more fibre-rich food, you will probably already be eating more complex carbohydrates. Make sure that you eat plenty of bread, particularly wholemeal, although you should not neglect white bread, pasta, rice or breakfast cereals if you don't like the wholegrain alternatives.
* Plan meals around the bulky staples like potatoes or rice and not around meat, fish, etc.
* Cut bread slices thicker and try to eat bread with meals without any butter or margarine. Take care not to increase your fat and calorie intake substantially simply by eating more bread and butter.
* Eat plenty of potatoes, either boiled or baked in their skins. If chips are a favourite, choose thick-cut oven varieties in order to reduce the proportion of fat, and do not eat them too often.
* If, in addition to improving your diet, you want to lose weight, you should increase the proportion – if not the actual quantity – of complex carbohydrates in your diet. Pasta or rice or pizza can be low fat, moderate calorie but reasonably bulky dishes. Including more complex carbohydrates in the diet is an alien concept. For years, we have been told that bread, potatoes and pasta are fattening. However it is the butter on the bread and the oil in the chips that provide the bulk of the calories and thus make such foods "fattening".

RULE 4: DECREASE FAT INTAKE, PARTICULARLY SATURATED FAT

At present fat accounts for about 40 per cent of energy. It has been recommended that in the UK 31-35 per cent of the calories consumed should come from fat, of which no more than 15 per cent should be from saturated fat. Other reports from other parts of the world have recommended that 10 per cent should come from polyunsaturated fatty acids.

CHECKLIST

* Try to grill food rather than fry it.
* Use a non-stick fry pan to brown meat and fish. This way you can use less fat but still capture the flavour.
* Use more low fat foods such as white fish, natural yoghurt, skimmed or semi-skimmed milk, pulses, lean meat, poultry and lower fat cheeses such as Brie, Edam and cottage cheese.
* Cut down on foods high in fat such as pastries, pies, sausages, fried foods, fatty meats like salami and fatty types of mince, cream, hard and cream cheeses, butter, coffee whiteners, hard margarine, full fat milk and ice cream.
* Use a small amount of polyunsaturated oil and margarine in cooking rather than saturated fats such as butter, lard and hard margarines.
* Use low fat spreads – but avoid the trap of spreading them twice as thickly.

❝

It has recently been proposed that all food purchased that contains more than 0.5 per cent fat should have to label and quantify the fat content. Such a move would help consumers to eat less fat, but it would still leave them in the dark about the fibre, sugar and salt content of the product.

❞

* Make casseroles or stews a day in advance and leave them to cool so that you can skim off any extra fat.
* If you do want to eat cakes and biscuits, make your own and use less fat or add more flour and extra ingredients like dried fruit.
* Try using natural yoghurt instead of cream. Full fat yoghurt may have a more acceptable taste than low fat yoghurt as a topping for desserts. Low fat yoghurt can be used to lighten mayonnaise or, when thinned, as a salad dressing in its own right.
* Buy low fat products such as low fat cheese and low fat sausages.
* Buy low fat, non-oily dressings for salads. Salad dressings can be a real fat and calorie trap.
* Look at the table below to see which foods are high in fat. Reducing fat consumption is one of the most difficult changes to make to the diet, partly because much of the fat eaten is invisible and so it is difficult to check how much you are having, and partly because the effects are not as immediate as, say, increasing fibre intake. Most people can usually manage to make a few alterations, like using skimmed or semi-skimmed milk, but find it harder to use less fat in cooking. This is partly because cooking methods have to be changed in order to use less fat. For example, browning foods, such as onions, may have to be done slowly in the minimum of fat. It can be hard to discard old recipes that are easy to prepare, but new recipes can become just as easy with practice, although they may need a bit of thinking about at the beginning.

How Much Fat?

It has recently been proposed that all food purchased that contains more than 0.5 per cent fat should have to label and quantify the fat content. Such a move would help consumers to eat less fat, but it would still leave them in the dark about the fibre, sugar, salt and saturated fat content of the product. Adults should not eat more than about 2¾oz (80g) of fat per 2,200 kilocalories (the average adult calorie requirement) a day. They may need to eat more or less, depending on their calorie intake. The chart below shows approximate 10g fat portions so that you can work out how much fat you are eating.

Food	Fat	Saturated Fat	Food	Fat	Saturated Fat
	grams	*grams*		*grams*	*grams*
275ml (½ pint) whole milk	10	5.9	15g (½oz) butter	10	5.9
1 litre (1¾ pints) skimmed milk	10	0.4	15g (½oz) polyunsaturate margarine	10	2.3
35ml (2tbsp) single cream	10	7.1	10g (⅓oz) lard	10	4.2
18ml (1tbsp) double cream	10	6.0	10g (⅓oz) sunflower oil	10	1.3
			30g (1oz) low fat spread	10	2.7

Food	Fat	Saturated Fat	Food	Fat	Saturated Fat
	grams	grams		grams	grams
30g (1oz) Cheddar cheese	10	5.8	100g (3½oz) eggs (2 small)	10	3.1
2.4kg (5lb 8oz) cottage cheese	10	NA but low	200g (7oz) roast potatoes	10	*
200g (7oz) lean ham	10	4.0	100g (3½oz) chips	10	*
60g (2oz) raw mince	10	4.2	30g (1oz) crisps (1 packet)	10	*
175g (6oz) grilled rump steak	10	4.2	20g (¾oz) peanuts	10	1.8
150g (5¼oz) roast leg pork (lean meat only)	10	3.9	150g (5¼oz) ice cream	10	3.8
125g (4½oz) roast leg lamb	10	4.9	45g (1½oz) sweet biscuits	10	5.2
75g (2¾oz) grilled liver	10	2.3*	40g (1½oz) Victoria sandwich (no icing)	10	3.7*
60g (2oz) grilled beefburger	10	4.1*	600g (20oz) white bread (20 slices)	10	2.3
40g (1½oz) grilled pork sausages	10	7.0	310g (11oz) wholemeal bread (11 slices)	10	1.7
40g (1½oz) pork pie (one quarter of an individual pie)	10	4.0	45g (1½oz) avocado pear	10	1.1
40g (1½oz) liver sausage	10	3.1	15g (½oz) mayonnaise or French dressing	10	*
50g (1¾oz) Cornish pasty	10	*	35g (1¼oz) chocolate	10	5.8
200g (7oz) roast chicken (no skin)	10	3.3	45g (1½oz) chocolate éclair	10	5.2
1kg (2lb 3oz) low fat yoghurt	10	0.2	65g (2oz) doughnut	10	*
850g (1.9lb) baked cod	10	1.7	30g (1oz) shortcrust pastry	10	*
100g (3½oz) fried fish	10	*	125g (4½oz) fruit pie with pastry top	10	*
75g (2¾oz) sardines	10	1.9			

*Indicates that the saturated fat content will depend on the type of fat used in cooking.

RULE 5: DECREASE CONSUMPTION OF SUGARY FOODS AND DRINKS

It has been recommended that the consumption of sugary foods and drinks in the UK should be cut by as much as 50 per cent. We know that frequent intakes of sugary foods and drinks cause dental caries, particularly in children.

CHECKLIST

* Identify the main sources of sugar in your diet and try to cut these down. The major sources of sugars, for most people, are the sugar added to hot drinks, soft drinks, sweets and biscuits.

* Only have sweets as an occasional treat. If you are given boxes of sweets or biscuits, don't undo the wrapping but keep them for bring and buy or jumble sales.

* Have fruit for pudding instead of sugary desserts. Fruit purées and fruit fools made with natural yoghurt or quark or unsweetened custard can make a pleasant alternative if you don't like raw fruit.

* Use a sweetener instead of sugar in hot drinks or try having them unsweetened. It will probably take a month to grow accustomed to the change.

* Home made cakes and biscuits can be made with wholemeal flour using less sugar and fat. Cakes can be eaten plain or with fruit or fruit purées instead of icing.

Children are often least keen to reduce their sugar consumption, so it is important not to put sweets and biscuits in lunch boxes and to keep them out of sight at home.

If you must eat sweet biscuits, choose high fibre varieties like digestives and muesli-type biscuits. Alternatively, choose crackers, bread sticks or wholemeal bread. If biscuits are eaten only because they are in the house, try to stop buying them.

* Squashes and fizzy drinks can account for a high proportion of the sugar in many diets. Try to have diluted fresh fruit juice or low calorie drinks instead. Diluted with sparkling mineral water fresh fruit juice makes a refreshing drink.

* Read food labels and watch out for words such as glucose, fructose, honey, sucrose, dextrose, brown sugar, corn syrup, etc. – as these all mean sugar in some shape or form.

* Choose a low sugar or sugar-free breakfast cereal such as muesli, porridge, wheat biscuits, Puffed Wheat or Shredded Wheat.

* Don't use sweets as a reward or bribe for children. If a word of praise won't suffice, give them little gifts, such as pencils or stickers. If they do have sweets, for the sake of their teeth they should be encouraged to eat them all at one time rather than in small quantities every now and then.

* Choose canned fruit in natural juice rather than sweetened syrup.

* Use "low sugar" products, but be careful as some of these include other sugars instead; remember to read the label.

* Look at the table on page 24.

Just as those who stop taking sugar in their tea and coffee wonder how they ever used to drink them with sugar, so those who reduce their sugar intake eventually prefer foods that are less sweet. However, it is not uncommon to go through a stage of compensating for cutting out puddings by eating chocolate instead!

Besides cutting down on your sugar intake, it is also important to eat foods containing sugar less frequently. Children are often least keen to reduce their sugar consumption, so it is important not to put sweets and biscuits in lunch boxes and to keep them out of sight at home. Tell them they can help themselves to fresh fruit juice, fruit, vegetables, bread, cheese crackers, nuts and dried fruit, and to the occasional diet drink but not the biscuit tin.

RULE 6: DECREASE CONSUMPTION OF SODIUM

We eat approximately 10 grams of salt a day. We should try to reduce this to about 5 grams. Although the link between sodium and high blood pressure is by no means conclusive, as nobody knows how to identify those who are sensitive to excessive sodium, it would certainly do no harm to avoid consuming too much sodium or salt.

Many people don't find it too difficult to reduce their salt intake, although it can take between 2 and 3 months to get used to low salt food. But, as 70-85 per cent of the salt eaten comes from processed foods, much of the responsibility for reducing salt levels lies with the food manufacturers. Salt confers a number of technological advantages in some processed foods and cannot, therefore, always be removed. However some low salt alternatives are available, but if all manufacturers reduced the salt level by only a small amount this would nonetheless help to reduce the over-all salt level in our diet.

CHECKLIST
* Always taste your food before you add salt.
* Be careful how much salt you add to cooking, and try to add herbs or spices instead.
* Sea salt is no healthier than ordinary salt, but if grinding salt helps you to use less then it may be an advantage. Compare how much you grate, shake or spoon on to an empty plate.
* Look out for low salt varieties of products.
* Replacing salt with salt substitutes is of doubtful benefit.
* Go easy on processed and fast foods as they are usually high in salt.
* Cut down on salty snacks such as crisps and salted nuts.
* The following foods are high in salt: cheese, bacon, ham, tinned and packet soups, snacks such as crisps, salted peanuts, smoked meat and fish, baking powder, tinned fish, foods that contain mono-sodium glutamate (MSG) or saccharin, soda water and yeast extracts.
* Eat plenty of fresh fruit and vegetables.
* Look at the table below.

SALT CHART

The quantities below give approximately 250mg sodium:

70g (2½oz) self-raising flour
50g (1¾oz) tinned spaghetti
45g (1½oz) brown, white or wholemeal bread (1½ slices)
15g (½oz) All Bran
20g (¾oz) Cornflakes or Rice Krispies
140g (5oz) muesli
65g (2¼oz) Puffed Wheat-type cereal or instant porridge
70g (2½oz) Weetabix-type cereal
40g (1½oz) cream crackers
110g (4oz) rye crispbread
60g (2oz) digestive biscuits
75g (2¾oz) ginger nuts
20g (¾oz) oatcakes
50g (1¾oz) water biscuits
70g (2½oz) Victoria sandwich cake
50g (1¾oz) rock cakes
65g (2¼oz) Madeira cake
100g (3½oz) fancy iced cakes
120g (4¼oz) rich fruit cake
425g (15oz) doughnuts
110g (4oz) jam tarts
75g (2½oz) mince pies
30g (1oz) scones
60g (2oz) Scotch pancakes

100g (3½oz) custard tart
120g (4¼oz) individual fruit pie
125g (4½oz) lemon meringue pie
70g (2½oz) treacle tart
40g (1½oz) Yorkshire pudding
0.4 litre (¾ pint milk
30g (1oz) margarine, except low salt varieties
30g (1oz) butter, except low salt varieties
20g (¾oz) Camembert, Danish blue cheese
40g (1½oz) Cheddar cheese
25g (1oz) Edam cheese
50g (1¾oz) cottage cheese
75g (2¾oz) pizza
25g (1oz) Welsh rarebit
10g (⅓oz) gammon, grilled
20g (¾oz) gammon, boiled
10g (⅓oz) bacon, grilled
70g (2½oz) stewed mince
25g (1oz) silverside
70g (2½oz) stewed steak
130g (4½oz) lamb's liver, grilled
90g (3¼oz) lamb's kidney, grilled
350g (12½oz) stewed oxtail, weighed with bones
25g (1oz) pork sausages, grilled
15g (½oz) salami
30g (1oz) liver sausage

20g (¾oz) black pudding, grilled
25g (1oz) ham
25g (1oz) tongue
30g (1oz) beefburger, fried
45g (1½oz) Cornish pasty or sausage roll
35g (1¼oz) pork pie
50g (1¾oz) individual steak and kidney pie
60g (2oz) salt cod, boiled
20g (¾oz) smoked haddock, poached
35g (1¼oz) bloater, grilled
70g (2½oz) pilchards, canned in tomato sauce
45g (1½oz) kipper, grilled
45g (1½oz) salmon, tinned
15g (½oz) smoked salmon
40g (1½oz) sardines, canned
60g (2oz) tuna, canned
70g (2½oz) crab
40g (1½oz) prawns in their shells
15g (½oz) prawns, peeled
7g (¼oz) cockles
90g (3¼oz) scallops
120g (4¼oz) mussels, boiled
50g (1¾oz) fish cakes, grilled
70g (2½oz) fishfingers, grilled
40g (1½oz) fish paste
50g (1¾oz) baked beans, canned in tomato sauce
90g (3¼oz) tinned carrots
110g (4oz) garden peas, tinned
95g (3¼oz) potatoes, tinned

95g (3¼oz) instant mashed potato, made up
45g (1½oz) crisps
80g (2¾oz) sweetcorn, tinned
10g (⅓oz) olives in brine
55g (1¾oz) peanuts, roasted and salted
70g (2½oz) peanut butter
95g (3¼oz) golden syrup
80g (2¾oz) toffees
25g (1oz) cocoa powder
100g (3½oz) drinking chocolate
70g (2½oz) malted milk drink
110g (4oz) tomato juice, tinned
50g (1¾oz) bread sauce
25g (1oz) brown sauce
55g (1¾oz) cheese sauce
25g (1oz) French dressing
70g (2½oz) mayonnaise
55g (1¾oz) onion sauce
20g (¾oz) piccalilli
30g (1oz) salad cream
20g (¾oz) tomato ketchup
55g (1¾oz) cream of tomato soup, canned
55g (1¾oz) cream of chicken soup, canned
60g (2oz) minestrone soup
60g (2oz) oxtail soup
2g (0.07oz) baking powder
5g (0.2oz) yeast extract
50g (1¾oz) curry powder
2.5g (0.09oz) stock cube
0.65g (0.02oz) salt

RULE 7: DRINK ONLY MODERATE AMOUNTS OF ALCOHOL

Excessive alcohol consumption has many detrimental effects on health. Those who drink little will not need to change, but probably everyone should rethink their attitude to offering alcohol to other people at social or business occasions.

CHECKLIST

* To keep within a safe limit, men should not drink more than 21 units a week. Women should not drink more than 14 units a week (see page 22).

* To help keep alcohol intake to a moderate amount, more non-alcoholic drinks, such as fruit juice, diet drinks or sparkling water can be drunk, or make your alcoholic drink into a long drink by adding any of the above.

* Don't use alcohol to help yourself relax – you are likely to drink more than you mean to.

* Offer non-alcoholic drinks to guests, not just orange and tomato juice. See the list below for some more interesting suggestions.

Low Alcohol and Alcohol-free Drinks:
Spritzer (white wine and mineral water)

Buck's fizz (sparkling white wine or champagne and orange juice)
Dry sherry mixed with lots of orange juice
Mulled wine
Dubonnet with lots of mineral water
Low-alcohol wine and lagers
Non-alcoholic punch
Mineral water with a slice of lime
Mineral water with fresh fruit juice
Mixer drinks like tonic water and ginger ale
Fresh fruit juices

RULE 8: MAINTAIN IDEAL BODY WEIGHT

If you keep to the other seven rules for healthy eating and take plenty of exercise, you should have little difficulty in reaching a healthy body weight (see the table on pages 74-5), but for further advice see Chapter 12.

When deciding to change eating habits and trying to follow these rules, the first step should be to analyse the quantities and types of food that you and your family eat. Eventually, like learning any new skill, this will become second nature and the analytical stage can be speeded up. For example, if you are planning to serve chilli con carne and brown rice you should ask yourself the following questions:

1. How much brown rice should I cook? This is partly determined by appetite but with the emphasis on eating complex carbohydrates (rule 3) the quantity will probably be larger than you would expect.
2. What type of fat and how much, if any, will I use?
3. What ratio of beans to meat should I cook?
4. How lean is the meat?
5. How much seasoning will I add?

—FOUR-STAGE PLAN FOR HEALTHY EATING—

Outlined here is a four-stage plan designed to help you on your way to healthy eating. Do not try to complete all the steps in each stage at once, but try to introduce a few changes every one or two weeks, or over a longer period if necessary, before going on to the next stage. If you decide to cut down on an item – sugary snacks for example – compensate by eating more of a healthy item such as fresh fruit. This way you will be eating more healthily but you won't feel you are missing out!

When you start to change your diet you may encounter one or two common pitfalls. Because you are cutting down on many items it is important to learn to cook and eat more of the bulkier foods such as rice, bread, potatoes and pasta. This will

> *Do not try to complete all the steps in each stage at once, but try to introduce a few changes every one or two weeks, or over a longer period if necessary, before going on to the next stage.*

ensure that you don't feel really hungry and end up eating snacks of unhealthy foods. It is also important not to cut down too drastically or you may again end up starving and eating unhealthy foods to satisfy your hunger. When you start to experiment with new recipes, don't be disheartened if they are not all a success.

You may find it helpful to make a list of all the changes that can be made to your diet. Tick off those you have already made and mark those that you are going to try next. As your list fills with ticks – but be honest and rub out those that you are not keeping to – you will feel encouraged.

Stage 1
* Grill food whenever possible.
* Replace white or brown bread with wholemeal bread.
* Cut out sugar in tea and coffee.
* Choose diet drinks or fresh fruit juice instead of sugary drinks.
* Use semi-skimmed or skimmed milk instead of whole milk, and yoghurt instead of cream.
* Use oils and spreads rich in polyunsaturates.
* Choose lean meat, poultry and fish.

Stage 2
* Start to cut down on the overall amount of fat you use in cooking. Browning vegetables and meats in a non-stick pan is a useful way of drawing out some of the fat in the meat and of changing the flavour of the vegetables without allowing them to absorb unnecessary fat.
* Replace rice, pasta and breakfast cereals with the wholemeal varieties. Use recipes in which rice, pasta or potatoes are the basis of a dish – for example, kedgeree, paella, risotto, stuffed baked potatoes and spaghetti bolognese.
* Cut down on between-meal sugary snacks like cakes, biscuits and sweets, and choose fresh fruit or bread instead. If you are really hungry eat a sandwich.
* Increase your consumption of fruit and vegetables. Try to have at least four pieces of fruit a day, including one citrus fruit; and four servings of vegetables a day, including one green vegetable, one yellow or red vegetable such as swede, carrots or tomatoes, and some salad.

Stage 3
* Eat more beans and pulses such as lentils, kidney beans, chick peas and haricot beans.
* Cut down on the amount of fatty meats, particularly processed meats such as pâté, salami, sausages and hamburgers.
* Cut down on between-meal salty, fatty snacks such as cheese, peanuts and crisps.
* Try to cut down on the amount of salt added to food, use more herbs and spices instead.

Stage 4
* Increase the quantity of high fibre foods that you consume, such as wholemeal bread, breakfast cereals and wholemeal products.
* Cut down on the amount of fatty cheeses consumed, choosing instead the low fat or medium fat varieties whenever possible, such as Brie, Camembert, cottage cheese, ricotta and Edam.

* Make sure that portions of meat and fish are not too large.
* Try to keep within the recommended limit when consuming alcohol.

——PLANNING MEALS——

The idea of eating three meals a day is a thing of the past. Unless you are entertaining, meals today are usually quick and easy. Whether this has brought about the increase in the amount of convenience foods and takeaways that we consume, or whether it is their existence that has encouraged the trend away from the traditional three meals is debatable.

There are many things to bear in mind when planning a meal. It's not only a question of the likes and dislikes of the members of the family. Meal planning may be determined by which foods you have in stock, whether you want to go to the shops, how much money you want to spend, how much time you want to spend in the kitchen and the type of kitchen equipment you possess.

The principles of planning a healthy meal or snack have been outlined in the rules for healthy eating (see pages 180-9). But in addition to the nutritional aspect of the meal, the aesthetic qualities should be considered. Colour, texture and flavour all help to make food enjoyable.

Colour is important and variety of colour will often make meals seem more attractive. Many meals can be improved by an interesting combination of colours. Fruit and vegetables, with their enormous range of colours, do the most to make a meal look colourful, but not all the impact has to be created by the food – it can also come from the plates and dishes used and the general presentation of the food.

Texture, whether it is chewy, crunchy, smooth, juicy or soft, is also important. Part of the trend towards eating high fibre foods is associated with the difference in texture between refined and unrefined foods. Many highly refined foods have very little texture and are bland to eat. Unrefined foods often have more texture and need more chewing. Fruit and vegetables, particularly when uncooked, come into their own when you are introducing a crunchy or juicy texture into the diet.

Flavour is the hardest quality to explain, and we know far less about it. We recognize the flavours we like and those we dislike, but why one person has a strong desire for one flavour over another is unknown. Smell is also important in determining the more subtle flavours of food.

TIMING OF MEALS AND SNACKS

The pattern of eating is a matter of habit, largely determined by the structure of each individual's day. Even those who are on nightshift have their own times of eating, perhaps having two meals on some shifts and three on others. Those who work odd shifts, like airline staff, often find it difficult to know when to eat. They usually try to stick to eating at regular intervals of 5 or 6 hours. The trend now is to eat all day long, and meals seem to fit around snacks, rather than the other way around. The main disadvantage of this is that we are more likely to eat too much fatty, sugary and low fibre foods, but if we can avoid this there is no reason to stick to the convention of three meals a day.

There are certainly no hard and fast rules for individuals about when to eat or even how much to eat. Diabetics may require snacks at certain times of the day to make sure that their blood sugar doesn't get too low. Other people, such as children and the elderly, may not be able to consume large quantities of food at one meal and need snacks to boost their calorie and nutrient intake. The individual variation between sizes of meal is as different as the number of different sized individuals.

Meals should fit our lifestyle, rather than the other way around, and if a person's lifestyle changes – perhaps because of a change in job or the arrival of a baby – what is provided as meals will be adapted accordingly.

Many families today own a freezer, and this provides an excellent opportunity to cook extra quantities of certain foods as useful standbys. Here are some ideas for foods that can be made in bulk and used twice in one week for different meals.

Tomato sauce can be used to help make a variety of dishes – such as pizza, bolognese sauce, tuna or white fish cooked in tomato sauce, chilli con carne, vegetables in tomato sauce – or it can be used as a basis for paprika sauce. To reheat tomato sauce on its own, place it in a microwave oven and reheat for 5 minutes on high (600 W) or simmer for 30 minutes.

Rice or pasta can be cooked when you are preparing a meal and the extra portion can be used for another meal. Rice and pasta can be made into salads or they can be reheated in a microwave oven, by simmering in a bowl or sieve over boiling water or in the oven in a casserole dish (cook for 30 minutes with some extra stock or water).

Vegetables such as green beans and peas can be cooked and later used for a salad.

Bread dough can be used to make a pizza or bread sausage rolls.

Grated low fat cheese is often acceptable in cooking and can be used on pizzas, in sandwiches, in sauces or in any topping that requires cheese.

Casseroles can be used later or frozen till required. Reheat as for the tomato sauce.

Beans and pulses can be used in a salad, puréed into a dip or used in a dish such as lentil bake.

Those who have a freezer will be well aware of their advantages. Everyone uses their freezer in slightly different ways but here are some suggestions for healthy foods to stock:

Meat such as lean mince or cubed, sliced fillets of meat; poultry such as turkey; chicken joints; liver and kidney
Fish such as cod, halibut or plaice fillets; trout; prawns; and fish steaks
Wholemeal bread, pitta bread, rolls and teacakes
Grated cheese
Fruit
Fruit juices
Vegetables
Cooked pulses
Ready-prepared dishes
Ready-prepared sauces
Herbs
Nut bakes, lentil roasts, etc
Fresh coffee beans

For those who have a microwave oven it is possible to prepare a meal from the freezer in minutes, and this allows great flexibility in eating habits.

DRINKING BETWEEN MEALS

The main rule is to avoid sugary drinks such as sugared tea, coffee, squash or any other drink containing sugar. As we saw on page 25, it is the frequency of sugar consumption that causes dental caries, so it is important to cut down on the number of occasions that sugary foods and drinks are eaten or drunk. It is better to use skimmed or semi-skimmed milk rather than whole milk or coffee whiteners as these are high in saturated fats. Alcohol should only be consumed within reason as outlined on page 20.

If you have a poor appetite, you may find it helpful to drink after a meal rather than before or with a meal. However, when you don't feel hungry but do need to eat, try to choose a milky drink, or lentil, minestrone or dried pea soup, or soup made with milk. Many other soups, although providing a comforting warmth, have little nourishment, compared with, say, a sandwich.

BREAKFAST

Breakfast has often been described by nutritionists as the most important meal of the day. However, research into its importance suggests conflicting conclusions.

Breakfast certainly seems to be important if you look at the derivation of the word: "to break the fast". There may be as much as 12 hours between the evening meal and breakfast. Some studies have concluded that missing breakfast leads to a loss of concentration and impaired performance during the morning. Steel workers and lorry drivers who didn't eat breakfast were found to be more accident-prone, and children who were reported to be apathetic, disruptive or unable to concentrate by their teachers were more likely to be those who have had no breakfast. A recent study of American children revealed that those who ate breakfast, particularly when cereals were included, managed to achieve a more nutrient-dense diet. They were less likely to be deficient in B vitamins and in iron, and yet their diet was lower in fat.

But other studies have contradicted these findings and suggested that going without breakfast does not affect a person's performance. One study showed that missing breakfast occasionally is much more of a problem than going without it regularly. They surmised that the ill-effects were caused when normal routines were disturbed. Therefore breakfast may be a psychological boost rather than a nutritional need.

However, those who go without breakfast may eat snacks that are high in fat and sugar and low in fibre such as chocolate, crisps and Danish pastries. People who are dieting often make the mistake of not having breakfast in an attempt to save on calories, but then wonder why they get hungry mid-morning. It makes more sense to start the day with a high fibre and low fat breakfast than to end up eating an unhealthy snack later. Conversely, if you don't feel like eating breakfast, plan to have a snack – like a sandwich or a piece of fruit – for mid-morning.

Many people no longer eat a cooked breakfast, in fact the trend has been towards the quick and simple breakfasts that consist of fruit juice, toast, breakfast cereal, tea or coffee. The nutritional benefits of this type of breakfast will

Breakfast may be a psychological boost rather than a nutritional need.

depend on the type of bread, type of milk and amount of fat spread on the toast. If these are well chosen, the meal can resemble the sort recommended by nutritionists – high fibre, low fat, low sugar and low in salt.

This change in the type of breakfast that is preferred now is one of the best things that has happened to our health as can be seen from the figures below:

Traditional Breakfast	kcals	Protein (grams)	Fat (grams)	Fibre (grams)
2 fried rashers back bacon	233	12.5	20.3	-
1 fried egg	116	7.3	5.9	-
2 fried halves tomato	7	0.5	3.0	1.5
2 rounds of toast (white)	140	4.7	1.0	1.6
Butter	74	-	8.2	-
Marmalade	26	—	—	—
TOTAL	596	25.0	38.4	3.1

Modern Breakfast				
Glass of fresh orange juice	50	0.6	—	—
1 bowl of bran flakes	106	3.6	0.4	5.3
¼ pint (150ml) semi-skimmed milk	75	5.2	2.4	-
2 slices wholemeal toast	130	5.2	1.6	5.1
Polyunsaturate margarine	74	—	8.0	—
Marmalade	26	—	—	—
TOTAL	461	14.6	12.4	10.4

The traditional breakfast provides 58 per cent of energy as fat whereas today's breakfast provides only 24 per cent of energy as fat. One government report has recommended that we reduce fat intake to 35 per cent of total energy, so the modern breakfast is certainly healthier. This breakfast also substantially increases the fibre content of the diet. As most of us in the West eat more protein than we require, it is extremely unlikely that the reduction in protein in the modern breakfast will cause any harm.

However, by reducing the intake of fat you often reduce the intake of calories. If you continued to consume fewer calories over a period of time you would probably lose weight. This would be fine if you wanted to lose weight, but otherwise you would need to increase your energy intake by eating more fibre-rich food such as wholemeal bread, rice, pasta and cereals.

One way to increase fibre intake or the quantity of food without increasing fat consumption is to cut thicker slices of bread. For this reason it is best to buy uncut or thick-sliced loaves. Wholemeal bread has a higher fat content than white bread, but this difference is trivial compared with the amount of fat often spread on a slice of bread. The extra fat in wholemeal bread is from the wheat germ part of the wheat grain, which also contains other valuable vitamins and minerals, including vitamin E and riboflavin.

Having fruit juice or fresh fruit for breakfast is a recent trend that is certainly welcome, particularly for those who are not fond of eating citrus fruit, as it will help ensure that enough vitamin C is taken.

In addition to the nutritional benefits of this type of breakfast, it is also more convenient to prepare. Mornings in most households can be chaotic times, and many people skip breakfast altogether because they feel they haven't got time or it's too early. Women who have to get ready for work or to take the children to school often do not have time to prepare breakfast for the rest of the family. Therefore breakfast has become an individual meal, both in terms of what is eaten and where it is eaten. But although there may not be much time to sit down, most of us could manage to have a glass of fresh fruit juice and a bowl of high fibre breakfast cereal or a piece of wholemeal toast.

A traditional cooked breakfast may still be cooked at weekends, and eating this type of breakfast once a week isn't going to do any harm, although foods such as bacon and sausages should be grilled rather than fried.

Teenagers often say that the idea of eating breakfast makes them feel sick, a statement that is extremely difficult to counter. However, you can encourage them to take a healthy snack to school to have at breaktime.

Today's standard breakfast of cereal and toast is fairly nutritious – and is even better if wholegrain cereal and wholemeal toast are eaten and if fat and sugar are used sparingly. Here are some suggestions for alternative breakfast menus:

Toast
> Wholemeal toast and peanut butter
> Wholemeal muffin and citrus spread such as lemon curd (made with low fat cheese, lemon juice and minimal sugar)
> Wholemeal bread and a slice of lean ham
> Wholemeal bread and cottage cheese and reduced sugar jam
> Wholemeal bread and small amount of low fat or medium fat cheese
> Wholemeal toast with mashed banana.

Cereals
> Porridge with chopped banana and semi-skimmed milk
> Dried fruit compôte, unsweetened muesli and semi-skimmed milk
> 1 bowl of unsweetened muesli and semi-skimmed milk
> 2 Shredded Wheat or Weetabix, chopped apple, raisins, walnuts and skimmed milk
> 1 bowl of Bran Flakes and semi-skimmed milk
> 1 bowl of jumbo porridge oats and skimmed milk.
> (In these suggestions sugar has been replaced with fruit as it provides vitamins and minerals as well as sweetness. However you can of course eat the fruit separately if you prefer.)

Cooked breakfasts
> Wholemeal toast with grilled mushrooms and poached egg
> Baked beans and egg pancake with wholemeal bread
> Wholemeal toast with grilled tomatoes and lean grilled bacon
> Boiled egg and wholemeal toast.

Late breakfasts
> Wholemeal and raisin muffin with a scraping of polyunsaturate margarine
> Low fat yoghurt with dried apricots
> Wholemeal teacake with low fat soft cheese
> 1 wholemeal scone with raisins and minimal sugar with a scraping of polyunsat-

'

*Today's family is changing not only
the food it eats but also the type of
life it leads, and even the traditional
Sunday lunch is disappearing.*

,

urate margarine

Sandwiches with either lean ham, medium fat cheese or boiled egg.

THE MIDDAY MEAL

Lunch, like breakfast is becoming less important. There is a tendency in many families, except perhaps those in which the mother or father works in the evening or in which there are young children, to let the evening meal be the main one of the day, although at weekends, lunch, particularly Sunday lunch, may resume its importance. But today's family is changing not only the food it eats but also the type of life it leads, and even the traditional Sunday lunch is disappearing.

As more people eat a cooked meal in the evening and have a quick snack for lunch, some concern has been expressed about whether a snack lunch is as healthy as a cooked meal. In fact, if you apply the principles of healthy eating, a snack lunch can be just as nutritious, as shown in the examples below:

TWO DIFFERENT TYPES OF MIDDAY MEAL

Cooked lunch	Kcals	Protein grams	Fat grams	Fibre grams
Roast chicken	148	24.8	5.4	—
Jacket potato	150	3.7	0.2	3.5
Carrots, boiled	14	0.5	Tr*	2.3
Green beans, boiled	7	0.8	Tr*	3.2
Gravy	28	0.9	1.8	—
Baked apple	56	0.5	Tr*	3.0
Custard	118	3.8	4.4	—
TOTAL	521	35.0	11.8	12.0

Snack-type lunch	Kcals	Protein grams	Fat grams	Fibre grams
Wholemeal bread (4 slices)	260	10.2	3.2	10.4
Chicken and tomato	148	24.8	5.4	—
sandwich filling	7	0.5	Tr*	1.5
Low fat spread	25	—	2.8	—
Banana	82	1.2	0.4	3.5
TOTAL	526	36.7	11.8	15.4

* = Trace amounts of this component are found in the food.

As you can see, these two lunches are similar, although the cooked lunch is slightly lower in fibre than the snack-type lunch. In both cases the fat content is approximately 20 per cent of total energy, which is below the recommended amount of fat. However it would take only a few changes to make both meals very fatty – a greasy gravy and a couple of knobs of margarine on the potatoes could more than double the fat content, as could a large portion of mayonnaise in the sandwiches.

What is eaten for lunch often depends on where you are. If the food that is available at school, at work, at home or in the pub is unhealthy, it may be possible to institute some beneficial changes. For example, a canteen might be asked to introduce healthier items, such as whole-meal bread and jacket potatoes with alternative fillings. Caterers are often more receptive to this approach than to being asked to cut out chips and pastries. It will also give them an opportunity to experiment with new dishes. Parents and teachers can bring pressure to bear on local authorities to provide healthier school lunches. In one authority lunches were recently altered to include more jacket potatoes with a variety of fillings. It was found that the consumption of chips subsequently decreased by 30 per cent.

> *In one authority lunches were recently altered to include more jacket potatoes with a variety of fillings. It was found that the consumption of chips subsequently decreased by 30 per cent.*

Lunch at School Government nutritional recommendations for lunches served by the schools were removed in 1980 as the DHSS felt they were no longer necessary, even though many nutritionists disagreed. At first, many schools continued to follow the old guidelines but these were gradually eroded as pressure to make financial savings increased. Now there is a greater use of convenience foods such as hamburgers, sausages and chips, which can be prepared by fewer staff. A recent DHSS report on the diets of British schoolchildren showed that they consume many processed foods, which are high in fat and sugar, and that much of this comes from school meals.

Although the removal of the nutritional recommendations was widely criticized, it has resulted in some beneficial changes in some parts of the country such as Leicester and Surrey. As interest in food and health has increased, many health authorities have now set up food and health policies to give guidelines about the food that should be provided in hospitals, schools and local industries. Although the health authority has no jurisdiction over the education authority, some education authorities are beginning to try and improve their menus in the light of these nutritional guidelines.

Parent-teacher associations and school governors have always been vocal in trying to improve the state of school meals and tuckshops, and they are often supported by both the teaching and catering staff. However, too many education authorities still don't regard food as a priority, and they are therefore unwilling to implement any changes. The situation is not helped by the provision of subsidized EEC butter, full fat milk and hard cheeses to the school meals service. (Although schools can have semi-skimmed milk, the subsidy on this is not as great as for full fat milk). Compare the catering service in your children's school with those in other authorities. Contact the dietetic department at the local hospital. The community dietitian may be able to give examples of financially successful, healthy catering to the school meals catering manager.

With the advent of cash cafeterias, the number of children having school lunches has risen. The ideal lunch should be cheap, nutritious and popular with the majority of children, but in

> *The situation is not helped by the provision of subsidized EEC butter, full fat milk and hard cheeses to the school meals service.*

reality this is hard to achieve. Below are some examples of foods that children should be encouraged to choose from what is likely to be on offer in their school canteen. How healthy these will be depends on the amount and type of fat used, the amount of wholemeal products in use and the amount of added sugar.

Foods to Choose at School:

Fish pie	Fishfingers
Shepherd's pie	Pizza
Jacket potatoes with fillings	Dhal with rice or chapati
Cauliflower cheese	Cheese salad with potato or bread
Mince and bean stew	Ham salad with potato or bread
Liver	Egg salad with potato or bread
Spaghetti bolognaise	Baked beans
Risotto	Vegetables
Hamburger in a bun	Fresh fruit
	Fruit and custard

Packed lunches Many children nowadays take packed lunches to school because parents (probably wrongly) believe them to be cheaper and because they think they can maintain control over what their children eat.

When preparing a packed lunch try to choose some form of pasta, rice or bread (preferably wholegrain), as the basis of the meal. Add some salad such as tomatoes or cucumber. If your children don't like salad in their sandwiches offer sticks of carrot or celery. Then choose something in the way of lean meat, fish, poultry, eggs, cheese, nuts or beans. Finally put in some fruit or fresh fruit juice. (Some schools will allow their pupils to have only water.) A low sugar cake such as a wholemeal teacake or a wholemeal sultana scone or a packet of low fat, low salt crisps or similar can be added for a treat provided that the sandwich and salad are generally eaten, not just left.

Here are some possible menus for varied and nutritious packed lunches:
Ham and cucumber wholemeal rolls; raspberry yoghurt; fresh orange juice.
Leek and potato soup; cheese sandwiches; carrot sticks; tangerine.
Wholemeal pitta bread stuffed with salad and chicken; banana; fresh apple juice.
Tuna and salad wholemeal sandwiches; apple; wholemeal teacake.
Cheese roll; egg and cress wholemeal roll; pear; fresh orange juice.
Peanut butter and grated carrot sandwiches; apple; date and apple slice.
Ham, cucumber, low fat cheese, tomato and brown rice salad; peach; fresh orange juice.
Lentil soup; chicken and lettuce sandwiches; orange.
Pitta bread stuffed with salad and tuna fish; wholemeal sultana scone; fresh apple juice.
Cheese and celery wholemeal sandwiches; banana; fresh orange juice.

It might be worth stocking your freezer with some ham, chicken or cheese sandwiches to use in an emergency.

Lunch at Work The lunch that is provided at work will depend to a certain extent on the number of people in a company and on the company's policy towards the provision of catering and dining facilities. Works' canteens range from those that offer a menu with one or two choices of food to more elaborate set-ups with one or two restaurants. Sadly there are still very few canteens that actively help their employees to make healthy choices. Where some attempt has been made, nutrition information has been given out to the workforce to help them switch to healthy eating.

> *There are still very few canteens that actively help their employees to make healthy choices.*

Labelling dishes has been one useful way of giving guidance.

As an employee may eat as many as three hundred meals a year at work, it is vital that he or she should be provided with the choice of eating healthily. It is sometimes argued that employees are not ready for this type of change. This may be true in some cases, but the current interest in food and health suggests that many obviously do want to change, and they will be unable to do so if they are not given healthy choices. Caterers have an important role to play in helping to improve the diet. As a first step, they could start by modifying some of their recipes: for instance a fruit crumble could be made with wholemeal instead of white flour, a polyunsaturate margarine instead of butter or a hard margarine, and by reducing the quantity of sugar.

As vegetables are often overcooked in canteens, it is important that canteen food is not relied upon as a source of vitamin C. For those who have their main meal in a canteen it might be advisable to have some salad or citrus fruit as well.

Lunch Outside Work Many people do not have a works canteen or dining facilities and therefore buy their lunch locally or take something to eat at work. If bought, the choice of food is determined by what is available in the shops, cafés, sandwich bars and pubs in the vicinity. It is certainly possible to buy a healthy type lunch, although most of the food provided in these places is often high in fat and low in fibre.

Taking your own lunch to work is the most effective way of controlling what you eat at midday. Besides sandwiches, add variety by taking salads or soups to work. If the office has a fridge and a microwave, this will further increase the range of food that can be eaten at work.

Some people do not feel that lunch is important, or they find that it makes them feel sleepy and so try to work through the day without stopping to eat. This is bad for you nutritionally, especially if it leads to snacking on unhealthy items throughout the afternoon. It is much better to eat a sandwich, either at lunchtime or perhaps earlier when you start to feel hungry.

Some healthy lunches could include the following (for further ideas see the packed lunches section on page 198).

Sandwiches:
   Mashed sardine and cottage cheese granary bap
   Ham and watercress wholemeal sandwich
   Peanut butter wholemeal sandwich
   Tomato and mozzarella salad with a granary bap
   Peanut butter, celery and curd cheese granary roll
   Grated low fat hard cheese, chopped celery and wholemeal sandwich
   Pitta bread filled with cottage cheese with prawns and lettuce
   Mashed sardine and cucumber wholemeal sandwich

Lean roast beef and salad wholemeal sandwich
(Remember that with all sandwiches you need to watch how much fat is spread or mayonnaise that is put into the sandwich.)

Salads:
Brown rice salad with ham, Edam cheese, tomato, cucumber, raisins, cress
Haricot bean and tuna salad
Wholemeal pasta, roast chicken, cucumber, cooked sweetcorn, cooked kidney beans, peanuts and lettuce salad
Salad niçoise
Brown rice with nuts, grapes, roast chicken, apple and lettuce salad.

Cooked items:
Wholemeal pasta with tuna and tomato sauce
Wholemeal pizza
Jacket potato with ratatouille and cheese
Wholemeal pasta with mushroom sauce
Brown rice and tomato sauce with Parmesan cheese
Grilled mushrooms and lean ham on wholemeal toast
Grilled hamburger in a wholemeal roll with salad
Leek and potato soup
Cheese and tomato sandwich in wholemeal bread
Celery soup
Hummus and wholemeal pitta bread.

CHILDREN'S TEAS

For most of us "tea" is now probably nothing more than a cup of tea and perhaps a slice of cake on special occasions. However for children under the age of twelve it can still be an extremely important meal. Young children are often immensely hungry at this time of the day, and it may well be more convenient to make this their proper main meal. It is also sensible if they are small eaters, as a biscuit or bun an hour or two before supper will probably spoil their appetite.

Whatever you give children at teatime should ideally complement what they have had to eat for the rest of the day. Many children will not eat vegetables at school, so it is important to try to provide some at teatime. You could make home-made soups, cook vegetables in cheese sauce or serve raw vegetable sticks. Try to include some fruit too.

Instead of fruit squash, offer milk, fresh fruit juice or even water. Don't put out the biscuits and cakes until after the savoury food has been eaten, and every now and again, when you know they have eaten enough, don't give them any cakes or biscuits at all so that they don't always expect them. Always provide plenty of bread, preferably wholemeal, as it is certainly much healthier than eating lots of cakes and biscuits. Only allow crisps occasionally.

Don't allow more than two biscuits or pieces of cake (depending on their size), and sometimes one piece will suffice. Try to make your own low fat, low sugar, high fibre cakes and biscuits – yeasted cakes can be made without sugar – and use fruit as cake decorations instead of icing or sweets.

The following are some possible tea menus:

Vegetable soup; jacket potato filled with grated cheese; date and wholemeal fruit loaf; slices of fresh fruit.

Hamburger in a wholemeal roll; low fat cheese sandwiches in wholemeal bread; carrot and celery sticks; low fat and low sugar fruit yoghurts.

Peanut butter sandwiches made with wholemeal bread; slices of pizza; salad; fresh fruit salad with natural yoghurt.

Cheese dip with vegetable crudités such as carrots, cucumber, tomato, radish celery, mushroom, etc.; baked beans on toast; wholemeal fruit scone.

Egg on toast; wholemeal and fruit tea cake; banana milkshake made with bananas and skimmed milk.

Potato layer bake (thinly sliced potatoes layered with onions, ham and cooked in stock. Put some cheese on the top layer and cover. Cook for 1½ hours at Gas Mark 5, 190°C, 375°F; slices of fresh fruit.

Chicken drumsticks; wholemeal rolls; salad; wholemeal carrot cake or low fat and low sugar fruit yoghurts.

If you and your children prefer to eat your evening meal together, offer half-portions of some of the meals suggested below. You will then not have the extra work involved in preparing, and cleaning up after, two separate meals. Among those that may be enjoyed by children are shepherd's pie, Lancashire hotpot, lasagne, spaghetti bolognese and fish pie.

EVENING MEALS

For most people, the evening meal is the main meal of the day. Most effort is concentrated into preparing the main course, and the evening meal may be the only time vegetables are eaten during the day. Fewer and fewer families have a traditional pudding and instead eat fruit, ice cream, cheese or yoghurt.

Here are some suggestions for healthy evening meals:

Shepherd's pie (some supermarkets label mince with their fat content); broad beans; carrots.

Roast chicken (remember that most of the fat is contained in the skin); stir-fry vegetables; jacket potatoes.

Watercress soup; pork goulash; wholemeal pasta; green salad.

Lancashire hotpot; peas; mashed swede.

Chicken baked with herbs, garlic and lemon juice; rice and kidney beans; leeks; green beans with almonds.

Vegetarian lasagne; cauliflower, watercress, pepper and walnut salad; mushroom and chive salad; wholemeal rolls.

Barbecued trout served with lemon; new potatoes; French green beans.

Beef and vegetable kebab; brown rice; salad.

Grilled pork chop; unsweetened apple sauce, new potatoes; French beans; carrots.

Vegetable chick pea hotpot; brown rice risotto; mixed green salad.

Paella made with brown rice; salad.

Plaice in tomato and paprika sauce; peas; potatoes.

Fish pie; courgettes; green beans.

Chicken curry; masur dhal; cucumber raita; brown chapatti.

Desserts for special occasions:
Baked apple with raisins and yoghurt
Fresh fruit such as pineapple; fresh fruit salad; orange slices; strawberries
Fruit fools made with stewed fruit puréed with natural yoghurt or quark or custard
Oat-topped fruit crumbles
Summer pudding
Prune and yoghurt mousse
Low fat cheesecake using yoghurt and low fat cheese
Raspberry sorbet
Plums cooked in orange juice and served with natural yoghurt
Baked bananas in liqueur served with natural yoghurt.

EATING OUT

In the past, eating habits tended to be more regular as most meals were consumed at home. Today we consume food in and from a variety of places at a variety of times. For example, commuters might find themselves eating breakfast on the train, lunch in a restaurant and evening meal at home. The range of foods available and where and how they are eaten have increased enormously over the last ten years. The traditional take-away meal of fish and chips has now been joined by, among others, jacket potatoes, croissants, pizza and Indian and Chinese dishes. With this increased access to different types of food at all hours of the day we need to think particularly carefully about what we eat. Below are some guidelines to help you choose healthy food when eating out.

Pubs More and more pubs are providing food. Today it is not just a question of a ploughman's lunch or sandwiches, but of finding comprehensive menus. As food in pubs is usually cheaper than in restaurants, they are gaining in popularity. The microwave oven has also helped pubs to offer a more extensive menu.

Pub food varies enormously, but much of the food provided is high in fat, particularly the pies and fried foods. Even the ploughman's lunch usually has large wedges of cheese and butter but little bread to go with it. Without nutrition labelling, it is hard to tell how much fat is in any particular food, but try to choose items like chilli con carne, toasted sandwiches, sandwiches and ploughman's lunches. The extra butter or margarine that is provided with pâté and cheese is often unnecessary, so ask for an extra portion of bread instead. Many pub meals are low in fibre – unless, of course, wholemeal bread is offered instead of white – and many pub meals contain little fruit and vegetables, so it is important that during the remainder of the day extra fruit and vegetables are eaten.

> *In the past, our eating habits tended to be more regular as most meals were consumed at home. Today we consume food in and from a variety of places at a variety of times.*

Restaurants Despite the introduction of new French cuisines, the food offered on many restaurant menus is still relatively high in fat, mainly because of the amount of butter, cream and pastry that is used but also because very little bread, pasta or potato is offered. More restaurants should offer the option of having sauces, butter or dressings served separately so that the customer can put them on if he chooses. Don't be afraid to ask the waiter if the vegetables or meat or fish could have all the butter or dressings or sauces served separately.

Many restaurants are now providing a selection of vegetarian dishes. In fact some of the best restaurants for healthy eating are vegetarian, although these are still hard to find in some parts of the country and are not always open in the evening. However not all vegetarian food is healthy, especially if lots of cheese, milk and fat has been used in cooking.

> *While the restaurant market declines, the take-away continues to grow and now accounts for one-quarter of all meals.*

Take-aways Now that meals have become less rigid, it is not surprising that the take-away market has increased substantially. While the restaurant market declines, the take-away continues to grow and now accounts for one-quarter of all meals. Many take-away meals are low in fibre or high in fat, but jacket potatoes, pizza, kebabs, chicken tikka and many Chinese and Indian dishes if chosen carefully are all acceptable.

Some recent research into the sodium and fat content of take-away items produced some interesting results. It showed, for example, that thicker chips contained less fat, so the recent trend towards the thin *pommes frites* is not desirable. It was also found that in London there was a greater chance of polyunsaturate oil being used in cooking than in the rest of the country and that chips that had been part-fried in advance contained a higher level of fat because they absorb more when they are cooked twice.

Although the fat content of take-aways varied, the research showed that the sodium content of many of them, notably beefburgers, Chinese dishes that use soy sauce and Greek and Italian meals, is high. Now that many people are demanding less salty food, it would be advisable for the owners of take-aways to use less salt. Those customers who want extra can always add it for themselves.

There is still far more that could be done to improve our food, particularly in the expanding areas of take-aways or fast food. Trends in the United States, where juice bars, vegetarian dishes and Indonesian and Vietnamese take-aways are increasingly popular, may prove to be the growth area in the UK too.

Below are some suggestions for the sort of healthy dishes you might select when you are eating out.

Starters:
Melon or other fruit;
Salad – ask for the dressing to be served separately so that you can add as little or as much as you like;
Soup – choose a non-creamy variety such as carrot, watercress, minestrone, leek and potato, and check with the waiter that no cream is added to the soup before serving;
Fish, vegetable or chicken terrine/pâté – this may not be suitable if lots of cream, butter or margarine was used;
Mushrooms or vegetables à la Grecque – although this may have used some oil in cooking the quantity is usually not too large;

Crudités – eat more of the vegetables and less of the dip;
Smoked salmon – ask for the butter to be served separately;
Seafood salad – ask for the dressing to be served separately;
Pasta – choose one with a tomato sauce such as *con vongole* (with clams) and go carefully with the Parmesan cheese as it is high in fat;
Moules marinière;
Tjatziki;
Hummus;
Asparagus or artichokes – ask for the dressing to be served separately;
Corn on the cob – ask for the butter to be served separately.

Main Courses:
Choose meat or fish that is grilled and not served with extra fat. If you choose a dish with a sauce, try to select one that is not obviously high in fat. If you're unsure, ask the waiter. Don't go for pastries or pies as these are bound to be high in fat. Try to choose foods that are high in fibre, such as jacket potato or wholemeal bread or brown rice, to eat with your main course. The same principles apply to eating out as choosing food at home.

Indian food If a lot of fat or cream is used in cooking eat a minimum of the sauce. Many restaurants will indicate which dishes contain cream – for example, korma and massala. Tandoori cooked food, particularly chicken, is probably the best as little fat is used. Rice dishes such as biriani and pilau are fine unless they have been refried. The best breads to choose are nan and chapati, especially the latter as wholemeal varieties may be available. Dhal and raita are also healthy choices.

Chinese food Avoid the deep fried items such as pancake rolls, sweet and sour dishes and fried rice. Try to choose a variety of dishes, for example two or three plain boiled rice or noodles, one chicken, one fish and one vegetable dish should be enough for two people. Chinese food can be extremely healthy depending on what you choose.

Italian food Avoid those dishes with lots of cream or cheese sauce and try instead the tomato-based dishes. Choose pasta for either a starter or the main course. If you have a plain meat or fish dish for the main course make sure it is not served with lots of butter. The same rule applies to the vegetables. If all the potatoes seem to be fried, choose some extra bread. Pizza is another good healthy alternative, but if it is made with salami, pepperoni or extra cheese it will tend to have a very high fat content.

French food It is often easy to find a fish or vegetable starter in French restaurants. Watch out for creamy sauces in the main course and try to choose one with a meaty sauce, for example *boeuf bourgignonne, coq au vin* or lamb with haricot beans. As with Italian food, watch that seemingly plain meat or fish is not served with lots of extra butter.

Desserts Try to choose fruit-based desserts such as fruit sorbet (which is rather high in sugar but low in fat); fruit crumble (especially if it is wholemeal although it could be high in sugar and fat); fresh fruit salad; fruit marinated in liqueurs; pancakes filled with fruit; fruit compôte; baked fruit; summer pudding.

SNACKS
Contrary to what many people believe, snacks are not a 20th-century phenomenon.

They have been an important part of many cultures for centuries, and the word itself dates from at least the 15th century. Initially snacks were thought of more as a gift than as a small meal. In many countries, even today, it would be regarded as discourteous to refuse a snack. They are given not only as a form of welcome and friendship but as a sign of prosperity.

> *Contrary to what many people believe, snacks are not a 20th-century phenomenon. They have been an important part of many cultures for centuries, and the word itself dates from at least the 15th century.*

However, the word "snack" is used loosely: it can apply to a piece of cake or a biscuit or to almost a full meal. A snack can mean sweets, cakes, biscuits, a piece of cheese or baked beans on toast. None of these would constitute a meal but might satisfy our desire to eat. Most of us feel that a snack involves little preparation and is easy to clear up. It doesn't involve much planning as it is usually made from items that are already available at home. There are not only international differences in what one is offered as a snack but also national ones. If people come to tea in the afternoon in certain regions of the country or with older people, they would be offered sandwiches and cake; in other regions they would be offered only a piece of cake or a biscuit, and elsewhere a cooked meal.

What constitutes a snack will depend on: when you eat; where you eat; how complicated or lengthy the preparation has been; what sort of food it is; whether the food is cooked or raw; and how much planning has gone into the event.

For example, to some people a ploughman's lunch is a snack; to others it is a meal. Whatever you call it, it should still conform to the rules required for choosing a healthy meal. That is, it should be high in fibre, low in fat and sugar and contain some fruit or vegetables. Recent research suggests that people are eating their food in snack form rather than as meals, but this is still no reason to eat unhealthily. A healthy snack could be beans on toast with tomato followed by low fat yoghurt, or low fat cheese on wholemeal toast with an apple.

JUNK FOODS

"Junk" food is a term much used today, but it is rarely defined. The expression is used mostly to describe food that is seen to have little nutritional value and that is not considered healthy, especially if it constitutes a large percentage of the diet. Manufacturers prefer to call it "fun" food. It is also often called "fast" food because it is quick and easy to obtain. It is an umbrella term, covering a range of foods, including: sweets, chocolate, instant desserts, hamburgers, chips, doughnuts, instant noodles and fizzy drinks. Public opinion seems to range from those who feel that these foods are virtually poisonous to those who consider them totally harmless which is, in any case, their own business if they choose to eat them. Here the problem is deciding where to strike a reasonable balance between the two. Junk foods are unhealthy only when they are eaten to the exclusion of all others or as a major component of the diet, which is more likely to happen to children and young people. It is not difficult for a parent, worried that a child is not eating enough, to fall into the trap of allowing the child to eat anything at all. And as adolescents gradually take more responsibility for feeding themselves, they may well start eating whatever they like. The main problem is that the fat, salt, sugar and additive content of many of these foods (and therefore of the overall diet) tends to be high.

Junk foods have become popular for several reasons. They are quick and readily available to eat. They may be bright, gaudy colours and be eaten in an informal atmosphere where nobody minds if you eat with your fingers. They are heavily advertised, with their appeal carefully targeted to reach the prime audience (often children and teenagers). And they are fairly cheap to buy, especially if they are not being bought for a family. However, they may still cost about double what it would cost you to prepare the same food at home. For example, a meal for four people of quarter-pound hamburgers with chips costs about £6.00. Making the equivalent meal at home would cost about half this amount.

Diets that include a large proportion of junk foods can be slightly deficient in some nutrients, particularly vitamin C, iron, folic acid and riboflavin, often because of the limited variety of foods chosen by the consumer. Junk foods also tend to be high in calories, fat (particularly saturated fat) and sodium and low in fibre. However, much depends on the total diet. Some of the sugar can be avoided if diet drinks or fresh fruit juice (now available in many fast food outlets) and the savoury part of the meal only are chosen.

The chart below shows the nutritional value of some junk and fast foods so that you can decide for yourself whether they should be included in your diet.

THE NUTRITIONAL VALUE OF JUNK FOODS

In the following table fat is given as a percentage of the total kcal value, as well as in grams, because the government now officially recommends that we look at the percentage of fat in our foods.

Food per portion	kcal —	fat g	fat %	sugar g	fibre g	sodium mg
Fried fish (shop bought; 180g (6½oz))	358	18.5	46	—	—	180
Chips (no salt added; 150g (5¼oz))	378	16.4	39	—	4.5	18
Crisps (1 small pkt; 28g (1oz))	149	10.0	61	—	3.3	154
Masur 100g (3½oz)	193	16.1	75	—	—	NA
Meat samosa 110g (3½oz)	329	30.5	83	—	0.8	20
Small hamburger	253	9.9	35	—	0.9	396
Quarter-pound hamburger	413	20.7	45	—	1.3	717
Fried chicken 150g (5oz)	351	22.9	59	—	Tr	142
Cola drink 330ml (11½ fl oz)	129	—	—	35	—	26
Toffee/chocolate bar 70g (2½oz)	265	11.3	38	39	—	90
Milk chocolate 30g (1¾oz)	265	15.2	51	28	—	60
Cornish pasty 140g (5¼oz)	498	30.6	55	—	Tr	885
Pork pie 125g (4oz)	470	33.8	65	—	—	900
Sausage roll 75g (2¾oz)	359	27.2	68	—	—	412
Steak and kidney pie 180g (6½oz)	581	38.2	59	—	—	918
Pork sausage 100g (3½oz)	318	24.6	70	—	—	1000
Fruit yoghurt 150g (5¼oz)	143	1.5	16	22	Tr	220
Fruit pie 110g (4oz)	369	15.5	38	31	2.6	210
Doughnut 75g (2¾oz)	262	11.9	40	11	Tr	30
Jam tart 50g (2⅓oz)	192	7.5	35	19	0.9	115
Ice cream 75g (2¾oz)	125	5.0	47	11	—	60
Milkshake 300g (10½ fl oz)	380	12.1	29	46	—	242

NUTRITIONAL VALUE OF SOME TAKE-AWAYS

Food	kcal —	fat g	fat %	sugar g	fibre g	sodium mg
Prawn cocktail 100g (3½oz)	278	24.8	80	—	Tr	1015
Liver pâté 85g (3oz)	172	12.6	66	—	—	333
Smoked mackerel pâté 85g (3oz)	309	30	86	—	—	276
Hummus 85g (3oz)	157	10.7	61	—	—	565
Taramasalata 85g (3oz)	292	26.4	81	—	—	63
Chicken tikka 100g (3½oz)	173	6.3	33	—	—	97
Fried rice 200g (7oz)	318	13.9	39	—	—	NA
Lasagne 225g (8oz)	340	19.4	51	—	Tr	668
Chilli con carne 225g (8oz)	346	20.1	52	—	7.5	562
Ratatouille 85g (3oz)	64	5.4	76	—	1.8	165

(Some of the information for these charts was supplied by the Nuffield Laboratories of Comparative Medicine; the quantities were originally calculated in grams.)

CONVENIENCE FOODS

The term "convenience food" in its broadest sense could apply to items like bread, jam, milk and even vegetables. In the past these things were all made or prepared by the family. Today's interpretation of convenience food is food that has been processed in some way and needs little preparation. It is often applied to manufactured foods like frozen or cooked, chilled and ready-prepared meals, instant mixes and canned dishes. Most people could prepare these dishes or meals for themselves but either don't have the time or the desire to do so.

The demand for ready-prepared meals, particularly chilled foods, has increased over the last five years. At the same time the consumer has demanded more flexible portion sizes, which has resulted in more dishes being made available in serving sizes for one and two rather than for four.

Many manufacturers are responding to the interest in healthy eating by modifying their products. Foods are now available with less fat, high fibre and so forth, but until detailed nutritional labelling is required by law it is hard to compare the saturated fat, salt or fibre content in one brand with that in another. However recent analysis of manufactured ready prepared meals shows that they tend to be high in fat, particularly saturated fat.

CHAPTER 10

SPECIAL NEEDS

*A*t different stages of life there are different nutritional requirements. This chapter looks at our needs at every age, from pregnancy, through childhood to old age.

——*PREGNANT WOMEN AND BABIES*——

Ideally, a healthy diet should be eaten even before the baby is conceived. The baby's health is determined long before the fertilized egg becomes implanted in the uterus. Medical evidence makes it advisable for the mother to be well nourished and preferably of normal body weight, to give the baby the best chance of a healthy start in life.

Pregnancy is often a good time to practise preventative medicine, as not only do the mother and doctor see each other regularly but women realize that they must now take greater care of themselves. As motivation is likely to be high, pregnancy is a good time to give up smoking and to make progress with developing healthy eating habits.

WEIGHT AND PREGNANCY

It is not easy to control the amount of weight gained in pregnancy. As soon as pregnancy begins, the body sets about saving all the nourishment, including energy in the form of fat, that it needs. Although the baby accounts for only about 6-9lb (2.7-4kg) of the total weight gained, the rest is not all fat: the tissues of the breasts and uterus get bigger and the blood supply increases. In addition, the weight of the placenta and the sack of membranes and fluid that holds the baby also increases.

The usual medical recommendation is that a woman should put on approximately 22-28lb (10-12.7kg) during the whole pregnancy. Mothers whose weight is normal before the pregnancy, will have an optimal weight gain of about 8lb 8oz (3.8kg) at 20 weeks, 19lb (8.6kg) at 30 weeks and 28lb (12.7kg) at term. However, perfectly healthy babies can be born to women who put on only a very small amount of weight as well as to those who put on over 3 stone (19kg).

More important than the quantity of weight gained is the rate at which it is

> *The baby's health is determined long before the fertilized egg becomes implanted in the uterus.*

gained. A sudden weight increase may indicate that extra fluid is being produced. Fluid retention or oedema, while not in itself harmful as far as the baby is concerned, does indicate that a closer watch on the mother's health may sometimes be necessary.

> *Pregnancy is not such a cause of weight problems as it is commonly believed to be,*

In fact, only 20lb (9kg) can be accounted for by the growth of the unborn baby and the supporting tissues and fluids together with any changes in the mother herself. A few extra pounds of body fat are put on as reserves against the times when the mother might go short of food before or after the birth.

Pregnancy is not such a common cause of weight problems as it is often believed to be, but those who are already overweight require especially careful monitoring if there is a disproportionately large gain in weight. On the other hand, those who are underweight have a tendency to put on less weight than average during pregnancy, which may result in the birth of a baby that is small for its dates. An underweight mother will, therefore, be monitored as closely as an overweight mother. Underweight mothers are often encouraged to boost their calorie intake as they have a tendency to lose weight at the first sign of any stress.

Overweight mothers should not restrict their food intake, as they may also restrict their intake of essential vitamins and minerals. Medical experts are of the opinion that the overweight mother should lose weight prior to conception.

DIETARY REQUIREMENTS DURING PREGNANCY

Being pregnant doesn't necessarily mean having to make radical changes in your eating habits, unless, of course, you tend to eat lots of sugary and fatty foods, in which case pregnancy provides an excellent opportunity to start to eat more healthily. During pregnancy the body is much more efficient than at other times: there is increased efficiency in the metabolism of protein, and in the absorption of iron and calcium. Some of the nutrients that are particularly important during pregnancy are discussed below.

Calories Recent surveys have shown that most pregnant women do not require any extra calories as the metabolism seems to become more efficient. There is certainly no justification for eating for two during pregnancy.

Protein Most people in the UK eat more protein than they require, and so the extra needed during pregnancy is unlikely to be a problem. During pregnancy, protein needs increase from about 1.9oz (54g) a day to 2.1oz (60g) a day. The average daily intake of protein in this country is approximately 2.9oz (82g), so most people will be well above these recommendations. Women whose protein (and calorie) intakes were adequate before pregnancy are unlikely to suffer any short-term restriction of protein intake, caused, for example, by morning sickness, that would harm the baby or the mother.

Iron Anaemia due to lack of iron can occur during pregnancy but it is less common than was once thought. The expectant mother will have stopped menstruating, and this helps to compensate for the increased demands for iron. Only women with a severe drop in haemoglobin levels are likely to be advised to take iron (and possibly folate) supplements.

Whether iron tablets are prescribed by the clinic or not, it is still important to ensure that your diet contains enough iron. Iron is found in a variety of foods such as meat, fish, eggs, offal, lentils, baked beans, wholegrain cereals, wholemeal breads, nuts and dried fruits. If you like offal, try to have liver or kidney once a week. Vitamin C from fruit and vegetables is also an excellent way of boosting the absorption of iron from foods in the diet.

Calcium Although calcium absorption becomes more efficient during pregnancy, women are sometimes recommended to obtain extra calcium from their diets as a precaution. The easiest way to get extra calcium is from milk, cheese and yoghurt. Dietitians recommend a daily intake of 1 pint (0.5 litre) of milk, or three 5oz (140g) cartons of yoghurt, or 4½oz (125g) cheese during pregnancy. However, if adequate dairy products are usually eaten, it is unlikely that any special efforts need be made to increase the calcium in the diet. On the other hand, suddenly cutting down on the intake of milk and dairy products during pregnancy, in the hope of preventing allergies in the baby, should not be done without medical supervision. Although the body can adapt to reduced states of calcium, the process takes a few weeks, and no one really knows whether a pregnant woman – whose calcium requirements are greater than normal – might suffer as a result of a sudden drop in calcium intake. If you are a vegan, you should consult your doctor who may decide to give you calcium supplements.

Vitamin D During pregnancy four times the normal amount of vitamin D are needed so that the body can use the extra calcium to strengthen the baby's bones. As this vitamin can be made by our bodies when it is exposed to sunlight, it is unlikely that we will be deficient in vitamin D. Most women already have sufficient stores to cope should extra demands be made by pregnancy. However, a few women such as the housebound or those of Asian origin may need to take supplements during pregnancy.

Folic acid or folate Folic acid is needed for the rapid development of a baby's cells particularly in the weeks immediately after conception. The mother also requires extra folic acid during pregnancy to prevent a form of anaemia, which can occur as a result of a large increase in the blood supply. Although this disease is rare in Britain, it is potentially serious. It has also been suggested that folic acid may play a protective role in preventing neural tube defects such as spina bifida. For these reasons some doctors will advise a folic acid supplement during all or part of the pregnancy. Such a supplement should not be taken except under medical advice. Folic acid is also found in liver, oatmeal, oranges, nuts, wholemeal bread, spinach, broccoli, kidneys and brown rice.

Vitamin B$_{12}$ Vegans' diets are likely to be deficient in vitamin B$_{12}$ and possibly in calcium, and they should take supplements during pregnancy. They are also usually advised to continue to take supplements during breastfeeding.

Overall, the best guide to healthy eating during pregnancy is to cut down gradually on fatty and sugary foods while making sure that you make up the calories by eating plenty of fresh fruit and vegetables, bread and cereals (which should be wholemeal whenever possible), milk (which can be skimmed or semi-skimmed) and some lean meat and fish. Eat offal too if you like it. Although pregnancy provides the opportunity to improve your eating habits, don't let over-enthusiasm to cut out unhealthy foods cause you to end up being hungry and going short of food.

Problems with Diet

Constipation The intestines can become sluggish when "relaxed" by pregnancy hormones, so to prevent constipation you should eat fibre-rich foods, particularly wholegrain breakfast cereals, wholemeal bread, baked beans, peas and lots of fruit and vegetables. You should also drink plenty of fluids, but try to drink extra water or fresh fruit juices rather than increasing your consumption of sugary drinks. Exercise will also help. Iron tablets can also be a common cause of constipation, and if you have been prescribed them, ask your doctor if you can stop taking them or change to a different brand.

Heartburn Heartburn or indigestion in pregnancy is partly caused because the growing uterus presses on the stomach and makes it uncomfortable and partly because small quantities of food and stomach acid are more easily refluxed (thrown back up) during pregnancy, causing heartburn. For this reason, eat several small meals rather than fewer larger ones. Fried or spicy food can sometimes cause problems, but there are no hard and fast rules. Don't eat just before going to bed when the digestive process tends to slow down. Instead, allow plenty of time for your food to digest. Your doctor may prescribe an antacid if your heartburn persists.

Morning sickness This can occur at any time of the day, not just in the morning! Most women suffer from it only in the first few months, but others find it continues throughout their pregnancy. The cause of morning sickness is unknown, but it is thought to be due to metabolic or hormonal changes brought about by the presence of the baby or the placenta. It does not always occur with each pregnancy.

Some women suffer from nausea so badly that they find they can eat only a little food. Taking a dry biscuit before getting up in the morning can help a few expectant mothers; others may find it more helpful to eat small amounts of food at times of the day when they are not feeling too sick. If you are well nourished before the pregnancy, problems like repeated vomiting will not cause the baby to go short of nourishment, however much it may distress you. A stay in hospital may be recommended if an expectant mother is vomiting severely.

Pre-eclampsia Pre-eclampsia is a disorder that can arise in the latter half of pregnancy. It is characterized by high blood pressure and an accumulation of fluid in the tissues, making them puffy. Sometimes the kidneys are affected as there is a leakage of protein into the urine. Because this disorder can put both the mother and baby at risk, doctors and midwives keep a watchful eye for any tell-tale signs. Both the cause and the treatment of this disorder remain a mystery. Bedrest sometimes works, but by no means always. Every now and again dietary treatments have been recommended, but it is worth noting that trying to restrict weight gain, a treatment that has been around since the beginning of the century, rarely works.

Fatigue Some women become so tired during pregnancy that they no longer feel like eating or preparing food. If there is someone else to help take over the cooking, this can help; alternatively make sure you keep a good stock of ready-prepared dishes. If you have no help, try to set aside some time for a rest with your feet up or for relaxation exercises, which can be of great benefit.

If you have a demanding toddler, then you may only be able to rest if the child is at playgroup or watching a favourite television programme.

Bleeding gums During pregnancy the hormones in the blood cause the gums to become softer and spongier so that they bleed easily. Bleeding, sore gums are one

❝
*The only safe solution is not to drink
any alcohol during pregnancy.*
❞

of the signs of gum disease, which can eventually result in the teeth working loose. Good dental hygiene, such as brushing the teeth well and using dental floss, can help, but you should take advantage of free dental treatment, available while you are pregnant and for a year after the baby is born.

Food cravings and aversions Cravings for certain foods are less common nowadays. It is more usual for women to develop an aversion to or be turned off by certain foods and smells. Common aversions are tea, coffee, alcohol and tobacco smoke. Since none of these substances is necessary or even desirable, this is an advantage. However, if you do "go off" tea or coffee, remember to keep up your fluid intake with water or fruit juice.

PROTECTING THE BABY

Alcohol There has been much interest in this subject recently, and a number of studies of alcohol and pregnancy have been carried out. Many of the early studies published results of what happened to the babies of alcoholic mothers. However, as the vast majority of women are not alcoholics other studies have looked at those women who drink small or moderate amounts of alcoholic drinks. Some researchers concluded that an expectant mother should not drink at all during pregnancy; others have suggested that you can drink a small amount during pregnancy without harming the baby or yourself. Since nobody has been able to work out how small is small, the only safe solution is not to drink any alcohol during pregnancy.

Smoking Smoking is dangerous to you and the baby. Babies of mothers who smoke in pregnancy are often smaller and weaker than those of non-smokers. A smoky atmosphere can also aggravate any coughs or chest infections. Therefore it is important for you and for anyone else living in your house to give up smoking while you are pregnant and preferably for good.

Pills and medicines If you have previously been prescribed drugs or medicines, check with your doctor and chemist to see if it is safe for you to take them while you are pregnant or are trying to conceive. Vitamin supplements should not be taken unless you are advised to do so by the doctor.

FEEDING THE BABY

Today more than half of the mothers who leave hospital are breastfeeding. Although doctors, dietitians and midwives would like to see an even greater proportion being breastfed, this figure is a vast improvement on the situation in the late 1960s and early 1970s. Then, bottlefeeding was portrayed as offering more freedom for the mother and giving her more control over the amount the baby was consuming. Since then, new research into the unique properties of breastmilk and the testimony of many mothers who feel that breastfeeding is a much simpler method of feeding (once any initial difficulties have been overcome) have done much to encourage new mothers to

❝
*Babies of mothers who smoke in
pregnancy are often smaller and
weaker than those of non-smokers.*
❞

breastfeed rather than bottlefeed their babies.

Breastmilk The biggest difference between human milk and infant formula milk is the immunological one. During the first few days of breastfeeding, the mother does not produce milk but a highly nutritious substance called colostrum, a thick, creamy liquid that sometimes looks quite yellow. Colostrum, being rich in antibodies, helps the baby to fight many infections. Breastfeeding is an important way of helping to reduce infant mortality and disease. Even if you would prefer to bottlefeed your baby, you might at least consider breastfeeding for the first few weeks.

Breastfeeding is an important way of helping to reduce infant mortality and disease. Even if you would prefer to bottlefeed your baby, you should at least consider breastfeeding for the first few days.

Frequent suckling, particularly during the first few days, not only increases the amount of colostrum produced but also stimulates the breast to produce milk. After a few days, colostrum is replaced by mature milk which will supply the baby with all its nutritional needs up to the age of about 6 months as well as continuing to supply anti-infective properties.

Human milk (breastmilk) has evolved to meet the needs of the baby, just as a cow's milk meets the needs of a calf. Manufacturers of bottlefeeds (which are based on cow's milk) can make the composition of their milks resemble breastmilk, but not all modifications are possible, and bottled milk can only approximate the nutritional content of breastmilk. Nor can it supply the antibodies.

Infant milk formulae are highly modified versions of cow's milk. For example, the proportion of protein in breastmilk is three times lower than in cow's milk The nature of the protein also differs. Breastmilk is rich in the protein lactalbumin rather than casein. Not only is lactalbumin easier to digest, but it contains a higher proportion of the amino acids cysteine and taurine. Studies suggest that these amino acids play an important role in the development of the brain. Taurine also helps aid fat metabolism.

The fat in cow's milk contains a high proportion of saturated fatty acids, whereas breastmilk is made from essential polyunsaturated fatty acids, mainly linoleic acid, and these fats have been found to be an important component of the brain and the nervous system. Polyunsaturates are found to be more easily digested by the baby than saturates. Breastmilk is also rich in an enzyme, lipase, which predigests the fats for the baby. Cow's milk does not contain much lipase, and, as a result, some of the fat combines with calcium and is excreted undigested, leading to a loss of both calcium and calories. Although vitamin D usually needs the presence of fat in order to be absorbed by the body tissues, a water-soluble form has been found to exist in breastmilk. Unlike breastmilk, cow's milk is a poor source of vitamin D, having only one-fifth as much as human milk. Therefore, infant formulae, which are made from cow's milk, need to have added vitamin D.

Concentrations of sodium and potassium are lower in breastmilk than in cow's milk. The kidneys of young infants are not able to cope with the extra sodium and potassium in unmodified cow's milk, which is why it is not introduced into their diet until they are six months old. Although breastmilk has less calcium and phosphorus

❝

*Babies that are fed on breastmilk
have been shown to suffer less from
respiratory and gastrointestinal
diseases.*

❞

than cow's milk, it is thought that babies absorb these minerals more efficiently, and just as too little calcium can be harmful so, too, can excess amounts. Some nutrients, such as iron and zinc, are better absorbed from breastmilk. All infant formulae milks are modified so that they contain lower proportions of sodium, potassium, calcium and phosphorus than cow's milk.

The composition of breastmilk also changes during the course of a feed – which infant formulae cannot. At first, breastmilk is high in protein and in water and hence thirst-quenching. But the protein decreases as feeding continues, and as the protein and water content begins to decrease, the fat and calorie content increases. The high fat and energy content helps to satisfy the baby's appetite. It is important that the baby gets this milk as it is rich in essential polyunsaturated fats and calories.

Babies that are fed on breastmilk have been shown to suffer less from respiratory and gastrointestinal diseases. As a baby's immune system is incompletely developed during the first months of life, it is provided with immunological protection from the mother's milk. For this reason breastmilk may protect the baby against allergies or help make the allergies less severe.

Infant formulae Modern formula feeds are not replicas of breastmilk, but they are a great improvement over cow's milk and the old-fashioned formula feeds. All non-breastfed babies should be given a modified formula milk. Overall, there is little difference between one brand and another of these modified formulae. Different brands are based either on milk casein or on whey; some of the protein may be partially broken down and some may have extra amino acids added. In addition they have added vitamin D, a low proportion of sodium potassium, calcium and phosphorus so that they are similar in composition to breastmilk. These modified milks should be given for at least the first six months and continued for 12 months or until your baby is well on to solids.

One advantage of bottlefeeding is that the father can enjoy feeding the baby as well as the mother. But whether you breast- or bottlefeed or do both, it is important that you feel relaxed while feeding the baby.

Vitamin drops and fluoride Vitamin drops, which include vitamins A, D and C, can be given from the ages of about one month until two years and they are sometimes recommended until five years.

Fluoride does not seem to be passed into breastmilk from the mother's diet, so tablets or drops containing fluoride will strengthen a baby's teeth. However, a mother who is feeding her baby a varied diet may decide, after discussion with the health visitor or doctor, that vitamin drops are unnecessary.

AFTER THE BABY IS BORN

Many women decide whether they will breastfeed or not before the baby is born. Some worry that their breasts are too small or that they will find breastfeeding distasteful. However, more than 95 per cent of women are physically able to breastfeed their babies successfully. It is important that breastfeeding is encouraged as soon as possible after the birth to help establish the suckling action.

Anxiety or tiredness can mean that a mother fails to produce enough breast-milk. It is important to relax and adopt the position that you find most comfortable. In the early days, the support of an experienced friend or midwife may also be helpful, although others may prefer the peace and quiet of their own thoughts. If you continue to doubt that

It is wise to keep the consumption of alcohol down to the minimum because a small proportion of the alcohol you drink will reach your baby through your milk.

your supply of milk is adequate, you should consult your health visitor or doctor who can check your baby's weight gain and tell you whether your baby is thriving.

Besides feeding the baby, you should ensure that you are receiving enough food yourself. You require the same type of food as during pregnancy but more of it, because you need more calories, protein, thiamin, riboflavin and vitamin A. In fact, many women are amazed at how much they can eat and drink. Some find it helpful to have a sandwich or drink such as milk after they have given the night feed.

If this is your first baby, you will probably find you get particularly tired, and you may well have little time, let alone the energy, to prepare meals yourself. To ensure you get enough to eat you should lay in some stocks of food before the birth. If you have a freezer you could make double the portions of meals such as stews and casseroles and freeze half for when you come out of hospital. Otherwise try to get family or friends to help you prepare some meals.

You will probably be 7-10lb (3.2-4.5kg) overweight after the baby is born. The surplus may well disappear of its own accord over the next few months, whether you are breastfeeding or not. However, not all women manage to lose the surplus pounds. and if you want to lose weight you should be careful not to restrict your food supply while you are breastfeeding because you are likely to restrict your milk supply as well. It is important to get breastfeeding established first, before trying to eat less, and to leave dieting until after the baby is on solids.

Instead of eating less, why not get back into shape with some gentle, regular exercise? If your nearest health centre does not provide a postnatal exercise class, you could buy a cassette tape with exercises specially adapted for new mothers. Teaming up with someone else may give you both company and encouragement.

Drugs and breastmilk It is wise to keep the consumption of alcohol down to the minimum because a small proportion of the alcohol you drink will reach your baby through your milk.

Researchers have found recently that babies and children of parents who smoke are more likely to suffer from respiratory diseases. It is also known that nicotine and other chemicals from cigarettes accumulate in breastmilk but it is uncertain what effect this has on the infant.

If you are taking any medication discuss with your doctor whether you can continue to do so while you are breastfeeding.

CHECKLIST

* Try to learn all you can about breastfeeding beforehand. You may find it useful to watch a baby being breastfed. Ask your midwife and talk to women who have enjoyed breastfeeding – they won't mind being questioned.

* Gather as much support as you can from your husband, family and friends, as well as from the midwife who looks after you.
* The baby should be put to the breast as soon as possible after the delivery.
* Consider the first two to three weeks to be the learning period but don't be discouraged by any difficulties you might encounter.
* Contact the National Childbirth Trust or La Lèche League to gain support from others (see address list on page 326).
* Mothers often find it easier to breastfeed in privacy as they will feel more relaxed.
* Make sure your back is well supported when breastfeeding. The most comfortable position may be found by sitting on the sofa, bed or by leaning against a bean bag on the floor.
* Help to establish breastfeeding by putting your baby to the breast whenever he is restless during the first few weeks. If your nipples are sore, make sure that the nipple is well inside his mouth and feed him for only 5 minutes on each side in the first few days, making up the feeding time with more frequent feeds. Feeding before he gets ravenous will also be easier on your nipples. Suckling thereafter can be as long as required. As the baby develops a stronger suck and the nipple becomes softer, the feeds should become shorter.
* Always start feeding on alternate breasts.
* If you are advised to top up with a formula feed, use this only as an emergency measure. If you offer the bottle too frequently, it may be counterproductive as less milk (because of reduced stimulation) will be available from the breasts. Instead, you will need to concentrate on feeding for longer and much more frequently for two or three days to stimulate the supply.

Tips about bottlefeeds:
* Measure the feed out carefully as instructed by the manufacturer and never add an extra scoop of powder or granules. If the mixture is too weak the baby will go short and may become underfed, and if it is too concentrated the feed will make him thirsty and the baby may become dehydrated.
* Always sterilize the bottle and equipment to which the feed is to be added.
* Don't insist that the baby finishes every bottle. Breastfed babies control the amount they take and so should the bottlefed baby.
* A whole day's feed can be made in advance if it is kept in the refrigerator and heated up over hot water prior to use or given cold.
* Babies will drink cold milk but some prefer it warm. Do not reheat a feed in the microwave: you might end up scalding the baby because the temperature that the milk reaches in the middle is usually too hot.
* Never add cereals or rusks to milk in the bottle as this over-concentrates the feed. A baby should not be left to sleep with the bottle in his mouth, as he could choke.

INTRODUCING SOLIDS
It is recommended that babies are not weaned until they are 3-6 months old. Breastmilk or formula milk, if given in sufficient quantity, will meet their needs until 6 months, but bottlefed babies should start to be weaned then, as their iron stores will be running low. Anxious parents often feel that milk cannot possibly be enough to sustain a baby's life, or they hope that the baby will sleep through the night if he is fed solids. Although some parents have weaned their infants before 3

months without the baby suffering any obvious harm, there are several good reasons why parents should wait until the baby is at least 3 months old, and preferably 4 months or older.

> *Weaning a baby is a golden opportunity for parents to rethink their own eating habits!*

A baby's digestive system cannot cope with some foreign proteins before 6 months. Egg and cow's milk should not be given before this age, when the digestive tract of most babies will be mature enough to cope with these substances. Some experts recommend not giving wheat before 6 months. If these foods are introduced too early, they are likely to make a baby more prone to allergies. Certain foods – spinach, turnip and beets, for example – are not advised before 6 months of age because they are rich in nitrate, which can cause a form of infantile anaemia. Other foods that can cause allergies are citrus fruits, nuts and berry fruit such as strawberries and raspberries, and these too are best avoided for the first 6 months. Salt should never be added to babyfood as the infant's kidneys are not yet sufficiently developed to cope with it. No sugar should be added as it will damage the growing teeth. Young babies should also not be given foods containing additives like colourants or artificial sweeteners as a safeguard against any unforeseen consequences at a critical stage in their development. The chart below lists suitable weaning foods.

As they get older, babies should gradually be given more chewy, fibrous foods and be gently weaned on to the sorts of foods the rest of the family ought to be eating. Weaning a baby is a golden opportunity for parents to rethink their own eating habits! Adult diets will change anyway as children increasingly partake in family meals, so it is worth taking this opportunity to make the change a positive one.

WEANING CHART
First Foods (about 4-6 months)
At first, the mixture should be thin; gradually thicken the first foods and increase the amounts as the baby tolerates more. When the first foods are well tolerated go on to the second foods.
Cereal-based purée such as rice flakes, oat flakes
Vegetable purées
Fruit purées or sieved banana
Cooked lentils or dhal (unspiced) plus full quantity of milk feeds
Puréed meat such as chicken, liver, etc.
Second Foods (6-8 months)
Gradually increase the second foods, decreasing the amount of milk given at these feeds. Fruit juice or water can be given if required.
Egg yolk (soft boiled or scrambled) but not before 6 months
Bread or chapatti
Breakfast cereals such as Weetabix or instant oats
Piece of cheese
Mashed potato with milk
Plain boiled rice
Mashed baked beans

Beans cooked till very soft and mashed with milk
Mashed fish or fish pie
Casseroles made with lean mince
Tender pieces of meat from a casserole
Pieces of fruit such as banana or apple
Natural yoghurt.

Third Foods (9-12 months)

A wide range of tastes, flavours and textures should be given so that baby will grow to enjoy a full range of foods.

Fish
Eggs
Meat
Any fruit and vegetables (however, either grate uncooked vegetables or give as
    finger food);
Baked beans
Breakfast cereals
Bread, rice, pasta or chapatti

When you start weaning, introduce solids gradually, slowly building up the variety of foods. If you are weaning because your baby is extra hungry, give him a cereal-based purée, such as rice flakes, which is more filling than fruit or vegetable purées. Introduce new items one at a time, about every four days. This will not only give the infant time to get used to new tastes but will also allow you to see if there is any reaction to the newly introduced foods.

Never give your baby skimmed or semi-skimmed milk as a milk drink or feed as these do not provide enough calories for a growing infant. They also contain too much protein, sodium and other minerals. Skimmed and semi-skimmed milk is also lacking in vitamin A and D.

Do not give foods with added salt. Besides salt, the only other foods that you must avoid using are hot, spicy foods, such as chillis. Don't forget that babyfood is not supposed to appeal to *your* tastebuds.

Sugar has been shown to encourage dental caries. Although your baby does not have any teeth at the moment, they will soon come through. It is advisable to give your baby water or diluted fresh fruit juices to drink. If he likes frequent sips, give water in between meals. If you're unsure whether a drink has sugar in it, read the label and look out for words like glucose, glucose syrup, dextrose, honey, sucrose and sugar.

Fruit juices should never be given at night. The saliva flow is less at this time of the day and the baby is more susceptible to dental disease from any form of sugar whether in fruit juices or any other kind of sweet drink. Give water or milk instead.

If you're unsure whether a drink has sugar in it, read the label and look out for words like glucose, glucose syrup, dextrose, honey, sucrose and sugar.

Consumer pressure has persuaded many manufacturers to produce baby-foods containing no sugar, no salt and no additives. However, although manufactured foods may be useful on occasions, they have no nutritional advantage over your own prepared food and are more expensive than home-made foods. To produce these all you need is a liquidizer, food mouli or food processor to grind up the food. If you have a freezer you can make extra portions to use when you are in a hurry or visiting friends.

Never push children into eating more than they want:

Never push children into eating more than they want: children will eat if they are really hungry, and there is no point forcing them to eat or, conversely, letting them fill up on sweetened foods when they have rejected a savoury item.

Try to use fresh or frozen fruit and vegetables whenever possible as canned fruit and vegetables are often high in sugar and salt solutions respectively.

Constipation can occur as the baby's digestive system adjusts to solids. It should be treated by giving extra fluid, such as water or diluted fruit juice. Once the infant is taking solids, fruit – particularly prunes – or vegetable purées should help to overcome this problem.

THE TEXTURE OF BABYFOOD

Purées of vegetables and cereals should be introduced to the baby first of all. It is advisable to sieve or mouli the purées you make the first few times they are given. Similarly fruit skins should be removed at least for the first 6 months. Those foods that have a strong flavour such as liver may need diluting with purées of potato or rice. Once your baby has mastered the sloppy purée you can begin to make it thicker.

Besides purées, babies like to put other foods in their mouth, especially when teething. You might like to try peeled and quartered apples, fingers of baked bread or peeled raw carrots. Try to avoid sweetened rusks, give pieces of baked bread. Even rusks labelled low in sugar can contain as much as 15 per cent added sugars. Whatever is given should always be under supervision in case the baby accidentally bites off too large a piece and chokes. They often only suck these foods leaving you to throw the mess in the bin.

At 8-9 months of age the baby can take lumpier food. Instead of puréeing food it is now possible just to mash it well. It is important to encourage your baby to chew, as this develops the muscle tone of the mouth and of the jaw.

At about this age you can start to give the baby high fibre foods such as wholemeal bread and cereals. However, foods with added bran or those fortified with fibre are unnecessary; indeed, because the extra fibre is more filling, it could cause a baby to eat insufficient food. Although this is unlikely to be a problem with healthy babies with good appetites, it is best not to give these foods all the time.

By about a year old the child can be eating much the same sort of food as the rest of the family. As children begin to eat more at mealtimes, they often begin to drink less milk. Vegan families are advised not to introduce a child to their way of eating until about 2 years of age, as it can be hard for a younger child to eat enough calories unless milk still makes up a large part of the diet.

Although it is possible to give hotter spices at one year of age, go carefully on the amount added to the child's food. Peanuts and whole nuts should not be given till 4 years of age as there is always a chance that young children will choke on them.

> *Most parents experience some feeding problems, but they seem to be less common among families that do not make food "an issue".*

However, foods like smooth ground peanut butter are suitable.

Over recent years there has been more interest in allergies particularly in children. The commonest foods to cause allergies seem to be cow's milk, eggs, citrus fruits, fish and wheat. This is why these foods should not be introduced until 6 months or even later, particularly for babies with a family history of allergies (see pages 93-4).

Artificial sweeteners such as aspartame and saccharin should not, like other additives, be given to babies and young children. This is a commonsense precaution at a time when a young child's development has not yet been completed.

CHILDREN

Parents usually have little trouble with feeding their child when it's under a year old. However, as the child gets older feeding problems can start, although at what age these occur and the form that they take will vary from child to child. Most parents experience some feeding problems, but they seem to be less common among families that do not make food "an issue".

The most important aims are to encourage the child to enjoy a variety of foods, to avoid tooth decay, and to enjoy as much exercise as possible. Although young children are naturally active, as they get older and enter adolescence they lose interest in exercise unless they are encouraged not to.

Until one year of age, a baby grows very rapidly and requires a substantial amount of food relative to its size. However, after one year the child grows less rapidly and will eat less. A weaning diet is usually a healthy balance consisting of fruit and vegetables and cereals with some meat or fish, and this should be encouraged to continue throughout life.

Try to keep any sweet food or drinks until mealtimes, remembering that they should never replace a main meal. There are many alternatives to offer between meals, such as fruit, wholemeal bread, fresh fruit juice, nuts (for those over 4 years of age) and dried fruit, diet drinks and wholemeal crackers. Some more healthy snacks are listed below. If between-meal eating becomes a problem, try adjusting the times of children's meals.

Giving three meals a day may seem easy at first until you realize that not all children conform to this pattern. It is not unusual to find that your child eats very little on some days while on others they will eat as the text books suggest they should – or even more. For a while you can let them live on snacks instead of trying to make them eat meals. If they are planned, snacks can form a nourishing diet. However this should be regarded as a temporary phase only.

Healthy Snacks for Children
    Wholemeal cracker biscuits
    Low fat cheese
    Wholemeal bread or rolls
    Pizza

Wholemeal cereals
Dried fruit* and nuts
Fresh fruit such as apple and banana*
Milk, either whole or semi-skimmed up to the age of five
Low fat yoghurt, preferably plain but if not flavoured with fruit juice
Wholemeal fruit buns
Fresh fruit juice*
Peanut butter.
*NB These are sweet foods and can be damaging to the teeth if eaten frequently between meals.

Encouraging good habits Exercise and fresh air can stimulate appetite. If a child is active and not allowed to eat in between meals, he is more likely to have a better appetite. Sweets, soft drinks, biscuits and other sugary snacks are bad for teeth as well as stopping a healthy appetite at mealtimes, so they should not be eaten between meals and should be kept to a minimum at mealtimes.

The proportions of different foods that should make up a healthy diet with a prudent degree of variety and balance, can be thought of in terms of a pyramid. You will be on the right lines if you try to encourage a child to eat mostly from the bottom two layers of the pyramid: bread and cereals; fruit and vegetables; milk, cheese and yoghurt; and lean meat, poultry, fish, pulses and eggs.

A child who enjoys trying out new foods is easier to feed, but forcing a child to try new foods will only make him resist. If he is used to being allowed to help himself from a serving dish and if his parents regularly try out new foods and recipes, he should be encouraged to experiment too.

Refusing food Many children are finicky eaters. This can be extremely tiresome for the mother who may be uncertain what to provide at the next meal. Whenever possible, offer children the same food as yourself, but if they refuse to eat it don't force them. Don't ask them what they want instead, or food will become a weapon – a way in which children try to control you. Children may refuse food once or twice, but you will probably find that over the course of a few weeks their diet balances out – provided you don't let them see you are either anxious or upset about what they are, or are not, eating.

If the problem persists here are a few things you might try:

* Stop giving any in-between meals or snacks as they may be filling them up or taking the edge off their appetite.
* Change the time of the meal – for example, try 5-hourly meals instead.
* Occasionally offer an alternative, but this should be another main course not a sweet.
* Offer drinks after food rather than before as these may be filling them up.

If your child still seems to be eating very little seek help from your local doctor or health visitor. They will most likely reassure you that your child is healthy and will give you the confidence to continue to provide a healthy balanced diet.

If your children refuse to eat vegetables, try offering some fruit instead. Or you can add vegetables to cooked dishes, such as home-made soups or casseroles. If they will only eat a few vegetables, serve these but also keep offering new ones from time to time without insisting that they're eaten. Growing your own vegetables and letting children help you pick and prepare them can help to overcome their refusal to eat vegetables. Or let them help you choose fruit and vegetables when you go shopping and encourage them to try new varieties.

Many children don't like drinking milk but they may still be happy to consume it in soups, milkshakes or sauces. If not, try to get them to eat some yoghurt or cheese, which should supply the calcium that their bodies need. Alternatively other sources of calcium are available from bread, oranges, soya beans, nuts and dark green vegetables.

Demanding too much food There are those children who eat anything they are offered and are always demanding food. This should not be allowed to get out of hand or you may end up with an overweight child. However, if your child is slim, he probably needs all the extra food he is eating, and, providing he is not filling up on sweets and biscuits, you can let him eat his fill of bread, crackers, fruit and so forth. If your child appears to have a weight problem you can help by making sure that you keep your stores of easily "borrowed" food to a minimum in both the cupboard and refrigerator and by making sure that you don't put out too much food at mealtimes. Encouraging children to exercise or play can often take their mind off food.

CHECKLIST

DO
1. Make the food look attractive.
2. Give small portions of food on the plate. If a child is hungry he can always come back for more. Preferably let children serve themselves.
3. Try to eat as a family as much as is possible. If this is difficult, invite their friends to eat with you as often as possible, as it is important that they learn about social eating.
4. Try not to fuss children while they are eating as a lot of concentration is required. Allow them to eat with fingers if they prefer, although encourage them to eat with a spoon and fork and eventually a knife.
5. Let them go without food if they seem tired. Make sure they get back to a regular sleeping and eating pattern as habits often slip as children get older.
6. Ignore food refusal as much as possible as most children go through a stage of not wanting to eat and it is important not to let your child see this as a potential battleground.
7. Seek professional help if any of these problems persist.
DON'T
1. Force them to eat what they don't want to eat.
2. Give them too much to drink with the meal as this may fill them up. They shouldn't need more than 1-1¼ pints (0.5-0.7 litres) milk a day. More than this and you may find they won't eat the other foods they require for health.
3. Make promises during the day with sweets or puddings. Much better to let them get down from the meal if they don't eat and make the next meal a bit earlier.

Children in the kitchen Children love helping in the kitchen. If your child is a faddy eater this is one way of overcoming his dislikes for certain foods. By helping prepare the food he becomes more interested in it – although he may take some time before he eats it. Don't encourage him to make just cakes and puddings, but involve him in helping you with main dishes as well. A child can put vegetables into a stew just as easily as he can put currants into a cake mixture.

Here are some items you can both prepare during a child's early years in the kitchen:

Sprout bean sprouts or mustard and cress

Make wholemeal bread and rolls in appropriate shapes

Make your own muesli

Make your own yoghurt

Make your own milkshake with fresh fruit such as banana or orange juice and milk

Cut bread up into shapes with animal cutters, etc. and toast these to have with cheese or sardines

Make wholemeal scones with added sultanas, apple or nuts or a combination of all of them

Make a savoury dip to eat with raw vegetables

Make salads

——*ADOLESCENTS*——

During this period the growth spurt occurs at different ages. For boys it is between 12-19 whereas for girls it is between 10-15. During this growth spurt the body requires more calories per kilogram of body weight than during any other period except infancy. Because of their different hormones, boys end up with a higher amount of muscle than girls, but whereas boys have only 8 per cent body fat, girls have 20 per cent, predominantly on the hips, thighs and breasts.

The eating habits of teenagers often become irregular, consisting of more fast foods than their parents approve of. This can mean that girls who are trying to slim may have a diet that is deficient in important nutrients such as vitamins A and C, iron and calcium. A recent nutritional survey on the eating habits of teenagers revealed that too much reliance was placed on the sort of processed foods that are high in fat, sugar and salt and low in fibre, and that quantities of soft drinks, chocolates, biscuits and white bread, which do not add up to healthy eating, were consumed. Teenagers, like everyone else, should be careful about the amounts of fatty, fried and sugary foods they consume. If they have small appetites or choose to fill themselves up on "empty calories" such as sweets, buns and sugary drinks, their intake of iron, calcium and vitamin C stores can often be inadequate.

Teenagers should try, therefore, to increase the amount of fibre in their diet by eating wholemeal or high fibre foods. Making sandwiches with wholemeal bread and eating baked beans, nuts, dried apricots and wholemeal breakfast cereals are all quick and easy ways of doing this. As many wholemeal products are also higher in iron than refined varieties, increasing fibre intake also ensures that iron intake is increased. Iron is needed for both the development of new muscle tissue and to cope with increased haemoglobin demands. (Haemoglobin is the blood

During this growth spurt the body requires more calories per kilogram of body weight than during any other period except infancy.

pigment that carries oxygen to the body's tissues.) Iron is particularly important during menstruation so teenage girls, who are still growing when they start their periods, need to have built up plentiful supplies. Some iron-rich foods are listed on page 48.

Excessive dieting can also be a problem at this age especially among girls, and the table below summarizes minimum acceptable weights for a range of heights. Weights below these may suggest the risk of anorexia nervosa, when the sufferer has a profound fear of putting on weight.

MINIMUM ACCEPTABLE WEIGHTS

Height in feet and inches	Height in metres	Weight in stones and pounds	Weight in kilograms
4 9	1.45	6 0	38
4 10	1.48	6 3	39.5
4 11	1.50	6 5	40.5
5 0	1.52	6 7	41.5
5 1	1.54	6 10	42.5
5 1½	1.56	6 13	44
5 2	1.58	7 1	45
5 3	1.60	7 3	46
5 4	1.62	7 5	47
5 5	1.64	7 9	48.5
5 5½	1.66	7 11	49.5
5 6	1.68	7 13	50.5
5 7	1.70	8 2	52
5 8	1.72	8 5	53

The principal nutritional risk for boys comes from drinking alcohol. Alcohol-related diseases are the leading cause of death in the 15-24 age group. Therefore it is important that they realize the dangers of alcohol and the importance of safe drinking habits.

Adolescents sometimes become very interested in food and decide that the "conventional way" of eating is not for them. They may want to try dietary customs that are radically different from those of their families, the most frequent change being a switch to vegetarianism. Unfortunately, many teenagers adopt a vegetarian diet with insufficient knowledge. Teenagers who become vegetarian just by cutting out meat and eating more vegetables may go short of iron unless they eat more pulses and cereals. Guidelines for a balanced vegetarian diet are given on pages 229-233.

Teenagers who move away from home for the first time to attend college or to work and go to live in digs or a flat can undergo a dramatic change in lifestyle, especially if they have had little experience of cooking and shopping for food. Initially, sharing accommodation with others can help to overcome some of the problems, and some sort of rota system to share the shopping and cooking can be organized. Buying larger quantities of food and sharing the fuel costs usually proves most economical.

> *Alcohol-related diseases are the leading cause of death in the 15-24 age group.*

Store cupboard for students:
  Pasta, preferably wholemeal
  Rice, preferably brown
  Flour
  Tinned tomatoes
  Tomato purée
  Cartons of UHT skimmed or semi-skimmed milk or powdered skimmed milk
  Breakfast cereals
  Herbs and spiccs
  Cans of beans or dried pulses
  Tins of tuna fish
  Potatoes (keep in dark cool place)
  Onions (keep in a dark place)
  Sunflower, saffron, corn or soya oil

In the fridge
  Cheese
  Eggs
  Milk
  Polyunsaturate margarine
Some simple meals that can be made even on a student grant are listed below:
  Cauliflower cheese with tomato salad and wholemeal bread
  Baked beans on toast and fresh orange juice
  Chilli con carne with brown rice
  Stir-fry liver and vegetables with brown rice
  Spaghetti bolognese
  Tuna in tomato sauce with pasta
  Risotto with chicken or chicken livers, pepper, onions, brown rice and salad
  Piperade with wholemeal bread
  Spanish omelette with wholemeal bread
  Potato layer bake with onions, bacon, low fat cheese and stock served with
    French beans
  Jacket potato with grated cheese and salad
  Grilled mackerel with mustard served with potatoes, white cabbage and carrots
  Meat, vegetable and haricot casserole served with jacket potatoes and cabbage
  Home-made minestrone soup with wholemeal bread and cheese
  Grilled home-made hamburgers made with lean mince plus salad and whole-
    meal rolls
  Fish pie with peas and carrots

DIET AND ACNE

Acne affects both boys and girls and is commonly believed to be aggravated by chocolate, fatty foods, soft drinks and beer, although there is little evidence to support the link with diet. However, it is probably not so much that these foods

> *Acne affects both boys and girls and is commonly believed to be aggravated by chocolate, fatty foods, soft drinks and beer, although there is little evidence to support the link with diet.*

cause acne as the fact that when eaten in large quantities they can crowd out other more important nutrients, such as zinc, polyunsaturated fatty acids and vitamin A, which have all been reported to improve skin health.

——THE ELDERLY——

Diet matters at any age, but as long as food is enjoyed and eaten with a reasonable appetite the older person is unlikely to have any special dietary needs. However, if the amount eaten declines substantially, health may be affected. A decline in food intake can often be associated with a number of factors such as poor health, a recent bereavement resulting in living alone and having to cook for one.

Elderly people who are also chronically sick are most likely to be at risk from nutritional deficiency. Pain, handicap, long-term drug therapy (including aspirin and laxatives) and badly fitting dentures, can all make getting, and eating, an adequate diet difficult. In such cases, especially adapted eating and cooking aids for the disabled, and possibly a curtailment by the doctor of some inessential drugs can do much to improve the appetite. The housebound may need a small supplement of vitamin D, although sitting in the sunlight by an open window can improve the body's stores of this vitamin.

The factors that might affect diet:
* Being alone – it is often easier "not to bother" cooking for one
* Difficulty in getting to the shops
* A sudden drop in income or sharp increase in living expenses
* Bereavement – widowers especially often don't know how to shop or cook
* Depression
* Anorexia – loss of appetite as a result of illness or as a side-effect of medication
* Disabilities such as arthritis or recent blindness
* Severe reduction in mobility or activity

The use of some common drugs can also lead to malnutrition: diuretics and laxatives cause potassium loss; aspirin may cause blood loss and so lead to iron deficiency; Digoxin lowers appetite; Phenformin or Metformin affect the absorption of vitamin B_{12}; and Co-trimoxazole affects the absorption of folic acid, one of the B vitamins.

But if less food is eaten – and this may be deliberate in the case of a weight problem – there is still the same need for nutrients like vitamins and minerals so the quality of the diet must be safeguarded. A diet of just tea, bread and jam or instant soup and crispbread will not benefit anyone.

TYPICAL REDUCTIONS IN NUTRIENTS MADE BY 70-80 YEAR OLDS

Calories and nutrients	Fall in intake %
Calories	19
Protein	24
Fat	30
Carbohydrate	8
Calcium	18
Iron	29
Vitamin C	31

The dietary guidelines for adults (see Chapter 9) continue to apply after retirement with only a few modifications.

Calories Keeping weight down is especially important as with age the less supple the body becomes and the fewer strains it can take.

> *Keeping your weight down is especially important as the older you are the less supple your body becomes and the fewer strains it can take.*

As the body ages the amount of lean muscle tissue usually decreases in proportion to the amount of fat. Fewer calories are therefore required to maintain weight, although the extent to which this happens depends substantially on the amount of exercise that is taken and exercising regularly keeps your muscles and bones in shape. One study showed that the food intake of those living in rural areas was substantially more than those living in urban areas yet those in rural areas were less likely to be overweight. There could be a number of reasons for this, but the study could indicate that those who lived in rural areas exercised more than those who lived in urban areas. Although you need fewer calories, the need for other nutrients does not diminish, and exercise can be a good way of stimulating the appetite.

Protein Although the requirement for protein diminishes with age as lean muscle tissue is reduced, so does the ability to digest and absorb food. Protein intake therefore needs to be adequate, but if a varied diet is eaten, protein intake is unlikely to be at risk.

Fibre People are now much more aware of the role that fibre plays in the diet. Constipation can be a problem for the elderly as their digestive systems do not function so efficiently, especially if they take little exercise. To help overcome this problem many elderly people turn to laxatives, and they may be abetted by their doctors who are used to prescribing laxatives instead of trying their patients on extra fibre first. Laxatives not only further decrease the limited muscle function of the digestive system but can – if taken for long periods – also prevent the absorption of many valuable nutrients, particularly vitamins and minerals.

Supplementing the diet with bran can help give temporary relief from constipation, although it should be avoided as a long-term solution whenever possible. Like laxatives, bran may interfere with the absorption of valuable nutrients such as calcium. Rather than using bran or laxatives it is much better to consume a diet that is high in fibre (see page 29). If you find that a bran or wholemeal cereal is not enough and you do need an extra supplement of raw bran to sprinkle on food, then drink extra fluid.

If it is not possible to bite into an apple, the apple can be cut up into pieces. It is important to chew food, as chewing stimulates the saliva flow. As we have seen, saliva has three important functions: it brings out the taste of food, it helps start the digestive process and it helps keep the mouth healthy. If badly fitting dentures are a problem, a dentist may be able to help. However, if there are any difficulties with hard fruit and raw vegetables, try to eat soft or stewed fruit and cooked vegetables, wholemeal bread and wholegrain breakfast cereals instead.

Iron There should be no need for iron tablets (which can also be a cause of constipation) unless you are severely anaemic. It is much more important to ensure that the diet supplies an adequate amount of iron. Many iron-rich foods, for example, liver, lean meat, sardines, spinach, wholemeal bread, nuts and dried fruit, wholegrain breakfast cereals and pulses such as beans and lentils, are also either high in fibre or protein or both.

Vitamin C Vitamin C is needed in increased amounts if the body is fighting infection or recovering from an injury such as a broken knee or a surgical operation. You should ensure that you eat one food rich in vitamin C each day. The easiest way to ensure an adequate supply of this vitamin is to have a glass of fresh orange or grapefruit juice each day, but other good sources of this vitamin are tomatoes, peppers, broccoli, cauliflower, brussel sprouts, strawberries, raspberries and blackberries.

Vitamin D Vitamin D is needed to transport calcium from the blood to the bones and back again. As the majority of our vitamin D comes from sunlight, the housebound should try to sit in the summer sun whenever possible, even if it means covering yourself with a cellular blanket that allows the sunlight through. Alternatively your doctor may wish to prescribe a vitamin supplement.

Cooking and shopping hints It is a sensible plan to keep a storecupboard of a few essential items for an emergency. A small freezer or fridge freezer can be a worthwhile investment. The sorts of foods you should store in your food cupboard should include: dried beans and pulses such as lentils; dried milk powder or UHT milk, which is useful for sauces, soups and making hot drinks; cartons of fresh fruit juice; tins of fish such as salmon, tuna or sardines; rice or pasta; porridge oats and other breakfast cereals; soups, especially lentil and pea soups; tinned tomatoes; tinned fruit in natural juice; tea and coffee. If you have a freezer, then packets of ham or bacon, fish in sauce, some sliced bread and grated cheese can be kept.

Although it is often a good idea to buy small quantities of fresh food so that nothing is wasted, it may be cheaper or more convenient to buy larger quantities for cooking and to freeze some in smaller portions.

If going to the shops is frustrating because they always seem busy, try Monday, Tuesday or Wednesday mornings when it is usually quieter. An assistant at the supermarket may be able to give a hand and may even be willing to fill a shopping basket from a shopping list. Ask a neighbour or family for a hand with heavy shopping once a month.

If you find preparing food tiring, take your time over preparation, and rest between stages. Ready-prepared dishes can be useful on occasions, but they usually cost more than dishes you make yourself.

If the appetite is small, then small nourishing snacks and drinks may be easier to cope with. Soups and drinks made with milk may be more palatable. A savoury milk drink, some bread and fruit is a nourishing alternative if a cooked meal is likely to be wasted.

Illness, disability and bereavement

Almost all malnutrition in the elderly is secondary to illness or disability. For instance, many drugs can interfere with the appetite, and if it is difficult to prepare or cook food it is sometimes easier simply to eat less. Widowers are also at particular risk of malnutrition if they have had little experience of buying, preparing and cooking foods.

If preparing food is difficult, perhaps because of arthritis in the hands, it is worth contacting the Disabled Living Foundation (address on page 326) for a list of suitable gadgets. The aids available include large-handled knives for easier gripping, non-slip mats to go underneath mixing basins, tongs, clamps and rubber grips for undoing screw tops. Some of these items are available from local shops, although others may have to be ordered from specialist shops.

Apart from these special aids, a sharp knife will be invaluable – blunt blades are not only difficult to use but are more dangerous. An electric or wall can opener and, maybe, a food processor for grating cheese or vegetables, could be helpful, while a microwave oven may also be worth considering. Microwave ovens do not involve bending, food can be thawed and reheated quickly, the controls are easy to operate, there is less risk of burns and they can save on washing-up. And if you don't know how to cook, buying a microwave oven may be more appealing than attending cookery classes.

——VEGETARIANS——

Over three million people are vegetarian in this country and the indications are that this number is rising. Many well-known people are vegetarian and nowadays vegetarians are certainly no longer thought of as cranks.

Vegetarianism embraces a range of different eating habits. Perhaps the most limited types of diets are those of the Zen macrobiotics and fruitarians. Vegans will eat a range of plant foods but no products of animal origin. Lactovegetarians will, in addition to plant products, eat dairy food such as cheese and yoghurt and will drink milk. This diet, with the addition of eggs, is also eaten by ovolactovegetarians.

In addition to the mainstream vegetarian movements, the recent interest in healthy eating has encouraged some people to become part-time vegetarians. Although this may be one way of saving money, the reasons are usually based on concern about health. Many people eat vegetarian food at home, but allow themselves to eat meat and fish when eating out.

WHY DO PEOPLE BECOME VEGETARIAN?

As we have seen, health is one of the reasons why people may become vegetarians, but there are a number of others. In recent years ecological considerations have become more important; many people feel a profound unease at the large amounts of land needed to produce meat compared with that required for cereals or other plant foods. It can take between 2 and 10lb (0.9-4.5kg) of grain to produce 1lb (0.4kg) of edible meat. A hectare of land, if planted, can produce ten times as much vegetable protein as the same land used for grazing cattle could produce in animal protein.

There is also a feeling that animals, being nearer the top of the food chain, may absorb undesirable levels of various pollutants. This has been dramatically demonstrated in Europe recently by the Chernobyl nuclear accident, after which several types of grazing animals, notably reindeer and sheep, were found to have unacceptably high levels of radiation even a year after the accident. Growth hormones used in meat production or rather the misuse of them are also seen as a potential problem by many and their use in many European countries has now been banned.

Others become vegetarian for religious or moral reasons. Many religions, for example Buddhism, Hinduism and Jainism, require their adherents to be vegetarian. Trappist monks and Seventh-day Adventists are also vegetarians. Some people become vegetarian because they are unhappy about the way that meat is produced and processed.

For others, adopting a vegetarian diet is simply an expression of concern about what they see happening in the world around them: the changes in the environment – the destruction of the countryside by the uprooting of hedges and the draining of land; property developments outside cities which leave inner cities to decay; concern about nuclear fuel; and concern about animals being used for experiments. The rise of vegetarianism can be seen as part of this questioning attitude towards the priorities and values of our society.

Are Vegetarians Healthier than Omnivores?

Vegetarians can be healthier than the general population, but this is not necessarily so. Vegetarians may have as fatty a diet as non-vegetarians, particularly if cheese and whole milk make up a large part of what they eat.

Much of the research on how healthy a vegetarian diet is has been carried out in the United States on Seventh-day Adventists, who suffer much less heart disease than their fellow Americans – approximately 60 per cent less. As they don't smoke or drink alcohol either, it is hard for researchers to determine whether it is the diet or the combined effects of a healthy, ascetic lifestyle. However recent research on vegetarians in the UK indicates that their diet is healthier as their blood cholesterol levels were considerably lower.

The fibre content of most vegetarians' diet is often 30 to 50 per cent higher than that of the average omnivore. A vegetarian's fat intake, particularly the intake of saturated fats, is usually lower than an omnivore's, provided the vegetarian does not eat an excessive amount of foods like full fat milk, hard cheese and eggs. Therefore, vegetarians should apply the same rules to choosing a healthy diet as anyone else.

Vegetarians are generally less overweight than omnivores, largely because their diet is much higher in fibre and lower in fat – or they may just be more health conscious than the rest of the population.

A Guide to Being Vegetarian

Like the rest of us vegetarians must ensure that their diet contains enough protein and enough calories for growth and the rebuilding of the body's tissues. It is, on the whole, easy to be a healthy vegetarian as long as you don't eat a restrictive diet. Experienced vegetarians do not usually find this a problem as they eat dishes containing a variety of items such as cereals, beans, nuts and vegetables, which not only ensures a good mix of proteins but also of the other nutrients needed for health.

It is rare for vegetarians not to eat enough protein, and the few cases that have been reported are usually associated with a failure to eat enough food of any sort – i.e., they didn't eat enough calories. Cereals, beans, pulses and nuts should predominate in the diet, particularly if few dairy products are consumed. Lack of iron can also be a problem, especially for teenagers or those on a restrictive diet. Increased amounts of beans and pulses, nuts and dried fruit or wholegrain cereals should help to overcome this problem, while fresh fruit and vegetables will provide the vitamin C to help the absorption of iron.

To ensure an adequate diet, whether it is vegetarian, vegan or macrobiotic, make sure that the diet includes something from each of the following groups:

Group 1
Pasta, bread, rice, cereals, preferably wholemeal.
Group 2
Fruit, fruit juice, vegetables including potatoes but not chips or crisps.
Group 3
Cheese, milk, yoghurt, soya milk, soya cheese.
Group 4
Eggs, beans, lentils, nuts and tofu (meat, poultry and fish).

CHANGING TO A VEGETARIAN DIET
Those who have been vegetarian for some time have usually learnt new cooking habits as well as introduced new foods into their diets. However, some people think that changing to a vegetarian diet means changing to the meat analogues like texturized vegetable protein (TVP). Although it is still possible to buy these substitutes, they never achieved the sales that their manufacturers hoped when they appeared in the mid-1970s. Although these meat substitutes are easy to store and contain only a small amount of fat, most vegetarians do not use them.

If you are about to adopt a vegetarian diet, here are some guidelines:

1. Use beans and pulses to replace meat or fish.
2. Go easy on the amount of high fat foods, particularly hard cheese and full fat milk.
3. Remember to include some salads in your diet. Vegetables that are cooked for a long time lose most or all of their folic acid.
4. Brown sugar or honey is no better for you than white sugar, so don't think that by using them you are gaining any nutritional advantage.
5. Only use the minimum amount of oil when frying, especially with vegetables like mushrooms and aubergines that soak up the oil. Instead use a non-stick frying pan, with the minimum amount of oil over a low heat.
6. Eat plenty of high fibre foods such as brown rice, wholemeal bread, wholemeal pasta and wholemeal breakfast cereals.

Vegetarians who don't want to rely on vegetarian convenience foods such as vegeburgers, vegetable pancakes and pasties often complain at first that there are no quick meals they can cook to replace the "meat and two veg". However, once they have established which new dishes they like, they can make double the quantity of those that are suitable for freezing. Here are some examples that you might find useful:

Tomato sauce can be used for pasta, pizza, ratatouille, to cook with beans or in lasagne
Wholemeal pancakes can be stuffed with stir-fried vegetables, vegetables in cheese sauce, ratatouille or with a bean sauce
Nut or bean rissoles or loaves can be frozen in portion-sized pieces
Home-made vegetable soup such as minestrone
Vegetable lasagne
Wholemeal quiche

Mushroom "burgers"
Stuffed vegetables
Vegetable curry
Vegetable goulash
Vegetable moussaka
Vegetarian stew

The recent interest in vegetarian eating has led to the publication of several good books. These will provide you with further ideas that will stimulate your interest in cookery.

YOUNGER VEGETARIANS

Many children have been brought up successfully as vegetarians. However, it is crucial that a child's diet is properly balanced because younger bodies require a higher percentage of protein and calories relative to their body weight. If a baby has pulses at least once a day, wholemeal bread or cereals two or three times a day and a pint of milk or its equivalent in cheese or yoghurt, plus fruit and vegetables, it will get sufficient of the vitamins, minerals and protein it needs. A baby will also need some fatty foods such as full fat milk, cheese or polyunsaturated margarine in order to get enough energy or calories. Provided a child's weight and growth are satisfactory and he or she is eating a variety of foods, he or she is getting all the calories and nutrients necessary. After a baby has been weaned there should be no need for any special food for a vegetarian child, providing that he is healthy.

The child of vegetarian parents may rebel against a vegetarian diet as he grows older. Although it is possible to ensure that he eats a vegetarian diet at home, it may be wise to let him eat meat or fish a few times at friends' houses so that he feels less socially isolated.

VEGETARIAN MENUS

Below are five daily menus – breakfast, lunch and evening meal – that will provide vegetarians with a balanced and varied diet.

Orange juice; peanut butter sandwich.
Pizza; green salad; fresh fruit.
Nut roast; jacket potato; steamed cabbage and carrots with cumin seeds; melon and
    orange fruit salad.

Wheatflakes and skimmed milk; toast and marmalade.
Cheese and tomato wholemeal rolls; fruit and nut bar; apple.
Green lentil and aubergine lasagne; cauliflower, walnut and watercress salad;
    grated carrot salad; orange.

Orange juice; cheese on toast.
Hummus with pitta bread and salad; fresh fruit salad.
Pepper and tomato quiche; jacket potatoes; French beans.

Muesli and skimmed milk.
Pasta with tomato sauce and Parmesan cheese; green salad; banana.
Stir-fried bean curd with vegetables and brown rice; fresh fruit salad.

Orange juice; wholemeal toast and poached egg.
Cauliflower cheese; wholemeal rolls; tomato and pepper salad.
Kidney bean and vegetable goulash; cooked cracked wheat; natural yoghurt; baked
  apple and custard.

—VEGANS—

A strict vegan diet is much bulkier than a vegetarian diet so people with small appetites such as children need to ensure they eat enough calories. There have been
some recent reports of children being malnourished because of extreme diets, but
these children were found to be on very restrictive diets indeed. This is not to say
that children cannot be raised on a vegan diet, but it must be done with the utmost
care. It is essential to make sure that no minerals and vitamins are lacking and that
they have enough to eat. The nutrients most likely to cause problems are calcium,
vitamin D and vitamin B_{12}.

The one vitamin that is not provided by the vegan diet is vitamin B_{12}. Deficiency
of this vitamin may take a long time to develop, but it can result in impaired blood
cell formation and nerve damage. This vitamin is found only in foods of animal origin with the exception of miso, tempeh, baker's yeast, brewer's yeast and fortified
soya milks. However, such foods may not be regularly eaten in sufficient quantities,
and it is recommended that supplements of this vitamin are taken. Vitamin B_{12} is
not usually required by the breastfed infant as long as the mother has enough vitamin B_{12} in her diet, but when weaning commences the infant should be fed on soya
milk containing this vitamin.

Folic acid, another B vitamin, which is in cereals and vegetables, is destroyed by
cooking. It is important that some raw vegetables should be included in the diet.

Lack of calcium may be a problem for vegans who don't consume milk or cheese,
but the following foods contain worthwhile amounts of calcium and may help: most
nuts (but particularly almonds); broccoli; soya beans; bean curd; soya milk or
yoghurt or cheese made from soya milk; dried fruit; and any dark green vegetables.
Pregnant women who don't like drinking milk may also find some of these other
sources of calcium useful.

Vitamin D should not be a problem if children have adequate sunshine or are
given the required dosage of vitamin supplements between 1 month and 5 years.
Milk-free margarines are also fortified by this vitamin.

Vegan meals could include:

Bulgar wheat paella; green salad with mushrooms; raspberry sorbet.
Mushroom and rice stuffed marrow; wholemeal bread; apricot crumble with soya
  milk.
Mushroom and barley loaf; tomato and aubergine bake; jacket potatoes; fresh
  fruit.
Black-eyed bean curry and rice; cucumber and tofu salad; tomato salad; baked
  apple.
Spinach soup; lentil rissoles; salad; wholemeal bread.
Vegetable crumble; brown rice risotto; peaches in orange juice.

FRUITARIANS AND MACROBIOTIC REGIMES

A macrobiotic diet is based on unrefined cereals, notably brown rice, and excludes or limits fruit and vegetables. A fruitarian diet consists of fruit, nuts and seeds. These diets tend to be rather extreme and cases have been reported of protein energy malnutrition, anaemia and vitamin deficiency. Every diet, whether unorthodox or traditional, should be checked to make sure it regularly includes something from each of the first two groups set out earlier (see page 231).

CHAPTER 11

SPECIAL DIETS FOR MEDICAL CONDITIONS

*M*ost people who eat a special diet do so as part of their medical treatment. However, the recent interest in healthy eating has been accompanied by an increase in the number of people following a special diet in the belief that this will alleviate a condition – such as recurring headaches. There is often no scientific proof that such a diet does help, but there is no reason not to follow it as long as it is nutritionally sound. Most problems arise when diets are too restricted and not nutritionally sound. Following a special diet can also create emotional strains within the family, and these must be carefully balanced against whatever benefits the diet may be thought to be bringing. Of course, when the diet is part of medical treatment it should always be followed. If there are any problems, a doctor can refer you to a dietitian.

As more people become aware of special diets and the reasons for them, there is much less stigma attached, although pressure from their peers can put considerable stress on children in this position. Some special diets are easier to stick to than others. Diabetic diets, for example, can be almost identical to a normal healthy diet. The diabetic who takes insulin will need to make other minor adjustments to his life, such as organizing the timing of the insulin and meals and snacks, but he will need to make little alteration to what he eats. Someone on a gluten-free diet, however, may need to reorganize his diet extensively.

In this section we will look at the major types of special diets and discuss some suggestions to try to make them more interesting.

—ALLERGIES—

With all the recent media attention given to food allergies one might think that they have become more prevalent. It may be true that allergies are more common than was once thought, but most doctors and nutritionists feel that now more people are aware of food allergies they are ready to blame all their symptoms on food (see pages 90-4).

Allergies seem to run in families. When both parents suffer from conditions like

Allergies seem to run in families. When both parents suffer from diseases like hayfever, eczema or asthma, they have a 60 per cent chance of passing this sensitivity on to their child, although the child may not exhibit the same symptoms or to the same degree.

hayfever, eczema or asthma they have a 60 per cent chance of passing this sensitivity on to their child, although the child may not exhibit the same symptoms or to the same degree.

An allergy may be suspected for various reasons: a rash that won't go away; bouts of headaches for no particular reason; feelings of being bloated; an irritable bowel; eczema and so on. You may even suspect which food is causing the trouble. Although it is possible to treat yourself if you are allergic to a minor item of diet such as chocolate or coffee, it is always wiser to seek professional help if more important foods are to be excluded. This is particularly true for those who suffer from multiple allergies or from allergies to foods that are a major constituent of our usual diet such as milk, eggs and wheat. However, allergic reactions can be temporary and may stop of their own accord. The individual in some way acquires a tolerance or "grows out of" reacting to the allergic stimulus.

A few years ago many doctors would have been dismissive of the suggestion that symptoms were caused by food, but today many are more sympathetic. If a doctor feels your symptoms are severe enough and that an allergy may be the cause, he can refer you to the local allergy clinic, or to a paediatric or dermatology department where extensive tests can be carried out.

If a hospital consultation indicates that someone is allergic to a food, he will probably be taken into hospital and tested with a range of different diets to assess the reaction. Alternatively the patient may be asked to eat something called an "elimination or exclusion diet" in order to discover which foods can and cannot be eaten without provoking allergic symptoms.

Although these diets have been published, they should never be undertaken except under medical supervision. They are so extreme that it is possible to make yourself ill, rather than better, by following them. Vegetarians, young children, pregnant mothers and the elderly should be especially careful about treating themselves because many foods that cause allergic symptoms, like eggs, milk and wheat, may be the mainstay of their diet.

The most common food-related allergies are usually those to foods that are taken frequently. As we have seen, wheat, milk and eggs are among the most well-known, but tomatoes and citrus fruits can cause food allergies too. The first three mentioned are particularly hard to avoid because they are often an integral part of another food. Eggs are often used in the manufacture of bread, quiches, pasta, soup, cakes and biscuits, while the nutritional consequences of eliminating a food, particularly one like milk – the largest provider of calcium in our diet – could be extremely serious.

It may take more than one hospital consultation to diagnose the food allergy, because some allergies, especially multiple food allergies, require extensive tests and research. Once the allergy has been diagnosed, a dietitian will translate the diagnosis into simple advice to be carried out at home. The dietitian will also have lists of branded goods which will be suitable for the patient. Although food allergy diets require a lot of work and effort, the benefits of such diets are soon felt.

——COELIAC DISEASE——

Coeliac disease is caused by the protein gluten which is found in many cereals. The disease is characterized by gluten damaging the tissue in the gut and preventing the absorption of fat. It is a wasting disease and causes a wide variety of additional symptoms, such as feeling bloated, anaemia, weight loss or failure to put on weight, and the failure to absorb certain nutrients, particularly the fat-soluble vitamins A and D.

Why one person should suffer from coeliac disease and not another is unknown, although it is thought that heredity plays some part. It is uncertain if the disease is due to the amount of gluten eaten before or after the onset of the disease. Nor is it understood why some get this disease as children and others as adults. It can also affect babies at the time they are weaned, and a perfectly healthy baby will suddenly "fail to thrive". It has been suggested that the disease occurs in babies who have been given wheat too early.

Some patients suffering from other conditions such as dermatitis herpetiformis or psoriasis find that a gluten-free diet helps to relieve their symptoms. Why such a diet should sometimes help is unknown, but medical advice should be sought before embarking on the diet.

Gluten is found mainly in wheat, but also, although to a lesser extent, in rye and barley. Most coeliacs can tolerate oats, but a few find that they have to avoid these as well. Gluten has particular characteristics that make it extremely useful in cooking. When mixed with water it forms a stretchy, elastic substance, not unlike chewing gum, and in bread-making gluten stretches to hold the gas produced in the dough and so enabling a light rather than a heavy, solid bread.

People suffering from coeliac disease have to keep to a gluten-free diet for life, but following the diet will enable them to lead an otherwise healthy life. Vitamin tablets may have to be prescribed initially, but, as the patient begins to respond to the diet, they can be stopped.

Although many foods do not contain gluten, keeping to such a diet requires an extensive knowledge of commercially prepared foods, for many of them use wheat for a variety of purposes, such as thickening, binding and as a filler. Thickened sauces and gravies served when patients are eating in hotels or restaurants are an obvious danger, but gluten is not, unfortunately, always clearly identifiable on labels. Descriptions that might imply that gluten is present include: cereal binder, wheat flour, wheat starch, rusk, edible starch, food starch, malt, cereal filler and hydrolyzed protein. A few manufacturers label their food in such a way (a crossed grain) that coeliacs can easily recognize gluten-free products.

The Coeliac Society, formed in 1968, is run by and for people with coeliac disease or dermatitis herpetiformis (see addresses on page 326). The Society produces an extremely useful list of

Descriptions that might imply that gluten is present include: cereal binder, wheat flour, wheat starch, rusk, edible starch, food starch, malt, cereal filler and hydrolysed protein.

manufactured goods that do not contain gluten. This list is updated yearly and at regular intervals in their newsletter.

GLUTEN-FREE FOODS

Meat All meat except sausages, beefburgers, meat paste, pies, canned meat and any rolled in flour or breadcrumbs.

Fish All fish except canned fish in sauce, fishfingers, fish cakes and any covered in batter or breadcrumbs.

Eggs Except those made into quiches or cakes.

Milk and milk products Cheese, skimmed milk, etc. are gluten-free but watch out, however, for cheese spreads, yoghurts and milkshakes.

Dried beans and lentils Except some canned bean products.

Cereals Such as rice, sago, maize, buckwheat, cornflour, soya flour, potato flour, rice flour, oats, oat flour and millet. Also all gluten-free flours of which high fibre varieties are now available. There is also gluten-free bread, pasta, cakes, biscuits, breakfast cereals and crispbreads. Avoid wheat, barley, rye, ordinary flour, semolina, pasta, breakfast cereals, cakes, biscuits, wheat germ and wheat bran. Go to the chemist for gluten-free biscuits, cakes and bread mixes.

Fruit and vegetables All except those made into pie fillings.

Fats, oils and cream All except suet.

Snacks Most nuts can be eaten except peanut butter and roasted peanuts. Some crisps can be eaten but no twiglets or cheese crackers.

Jam and preserves All except lemon curd, chocolate spread and mincemeat.

Sweets and chocolate Most boiled sweets, but consult the Coeliac Society list.

Puddings Home-made using gluten-free products to make crumbles and pies. Plus fruit sorbets, meringues, jellies and fresh fruit salads. Watch most manufactured puddings.

Drinks Tea, coffee, squashes all except barley water, tomato juice, vending drinks, cocoa and drinking chocolate.

Seasonings and sauces All except curry powder, mixed spices, stock cubes, chutneys and pickles, salad dressings, packet sauces and gravy.

Soups All home-made using gluten-free products but not canned or packet soups.

Alcohol All alcohol except beer, particularly draught beers.

Some gluten-free products are available on prescription, but as coeliacs are not classed as chronically sick or disabled these items are available free only to those exempt from prescription charges. Gluten-free cakes and fancy biscuits are not prescribable but are available for purchase.

It is possible to eat a gluten-free diet that is high in fibre, low in fat and low in sugar. However a newly diagnosed coeliac may not find this initially practical. The most important step is to regain any lost weight, which is helped partly by eating a gluten-free diet and also by eating enough food.

Maintaining a high fibre diet is much easier now than in the past as brown bread mixes are available. It is also possible to make high fibre bread using items such as brown rice flour, yellow split pea flour and ground almonds. Additional fibre can be incorporated into the diet by consuming beans and pulses, nuts, brown rice, buckwheat, millet, oats and fruit and vegetables.

Gluten-free food requires different techniques from normal cooking. Gluten-free pastry has to be kneaded thoroughly, otherwise it is difficult to handle, but sponge cakes made with gluten-free flour are usually extremely light. Making bread usually involves mixing the ingredients as a batter, and the new bread mixes are easier to make successfully.

Eating out can cause problems for coeliacs. However, it is important that they should try to lead a normal life, and they should tell their friends what they can and cannot eat and give them examples of dishes that are suitable. If they are eating out in a restaurant or going on holiday, it is sensible to try to contact the chef in advance to outline food requirements. However, if it is impossible or impracticable to arrange for special food, such dishes as fruit starters, grilled meat and fish, plain vegetables and fresh fruit are all acceptable. Airline or shipping companies are usually willing to provide gluten-free meals if they have plenty of warning, but it may be worthwhile to take some bread or bread mixes on holiday.

Children, particularly teenagers, may be a problem if they start rebelling against the diet. But once they realize how ill they feel without it, it is unlikely they will protest too much. Children with coeliac disease should be taught about their diet as early as possible. This doesn't mean they have got to make all the decisions about the diet themselves but at least if they go to a friend's house they will know what to choose. Parents of coeliac children might like to make all the foods for their parties gluten-free.

Sample meals:

Breakfasts
Gluten-free muesli
Low fat natural yoghurt and banana
Porridge
Brown gluten-free toast with mushrooms
Poached egg and gluten-free toast
Oat muffins made with gluten-free flour
Dried fruit compôte

Packed Lunches
Rice salad
Gluten-free sandwiches
Potato salad
Meat or fish salad
Gluten-free pasta salad
Salads
Fruit
Gluten-free biscuits
Gluten-free soup, e.g., lentil, minestrone
Home-made oat biscuits or cakes

Main meals
As normal, but use arrowroot, cornflour, potato, buckwheat or rice flour to thicken the sauces. Pastry such as shortcrust or suet can be made with gluten-free flour – but don't forget that all pastry is high in fat.

Chicken casserole (don't thicken with wheatflour)
Fish pie
Kebabs
Grilled meat or fish
Chilli con carne – don't forget to check the chilli powder
Vegetables and potatoes
Salad – always check the salad dressings.

Desserts
Sorbets and ices
Crumbles made with millet and oat flakes
Custard
Jelly
Fresh fruit

Sample menus
Chicken tandoori; dhal; nan bread made with gluten-free flour and yoghurt; raita; salad. Mango ice.
Curried chicken salad with banana and apple (made with fresh spices); green bean salad; tomato salad. Plum crumble – topping made with oats, oat flour and soya flour.
Trout with almonds; steamed green beans; steamed new potatoes; steamed carrots. Raspberry fool.
Boeuf Bourguignon – but don't thicken with wheatflour; jacket potato; peas; swede. Baked apples with almond paste and raisins and yoghurt.
Vegetable curry; nut risotto; salad. Oranges in caramel.

—*DIABETES*—

All forms of diabetes result from an inadequate supply of insulin (see page 85). Diabetes produces a variety of symptoms such as blurring of vision, loss of weight for no apparent reason, excessive thirst, frequent passing of urine, tingling of the fingers and lethargy.

MATURITY ONSET DIABETES
A maturity onset diabetic or non-insulin dependent diabetic (NIDD) usually produces insulin but is not able to use it properly, so the amount produced is not enough to stop the onset of the disease (see page 85). It is particularly important that an overweight NIDD loses weight as this will increase the efficiency with which the insulin produced is used. Many NIDDs find that this is the only treatment necessary, but some may require both diet and tablets. The recommended diet is similar to that for normal healthy eating: high fibre, low fat and low sugar. However, those who are taking large doses of tablets need to distribute their food intake carefully, and they should follow similar guidelines as insulin-dependent diabetics (see below).

JUVENILE ONSET DIABETES
The onset of diabetes can occur at any age but is most frequent among young

people. The initial symptoms are similar to, but often more pronounced than, those of the maturity onset diabetic. As the pancreas has completely stopped producing insulin, these diabetics need to inject themselves daily with insulin – hence the term "insulin-dependent diabetics" (IDD).

Until recently the diet of insulin dependent diabetics centred around a restriction of carbohydrate intake. Sugar was excluded and starchy carbohydrate foods were reduced. The diet was designed to prevent the insulin supply from being overburdened. In contrast, protein foods, such as meat, fish, eggs and cheese, and all foods containing a high degree of fat, such as oil, butter, cream and margarine, were allowed freely.

The reasoning behind the low carbohydrate diet was plausible but fallacious. As IDDM diabetics are reliant on an external insulin supply, it seemed logical to reduce the amount of carbohydrate foods eaten and so minimize the amount of glucose produced by these foods, thus reducing the demands on insulin in the body. However, it is now realized that much of the glucose in the blood does not come directly from carbohydrate foods but is released by the liver, and the extent to which this happens is dependent on the total number of calories consumed.

Recent research has shown that blood sugar (glucose) levels of diabetics are better controlled on a high fibre, high carbohydrate, low fat diet. Previously the carbohydrate (CHO) content represented approximately 40 per cent of the energy intake. It is now recommended that this is increased to at least 50 per cent of total energy intake. The carbohydrate units for each food are shown at the end of this section (see pages 244-5).

Daily Calorie Intake	CHO in g to provide 50% of Total Calories
3000	350
2700	330
2500	310
2200	270
2000	250
1700	210
1500	180
1200	150
1000	120

Research has shown that blood sugar levels do not rise as rapidly when a high fibre diet is eaten. If sugar – particularly in large quantities – is given on its own, in sweets or sugared drinks, the diabetic is less likely to be able to cope with the resultant increase in blood sugar. Starchy foods, which are rich in fibre, release their energy more slowly and allow a diabetic to have better control over the sugar. High fibre, starchy foods, particularly oats, beans and lentils, which contain a viscous (gummy) soluble fibre, are of particular importance in retarding the absorption of blood sugar. Some diabetics use guar gum, a soluble fibre that, when mixed with food, has been shown to bring blood sugar levels closer to normal.

Reducing the amount of fat eaten helps to reduce the calorie intake. Heart disease is extremely prevalent among diabetics, and it has been suggested that their fat intake should be reduced, although further research is required to determine which type of fat should be recommended in a diabetic diet. However, as we have already seen, evidence to date suggests that a marked reduction in total fat, particularly saturated fat, with a moderate use of polyunsaturates, helps to lower blood cholesterol levels in most people, including diabetics.

The recommendations for diets for diabetics outlined below are similar to those recommended for the whole population. Catering for the diabetic should be similar to, rather than different from, catering for everyone else in the family. However, there are a few additional rules to follow because the diabetic must also ensure that his insulin requirements are balanced with those of any activity and with the amount and timing of food.

1. Maintain ideal body weight. This should be done by controlling the intake of calories. Always discuss a weight-reducing diet with a doctor or dietitian as it may affect insulin requirements. Never go on a crash diet.
2. Eat a high fibre diet. Try to eat a diet that provides 50 per cent of the energy intake from complex carbohydrates that are rich in fibre.
3. Keep sugar intake to a minimum. Although diabetics can cope with small amounts of sugar, they should use foods that contain significant quantities only occasionally except in an insulin crisis.
4. Reduce your total fat intake. This will help to maintain ideal body weight.
5. Have regular meals and snacks. Eating at regular times will help to maintain good blood sugar control, particularly for those on tablets or insulin. The meal pattern can be worked out to fit in with individual lifestyles, and because the insulin will still be active at night a bedtime snack is necessary.

Special Advice Relating to Certain Foods
Unsweetened Fruit Juice Although unsweetened fruit juice can be included in small quantities on a diabetic's diet, it must be counted as part of the carbohydrate allowance. Too much fruit juice instead of fruit should not be relied on as it does not contain any of the fibre that is present in fruit.
Alcohol Unless contrary to medical advice, moderate amounts of alcohol may be consumed provided that its energy contribution is taken into account. However, diabetics on insulin or tablets should not count alcohol as one of their carbohydrate exchanges; it is preferable for these to come from food. Choose dry wines, beers and lager, but avoid beers and lagers that are low in carbohydrate and even some of those that are brewed specially for diabetics: these may have both a higher alcohol and a higher calorie content (see below). Drink spirits only occasionally, and if a mixer is used, make sure it is a low calorie one. The maximum recommended amount is three drinks a day, although it is better to drink less.

Overweight diabetics should not have more than one drink a day as part of their diet. Never drink on an empty stomach unless food is to follow shortly, and it is essential that any bedtime snack taken after drinking alcohol in the evening is of the high fibre variety. Sweet alcoholic drinks such as port or liqueurs are not recommended. If there are any doubts about whether alcohol can be drunk, ask a doctor or dietitian for advice.
Sweeteners Fructose is now being used by diabetics to make occasional cakes and biscuits at home. It is one and a half times as sweet (and four times as expensive) as sucrose, so only use about half the amount. Because fructose in small quan-

tities can be used by the body without insulin, it is less likely to upset the diabetic's blood sugar balance.

Sorbitol is not recommended. It is higher in calories and has a laxative effect if eaten in too large a quantity. Non-calorific sweeteners, such as saccharin and aspartame, can be used in drinks and cold puddings, but they are not always suitable for cooking. However they can be added to stewed fruit once it has cooled down. A new sweetener, aceslulfame K, tolerates heat and can be used in hot foods.

Special Diabetic Foods Except for the low calorie products like diet drinks, low fat and low-sugar yoghurts, many special diabetic foods are overpriced and, until recently, they contained more calories than their non-diabetic counterparts. Some low calorie drinks do contain sugar, so it is advisable to choose one without sugar. However, recent legislation has stated that foods that claim to have been made specially for diabetics must provide no more energy, no more fat and have a 50 per cent reduction in readily absorbable carbohydrates when compared with those foods not made for diabetics. Diabetic foods that have an energy value of more than 50 per cent of the normal comparable food will have to carry a label stating that the food is unsuitable for the overweight diabetic.

Exercise A diabetic on insulin needs to take extra exercise (over and above the amount normally taken each day), so it is usually necessary to take at least some extra carbohydrate. As exercise uses up blood sugar it needs replacing, but the amount you need varies from individual to individual. For prolonged exercise, such as windsurfing, skiing and climbing, it is best to eat extra starchy carbohydrates; for short bursts of strenuous exercise, such as swimming and judo, it may be necessary to choose sugary foods. Here are some examples:

Starchy Foods (20g CHO)
1 thick slice wholemeal bread with peanut butter or low fat spread
1 wholemeal fruit bun
1 fruit scone
1 bowl muesli and skimmed milk
1 extra potato
1 fruit snack bar

Sugary foods (20g CHO)
1 miniature chocolate covered Swiss roll
1 small Kit Kat
3 toffees
1 large scoop ice cream

Illness IDDs need to remember that even though they may not feel like eating, it is important to balance their insulin against some food. They may find that when they are ill they require more insulin to maintain control. If they don't feel like eating meals, milky or sugary drinks should be chosen and should be taken throughout the day to avoid either a high or low blood sugar developing.

20g CHO portions
1 5¼oz (150g) carton fruit yoghurt
4 fl oz (113ml) lemonade
4 small cheese biscuits

⅓ pint (0.18 litre) soup and 1 small slice bread and low fat spread

10g CHO portions
1 cup soup
1 cup milk
1 scoop ice cream
2 plain biscuits

SAMPLE MENUS:

Day 1	CHO	Calories (kcals)	Day 2	CHO	Calories (kcals)
Daily: ½ pint (0.3 litre) semi-skimmed milk for tea and coffees	15	130	Daily: ½ pint (0.3 litre) semi-skimmed milk	15	130
Breakfast:			*Breakfast:*		
4tbsp (70ml) muesli with milk from allowance	40	200	1 small glass fresh orange juice	10	50
Mid-morning:			2 large slices wholemeal bread	30	140
1 wholemeal and bran biscuit	10	70	Scraping of polyunsaturate margarine	—	35
Lunch:			No-added-sugar jam	—	10
Wholemeal bread and tuna sandwich (2 large slices bread)	30	270	*Mid-morning:*		
Celery, raisin and apple salad	10	75	1 digestive	10	70
1 small glass orange juice	10	50	*Lunch:*		
1 apple	10	50	1 large wholemeal bap filled with chicken and salad	30	290
Mid-afternoon			1 orange	10	50
1 wholemeal and sultana scone	20	160	1 low fat fruit yoghurt	20	130
Scraping of polyunsaturate margarine	—	35	*Mid-afternoon:*		
Evening:			1 banana	20	70
Chicken casserole	—	340	*Evening:*		
Rice and lentils (made with 2½tbsp (44ml) brown rice cooked together with 2tbsp (35ml) green lentils)	60	300	Trout cooked in white wine	—	285
Cabbage	—	10	1 large portion broad beans, 10tbsp (175ml)	10	70
Carrots	—	20	1 medium jacket potato	30	170
1 slice of pineapple	10	50	Courgettes with yoghurt and mint dressing	5	30
Bedtime:			Baked peaches in orange juice stuffed with ground nuts, wholemeal and bran biscuit crushed and some egg to bind	25	250
2 wholemeal and bran biscuits	20	140	*Bedtime:*		
TOTAL	235	1900	1 digestive biscuit	10	70
			1 apple	10	50
			TOTAL	235	1900

Day 3	CHO	Calories (kcals)		CHO	Calories (kcals)
Daily: ½ pint (0.3 litre)			Cucumber salad	—	10
semi-skimmed milk	15	130	1 large wholemeal roll	30	170
			1 large banana	20	120
Breakfast:					
1 large bowl porridge			*Mid-afternoon:*		
(9tbsp [160ml])	30	150	2 wholemeal and bran		
1 small glass fresh orange			biscuits	20	140
juice served with milk			*Evening:*		
from allowance	10	50	Bolognese sauce	—	305
Mid-morning:			served with 2½oz (70g)		
1 small slice wholemeal			pasta	70	350
bread	10	70	Green salad	—	10
Scraping of polyunsaturate			*Bedtime:*		
margarine	—	35	1 wholemeal and sultana		
Lunch:			bun	20	130
Ham salad with lean ham	—	100	Scraping polyunsaturate		
4tbsp (70ml) bean salad	10	75	margarine	—	35
Carrot salad	—	20	TOTAL	235	1900

—LACTOSE INTOLERANCE—

Lactose intolerance is found in people who are unable to digest the milk sugar lactose. As a result they get bloated and suffer abdominal pain and diarrhoea when they consume more than a certain amount of milk and milk products. In only a few populations in the world can adults fully digest lactose, among them the north Europeans. However, many of the world's population, including people from Asia, the Middle East and Africa, are unable to digest lactose because they do not possess the necessary enzyme.

Lactose is broken down by the enzyme lactase in the digestive system to form glucose and galactose (see page 23). Unless it is stimulated to stay in production by the consumption of milk, the enzyme disappears. The levels of lactase in the body are highest around the time of birth, but tend to decrease with age. Those with lactose intolerance have a deficiency of the enzyme.

Those with lactose intolerance, who may include, temporarily, newly diagnosed coeliacs, must avoid milk or foods to which milk solids have been added. Some can manage small quantities of milk (a couple of tablespoons) but cannot manage larger quantities. Lactose is found in cream, all milks, evaporated milk, yoghurt and ice cream. In some products a bacteria called lactobacillus has soured the milk, breaking down some of the lactose at the same time. Some people with this intolerance can, therefore, manage to consume yoghurt, most cheeses and sour cream without any ill effects.

It is now possible to buy milk that has the enzyme lactase added to it. This converts most of the lactose and makes the milk suitable for those with lactose intolerance. Those who are lactose intolerant, besides using this type of milk, should also consult a dietitian who will provide a list of brand foods that do not contain milk. For example, it is now possible to buy a high polyunsaturate margarine that contains no milk solids.

——THE RISK OF CORONARY HEART DISEASE——

The diet that is recommended for general healthy eating is also suitable in helping to prevent coronary heart disease.

It is recommended that the intake of fat, particularly saturated fat, be reduced as this will help to lower the amount of cholesterol in the blood. In the US the public are still advised to reduce their intake of dietary cholesterol as well as reducing the amount of fat, particularly saturated fat, that they eat.

In the UK only people with very high levels of cholesterol in the blood are recommended to reduce their intake of cholesterol as well as to reduce their intake of saturated fat. This means eating no more than 3 or 4 eggs a week and reducing the intake of shellfish and offal. Anyone identified as belonging to this particular risk category, should seek the advice of a dietitian.

Increasing the consumption of fibre may be beneficial for the heart because foods rich in fibre, particularly the soluble fibre that is found in beans, lentils and oats, have been shown to help lower the blood cholesterol level.

Other factors besides diet are also known to increase the risk of having a heart attack. These include smoking, the amount of exercise taken, being overweight, having high blood pressure, a family history of coronary heart disease, diabetes and feeling stressed at home or at work.

Sample daily menus:
Fresh orange juice; large bowl of porridge with skimmed milk.
Minestrone soup with haricot beans; wholemeal bread; chicken salad; apple.
Stir-fry liver with carrots, cabbage, spring onion and ginger; brown rice; salad; prune fool – made with natural yoghurt puréed with cooked dried prunes.

Wholemeal toast with polyunsaturated margarine and honey; muesli with skimmed milk.
Tuna fish, celery and apple sandwiches; fresh fruit.
Cod baked in Italian tomato sauce with black olives and capers; steamed French beans; steamed new potatoes; strawberries with natural yoghurt or on their own.

Weetabix with skimmed milk.
Wholemeal toast with polyunsaturate margarine and strawberry jam.
Large jacket potato with chilli con carne; salad; tangerine.
Ragout of lamb; boiled potato; broad beans; carrots; pears in red wine with natural yoghurt.

CHAPTER 12

SLIMMING

*A*s a nation we are, on average, becoming heavier, although millions of pounds are still spent each year on trying to slim. However, slimming for cosmetic reasons may not be the same as eating a healthy diet, and being slim is no guarantee of health, nor is it necessarily a sign of healthy eating.

Being overweight is due to the excessive accumulation of (adipose) fat, which is usually the result of excess energy, i.e. calorie, intake compared with energy expenditure. At any one time, about 60 per cent of the female population of the UK are trying to lose weight, although only 32 per cent of them are actually overweight. Together with the 30 per cent of men who are overweight, there are about 11 million overweight adults in the UK. Between 2 and 10 per cent of all children in the UK are overweight. Children of overweight parents are more likely to be overweight, but most people seem to gain excess weight in their mid-twenties and not during childhood.

——*DOES BEING OVERWEIGHT MATTER?*——

First, of course, you need to lose weight only if you really are overweight (see the chart on pages 74-5). But assuming that you are overweight, why should you change? If being slim improves your self-image, it can be of great benefit.

There are, of course, also some sound health reasons why anyone who is overweight should slim. Carrying excess fat around seems to make people more vulnerable to certain illnesses. Hypertension is much more common in the overweight, and it is often successfully treated by a reduction in weight. Maturity onset diabetes is more common among the overweight, and it too can be treated by going on a reducing diet. Other diseases such as angina, heart disease and osteoarthritis can also be helped by weight reduction. Those who are told to lose weight for health reasons often have the greatest chance of doing so successfully.

The social pressures to lose weight are enormous. Not only are we persuaded to conform by advertisements, magazines and television programmes, but also by those around us. The ideal person today is seen to be slim: slimness is associated

> *Between 2 and 10 per cent of all children in the UK are overweight.*

> *From childhood onwards food is often used as a means of manipulating behaviour.*

with success at work, success in the home and the ability to attract friends. This image of the ideal person puts considerable pressure on many people and, ironically, one of the dangers is that food can end up being used as a way of compensating for this pressure. This, in turn, may lead to people becoming more overweight, thus further increasing the pressure so that a vicious circle is started.

From childhood onwards food is often used as a means of manipulating behaviour. It can be withheld as a punishment or proffered as a reward, and eating patterns can be interpreted as signs of good or bad behaviour in children. Parents who have used food in this way could find that their child develops an eating disorder in later life, either over-eating, or refusing to eat.

However, some people do have a definite tendency to fatness that is metabolically based, although it must be said that such cases are rare. Middle-age weight gain is usually the result of taking less exercise and failing to adapt food intake to the lower amounts needed.

There is no doubt that losing weight usually makes slimmers feel happier or more attractive, but this is often merely because they have gained more confidence in themselves. It is no good promising ourselves that if only we could lose weight we would get a better job, or find a lover, or have more friends, because these factors are rarely related to weight, but to self-confidence. The best reason for losing weight is because you want to. Being bullied into dieting is unlikely to be effective, especially in the long term. A holiday on the beach or a wedding can provide a useful short-term incentive, but successful slimming is a long-term process, not an overnight miracle.

—— *WHAT LOSING WEIGHT IS ALL ABOUT* ——

If you read everything that has been written about losing weight you would probably become very confused. Dieters seem to clutch at straws and hope that each new wonder diet that is invented will help them. They may indeed lose weight in the short term on some of these diets, but few people can manage to stick to unfamiliar routines for long. Many diets are too anti-social. Grapefruit and eggs for two weeks may just be achievable, but it is hard to imagine, let alone stomach, keeping to that strict regime for any longer. Our tastebuds and our eyes tell us that we want to eat other foods.

Diets that promise quick weight loss are illusory. Weight loss should be slow and gradual to be effective. Energy requirements vary from individual to individual, and this in part explains the different weight losses of people on the same diet. The first 5lb (2.2kg) or so that is lost is water, not fat. Many diets suggest that 9lb (4.1kg) can be lost in seven days. But not all that weight will be fat. For a start only 4lb (1.8kg) of that loss will come from fat. Each 1lb (0.45kg) of body fat represents

> *Parents who have used food in this way may find that their child develops an eating disorder in later life.*

approximately 4,000 calories. To lose 1lb (0.45kg) of fat you must either expend more energy or consume fewer calories. If your body uses 2,000 calories a day and your dietary intake is 1,200 calories, you would have an energy deficit of 800 calories. After a week you would have a deficit of 5,600 calories, the equivalent of 1lb 8oz (0.7kg) of fat. Even with the water loss, this would still amount to only 6lb 8oz (2.9kg) in seven days.

Many dieters stop and start diets all the time with the end result that their bodies contain a higher proportion of body fat than when they first started dieting. This phenomenon has been called the "yo-yo" effect and may well be more harmful to health than remaining slightly overweight. Losing weight should mean losing fat and not other body stores, such as protein (sometimes referred to as lean muscle tissue) from the muscles. But fat is the body's long-term storage unit and is the hardest energy store to reduce.

The higher the proportion of fat to muscle in the body, the less energy is required. Women require fewer calories than men because their bodies contain about 20 per cent body fat compared with the 8 per cent of men. Any loss of lean muscle tissue, through too severe a diet – i.e. one that is extremely low in calories – can result in people looking fatter than they did before! Because fat is lighter than muscle it is quite possible to be the same weight as you were before dieting but to find that your measurements, especially hips, waist and thighs, have increased. This is part of the "yo-yo" effect.

There are several other influences on metabolic rate apart from the proportion of body fat and lean muscle tissue. Just as a car's fuel requirements are determined by how it is constructed, how much it weighs, its aerodynamics and how fast it is driven, so the calorific needs of the human body are determined by a range of factors.

The basal metabolic rate (BMR) measures how many calories the body requires when at rest to maintain vital functions and keep the heart, digestive system and lungs working. The following factors affect BMR:

Sex The BMR for men is higher than for women. This is for a number of reasons but partly because men have a higher proportion of lean muscle tissue and because women are usually smaller than men.

Weight The heavier a person is, the higher the BMR.

Fatness Lean muscle tissue uses more calories than fat.

Age As a person ages the metabolic rate slows down. It decreases as our lean muscle tissue is lost.

Sleep patterns There are indications that the BMR is fractionally lower during sleep.

Temperature The colder the surrounding air, the more heat the body generates and so the higher the BMR. Sudden fluctuations in temperature may also result in increased BMR and so someone who is ill with a fever may lose weight, both because of the increased BMR and because less food is being eaten.

> *Women require fewer calories than men because their bodies contain about 20 per cent body fat compared with the 8 per cent of men.*

Metabolic rate can also alter on a diet. When dieting some people may notice that after a while they seem to stop losing weight. This is because the body has reached *status quo*. The vital organs simply slow down and "get by" on less energy. The remedy is to increase the metabolic rate by exercising more.

——HOW MANY CALORIES ARE NEEDED?——

The Department of Health and Social Security recommends that an average woman requires 2,200 calories a day whereas an average man requires approximately 3,000 calories a day to maintain weight. However recent research suggests that these levels may be too high. From a total of twelve normal-weight women only one-third were found to require the level of calories suggested by the DHSS. The remainder required approximately 1,850 calories, with the exception of one woman who required only 1,470 calories. A similar picture seemed to be true for the men. A study of overweight women, however, indicated that they used up more energy than someone of normal weight. This is because being heavier, their bodies had a higher proportion of both lean muscle tissue and fat. The amount of energy needed to maintain their weight was nearer 2,440 calories a day.

Studies of overweight people show that the majority of women lose weight on a 1,000-1,200 calorie diet, whereas most men will lose weight on 1,200-1,500 calories a day. Certainly, these diets will, if sensibly chosen, ensure that the body obtains enough vitamins, minerals and trace elements. Calorie levels lower than this would require some vitamin and mineral supplements. The other reason why higher calorie allowances are being recommended in place of the 800 calorie diets of the past is that people are more likely to stick to them for a satisfactory length of time and they are socially much easier to maintain. However, some individuals need a lower intake of calories to lose weight and may have to adopt an intake nearer to 800 kilocalories.

——EXERCISE——

Exercising on a diet is now regarded as almost as important as the diet itself. That does not mean that those who do not exercise will not lose weight, but exercise certainly speeds up the process. Although exercise *per se* may only burn up a few calories, it has many other benefits.

Exercise tones up the muscles, which ultimately improves body shape. This enhances self-confidence and self-image so that the "comfort eating" that may result from feeling overweight becomes less of a temptation. Exercise also makes us more aware of our body shape, and this may help to control food intake. If exercise is taken for long enough, it prolongs the burning up of calories for several hours, and depending on the exercise chosen, it increases the suppleness, stamina and strength of the body. Some specialists believe that those people who carry out regular exercise are less prone to illnesses like colds and coughs. Many people also forget that the heart is a muscle and like most muscles needs exercise.

For those under stress 15-20 minutes of regular exercise also stretches the muscles and releases the endorphins, the pain-releasing hormones, which help to get rid of tension. This gives a feeling of well-being and calmness, which can encourage better eating habits. Exercise also provides something positive to do when losing weight, rather than just sitting around eating less! If you are one of the people who feels they must eat or drink after exercise, try to choose something that is permitted on your diet, for example, an apple or a cup of tea or coffee without sugar, or a low calorie soft drink.

A survey carried out by Heartbeat Wales showed that only 2 per cent of women in Wales take any regular exercise that would have a training effect on the body and heart.

Alternatively you could have part of a meal you would be going to eat later – e.g., eat one sandwich now and one later.

The most important point about the exercise chosen is that it should be enjoyable. Otherwise it will not be continued with on a regular basis. It need not, and indeed should not, be over-strenuous until you have gained sufficient fitness. It is no good doing the same exercise as a friend if you loathe that particular exercise. Decide whether you want to exercise on your own, in a group or with a friend.

Surveys carried out in the UK suggest that women find it hard to find opportunities to take exercise – or are just lazy. A survey carried out by Heartbeat Wales showed that only 2 per cent of women in Wales take any regular exercise that would have a training effect on the body and heart. On the other hand, 23 per cent of men find the time to do some regular exercise, that is 15-20 minutes' exercise at least 3 times a week, which makes the heart beat faster.

—FAD DIETS—

The slimming business can be a very profitable one. Since the 1960s the number of diets brought to the attention of the public has increased to such an extent that it seems hard to believe that anyone still needs to lose weight. Unfortunately, only a minority of these diets are sensible and even they often do not succeed, largely because of that human failing, lack of willpower! Some fad diets are nutritionally inadequate as they do not provide enough vitamins and minerals. Many others actually constitute a health risk.

FASTING

Fasting may mean consuming a pint of milk a day or it can mean going without food altogether, thereby approaching starvation. Drinking milk will at least help to spare the muscles and tissues from being wasted, as without the milk these, and not necessarily the body fat, will be used up more rapidly. Some people find this type of diet easy because they never have to face real food. It results in a build up of ketone bodies, which are produced when fatty acids are broken down in the liver to provide a source of energy, indicating that the body is relying on its own fat store for energy. If you know someone who has fasted, or even dieted very severely, you may have smelt these ketone bodies on their breath. The smell is similar to pear drops. An accumulation of ketone bodies in the blood is called ketosis which can result in nausea, vomiting, fatigue, dizziness and low blood pressure. Severe depression and irritability are not uncommon amongst those who fast because of the extremes of the diet.

PROTEIN SPARING DIETS

These are the liquid diets of about 400-600 calories. They are really only one step away from fasting except that extra vitamins, minerals and trace elements have been added to make them more nutritious. These diets were originally designed for use in hospital by the extremely obese, people whose degree of overweight is life-threatening rather than those who only need to lose a stone or two. Anyone wanting to lose weight should first make a determined effort to diet by conventional methods before trying a very low calorie diet. These have recently achieved popularity among those who have tried unsuccessfully to lose weight by all other methods. Many who follow these diets seek no medical supervision as recommended and this has led to some tragedies. They should certainly not be followed by the elderly, the young, the pregnant or those known to have a medical condition. These diets also fail to re-educate eating habits so, even if weight loss occurs, there is still no basis for a healthy diet in the future. They are only meant to be used for three to four weeks and therefore are really only suitable for those who are a bit overweight. The danger for the severely overweight is that they might be tempted to use them for much longer periods or at frequent intervals which may lead to undesirable loss of muscle tissue.

LOW PROTEIN DIETS

These are diets that rely on single food items, such as grapefruit or bananas. They contain almost nothing but carbohydrate-type foods, and are usually nutritionally inadequate, particularly in iron and calcium. As these diets are low in protein, they make the body rely on its own muscle tissue to meet its need for new protein. Body fat is lost, as is lean body tissue.

THE HIGH PROTEIN OR LOW CARBOHYDRATE DIETS

These diets have been among the most commonly prescribed, and they come under a variety of names. Because they are based on protein, these diets have helped to perpetuate the myth that carbohydrate foods are fattening. They are popular, especially with those who like to eat large portions of meat or fish. Although these diets are high in essential nutrients, they are very expensive.

They have other drawbacks too. Because they are proportionately high in fat, they are likely to raise the level of blood cholesterol and hence the risk of coronary heart disease. In the absence of carbohydrate, these diets use the body's fat for energy and this may result in ketosis. Low carbohydrate diets also overlook the importance of eating a diet high in fibre and complex carbohydrates. Many low carbohydrate diets do not distinguish nutritionally between sugar and starch.

Some of these diets are exceptionally high in protein and force the kidneys to excrete large amounts of nitrogen. In a healthy person this should not be a problem, but it may put a strain on someone with a marginal kidney problem. A few diets also restrict fluid intake, which may further overload the kidneys, although there is no medical basis for restricting fluid on a diet. The only reason that is suggested is to make dieters think they are losing more weight.

CALORIE-CONTROLLED DIETS

On these regimes you are allowed to eat whatever you like, provided it does not exceed 1,000 kilocalories a day. Although this type of diet provides freedom of choice, it will not necessarily re-educate eating habits. Another disadvantage is that many people underestimate portion sizes and therefore find they have eaten more than they thought, with the result that they do not lose weight. On the other hand, such diets can help to teach about the energy value of foods.

——OTHER AIDS TO SLIMMING——

SLIMMING CLUBS
Many slimmers can find it helpful to diet in a group. Not only can this offer group support and encouragement, but groups achieve good results with many of their clients. However they vary in quality, and depend largely on the leader and the type of diet advocated. Most slimming clubs today offer high fibre-low fat diets, and if you are thinking of attending a club you should look for one that provides this type of diet. Commercial slimming clubs can be expensive, although the monetary incentive can also help people to lose weight. In addition to the commercial slimming groups, health authorities sometimes run their own groups with the aid of a dietitian. These have most of the same benefits but are considerably cheaper.

SLIMMING PRODUCTS
Slimming products fall into two categories: meal replacements and alternatives to high calorie foods. Meal replacements usually take the form of biscuits or drinks and are supposed to replace two meals each day. They don't retrain eating habits because they resemble the type of foods that we should be learning to eat less often. Some higher fibre varieties are available, although over a whole day you are unlikely to have eaten more than 12g of fibre. However, some dieters find them useful if they only have a few pounds to lose or to help get them started on a diet.

The market for alternatives to high calorie foods seems to be constantly expanding. However these products are only of benefit if they are included as part of a calorie controlled diet. They range from yoghurts to drinks, low fat spreads and even lower fat sausages! Many of these products are reduced in calorie content by adding air or water or sweeteners – be sure not to end up eating twice as much.

WATER PILLS OR DIURETICS OR FIBRE TABLETS
Many patients request diuretics from their doctors, not for a specific health problem, but as a means of losing weight. Although this will achieve a loss of 3-7lb (1.4-3.2kg), it is a loss of water and not a loss of fat. As soon as the pills are stopped the weight returns. The use of diuretics for weight loss is not advisable. They can interfere with muscle function, disrupt the balance of body salts and cause heart rhythm abnormalities. If you do seem to suffer from water retention you should consult your doctor.

Fibre tablets are supposed both to provide bulk to the diet and also to get rid of any excess fluid. However, the evidence that they can help people lose weight is unsubstantiated.

APPETITE REDUCERS
These tablets are supposed to be eaten before meals to help control the appetite.

The methylcellulose in the tablet swells in the stomach, and this is supposed to make the stomach feel full. However, many people who use these tablets have found that they can still manage to eat their normal quantity of food, thus negating any benefit intended. These tablets are also expensive and the money might be better spent on a few treats in your diet such as a piece of steak or salmon or strawberries. The tablets have no nutritional value whatsoever.

LAXATIVES

Some cases have been cited recently of anorexics using laxatives to lose weight. Laxatives increase the water weight of the stool so that the weight lost is body water and not fat. Their use may also deter the absorption of food and hence some of the calories absorbed – but the amounts are only small. More importantly, they also interfere with the absorption of vitamins, minerals and trace elements by the body. If laxatives are over-used there may be problems with bowel function in later life, especially constipation.

APPETITE-SUPPRESSING DRUGS

Although these drugs may aid weight loss for a while, they are dangerous if taken for more than a short period. Most people rapidly gain weight when they stop taking them and may well end up heavier than before! These drugs do not help to establish good eating habits and they are also addictive.

——— OTHER CAUSES OF OVERWEIGHT———

WHY DO EX-SMOKERS GAIN WEIGHT?

Many ex-smokers return to smoking because they find that their weight increases. Smoking increases the metabolic rate, and the nicotine in cigarettes depresses the appetite and dulls the tastebuds. Smokers have also been found to produce higher than normal levels of an enzyme called lipoprotein lipase, which helps to use up body fat. A higher level of this enzyme is also found in those losing weight.

Ex-smokers should put on only an extra 4lb (1.8kg) on average. Those who put on more weight may be eating more snacks or sugary drinks in order to keep their fingers and mouths occupied. Food acts as a strong gratification stimulus, and it is important not to slip into bad eating habits while giving up smoking. Eating can easily become a reward for the loss of smoking, compensating for that denial by the pleasure it gives. If you are going to give up smoking, look at your eating habits so that you can notice if they change. Most people find it hard to diet at the same time as stopping smoking, but it is important to eat healthily. The addition of plenty of fruit and vegetables as snacks to a diet will help both to compensate the body for the lack of the gratification caused by not smoking and will replace the vitamin C in which smokers are often deficient. Learning breathing and relaxation techniques will also help to relieve tension from giving up smoking.

DOES THE PILL MAKE YOU PUT ON WEIGHT?

Many women find that they gain weight when they are taking the contraceptive pill and lose weight when they stop. This seems to be partly due to the levels of the hormones oestrogen and progesterone, which cause fat to develop around the hips, buttocks and thighs. The doses of synthetic hormones in the pill can affect the body in the same way and increase fat formation. Some women blame the pill for their putting on weight. Should you find that you are putting on a lot of weight, talk to your doctor, who may be able to prescribe a different pill. If the pill is not to blame, then take plenty of exercise and keep an eye on your weight.

GLANDULAR PROBLEMS
Although some specialized glandular problems (most commonly myxoedema and Cushing's Syndrome) do affect weight, the number of sufferers is very small. Most people who are overweight are those who do not balance their energy intake and output. People do vary in the amount of energy they need in order to live and be active, and although overweight people may not necessarily eat more than the average person, it is still more than they need.

DOES FIBRE HELP YOU LOSE WEIGHT?
It is unlikely that eating more fibre in itself will help you to lose weight. It has been suggested that as fibre can give a feeling of fullness it may act as an appetite suppressant, but as all food intake is reduced during dieting, it is unlikely to have this effect. On the other hand, foods that are rich in complex carbohydrates – including fibre – add bulk to a meal so that the plate does not look so empty. A large baked potato or a plate of pasta with a low calorie sauce can *look* more satisfying than smaller portions of meat and vegetables. Further research needs to be carried out to see just what effect fibre has on a weight-reducing diet. However, there is no doubt that fibre is beneficial to health as fibre-containing foods add a higher proportion of vitamins, minerals and trace elements than refined foods, as well as useful bulk for the intestines.

——*HOW TO LOSE WEIGHT*——
Like stopping smoking, dieting is easy to start but difficult to keep up. And, like stopping smoking, success will really be possible only if the new way of eating becomes part of a permanent change in lifestyle. First, you need to be convinced that such a change is necessary or at least worth a very determined try. Once you have made the decision to try, the change can be made harder or easier depending on how you approach it. The hard way is to think of yourself as going on a permanent diet. Diets are often depressing. They mean following a list of do's, but mostly of don'ts, which can seem like an unending form of punishment. On the other hand, if you view the change positively – as a way of helping yourself feel better – and are prepared to tackle the process of change one step at a time, the experience can be rewarding and you should find that you feel the benefits sooner than you perhaps imagine.

As you diet each achievement should be a spur forward towards your goal, not the opposite. First, set a realistic goal. Although you may know that you should really lose two stone, concentrate on the first stone before tackling the next. This way you will be more likely to achieve success.

Second, you need to boost your self-confidence. For most people looking good and feeling fit are great morale boosters. If you have not bought any new clothes for some time, you could think about buying something that will make you feel good. Don't buy anything too well fitting: your shape is, you hope, going to change again. Sweaters or sports clothes with elasticized waists can usually accommodate a range of sizes.

Next, you need to find a form of exercise that you will enjoy and not mind doing three or four times a week. If you find jogging boring, consider walking, swimming or cycling. An early morning or evening swim can be very refreshing and relaxing, and cycling to work can save time as well as money. There are cassette tapes and videos available with programmes of keep fit exercises. A limited amount of regular exercise lasting about half an hour, but hard enough to get you a *little* out of breath, makes many people feel fitter.

But before you start to change your eating habits, you need to develop awareness and understanding of your present eating pattern. You may find that keeping a food diary will help. Not only should you write down everything you eat and drink, but you should also write down where you had your meal and what sort of mood you were in. Be honest with yourself, and you may realize where you slip up.

FOOD DIARY

Time	Place	With Whom	Time of Day	Mood	Degree of Hunger	Actions	Food Eaten and Amount
7.00am	Kitchen table	Self	Breakfast	Happy	5	Listening to the radio	4fl oz (100ml) orange juice 1 slice wholemeal bread 2tsp peanut butter Tea, 1 sweetener
10.00am	Kitchen	Self	—	Fed up as gas man did not come to do the gas fire	0	Ironing clothes	4 biscuits Cup of coffee with sugar instead of sweetener
1.00pm	Lounge	Self	Lunch	Fed up as can't get hold of Gas Board	2	Watching TV	Pkt crisps (small) 2 white rolls 3oz (85g) corn beef Lettuce 1 piece apple tart (leftover) and double portion of cream

If you examine the reasons why you eat, you may understand what causes you to over-eat, and once you are able to recognize these situations you should be able to learn to control them. Some people who have only a small amount of weight to lose may find changing their behaviour alone will help them lose weight. For example, a mother who always eats up her children's leftovers rather than throwing them away may decide to use the leftovers to help make another meal or she may be able to learn to throw them away. Others with more weight to lose may find that behaviour modification combined with dieting will be of greater help. Look carefully at the behaviour modification chart on page 256.

If you cannot leave food on your plate, serve yourself small portions.

One behaviour pattern that is common to many dieters is always to eat food that is offered to them. This may be as a result of upbringing – for example, being taught always to clean the plate or that eating what is offered is being polite – but all dieters must learn not to always accept food that is offered and to learn to refuse it with polite firmness. If you cannot leave food on your plate, serve yourself small portions. If you feel it is impolite to refuse food, you can still show an interest in what is being offered. You can compliment it without having to eat it.

Slimmers seem to eat for many reasons. They may be tired, angry, harassed or cold, but they hardly ever eat because they are hungry! Dietitians have many stories to tell of patients who may give a wonderful history of what they have been eating but who never show a sign of weight loss. If asked if they ever felt hungry, the majority of patients would say no. However, it is almost impossible to diet without feeling hungry at some stage. Slimmers should listen to their bodies and feed them when they are hungry rather than because they fancy something. They should, ideally, learn to be hungry at mealtimes, and if you aren't hungry at a mealtime eat a bit less and perhaps have a little extra at the next meal.

Eating only at mealtimes may also help to stop you from eating chocolates, sticky buns or another high calorie snack. If you do tend to eat snacks, at least try to choose sensible low calorie snacks rather than the high calorie varieties.

If you do cheat, the most important thing is to go straight back to your diet and not get depressed about cheating. Feeling depressed will probably make you eat even more. Don't feel that all is wasted and embark on a binge of eating! Instead, start again at the next meal and, if you can, do something to compensate for the extra calories like taking some additional exercise. If your cheating still persists, complete another food diary to see where you are going wrong.

You might find it useful to take up a new hobby to help to get you over those moments when you might want to cheat. Some slimmers brush their teeth every time they want to eat; others play patience or knit. The more occupied your mind and hands are the less likely you are to worry about food. Try to find something that will occupy your mind – you never know, you may find new interests and skills you never knew you had!

WEIGHT LOSS

Although you will be keen to know how you have done on your diet, don't weigh yourself more than twice a week, preferably only once. Your weight will fluctuate throughout the day and during the week because of changes in water retention. Women may find that their weight fluctuates more than normal before a period, although this should settle down after a couple of days. Water retention can be discouraging to many slimmers.

After you have been dieting for a while (the timing will vary from person to person), don't be surprised to find that your weight will seem to stay stationary. This often happens as your body gets used to receiving less food and adjusts itself to a slower metabolism. If you haven't cheated you will find that you soon start to lose weight again. You may even find that after a stationary period your weight will drop dramatically. It is important not to further reduce your calorie intake, otherwise your metabolism will adjust to an even slower rate.

Finally, weight control is your own responsibility. It's *up to you*. Don't get someone else to be responsible otherwise you will cheat when they are not looking. You must look out for yourself.

Tips On Slimming

Each of you will value these tips differently, some will work for you and others won't.

* Instead of thinking so much about what you should eat less of, concentrate on what you should eat more of such as fresh fruit, vegetables, wholemeal bread, pulses and fish.
* Put all tempting items at the back of the refrigerator or cupboard. Keep all such items in a container so that they aren't obvious when you open the door. Don't keep biscuits, nuts or chocolates in the house.
* If you're still hungry after you've finished your meal, remember that it takes at least 20 minutes until the signal that your stomach is full to reach the brain. Even if you feel hungry just try to wait, and the feeling may go away.
* Serve yourself on a small plate so that your portions look larger.
* Try to include more high fibre foods in your diet.
* Remember that the food you eat doesn't have to be boring. Many people have given up dieting because they ate cottage cheese one meal after another. Don't forget to use herbs and spices to make your food more interesting. You could make chicken tikka or spicy home-made hamburgers or pears with ginger or buy low calorie speciality meals every now and again.
* Eat your food slowly. It is important to enjoy eating, but remember not to eat more because everyone else at the table is still eating.
* Many find it is better to eat food sitting at a table rather than slouched in a chair watching television. If you do two things at once your body may not be sure which it is trying to enjoy and probably won't succeed at either.
* If a certain routine is associated with eating try to change your routine.
* Drinking water with your meals can help you feel fuller.
* Watch out for foods high in hidden fat as these are likely to be high in calories.
* Don't eat leftovers. Give them to the dog but don't make him fat instead!
* Learn to say "no" to food. Many slim people are able to say no kindly but firmly without having to make long excuses. You are more likely to have unwanted food and drink pressed on you if you give the impression that you could be tempted!
* Only buy foods you require for your meals. This is harder if you have a family, but try not to buy tempting foods. Do not shop for foods when you are hungry.
* Always have a variety of low calorie foods such as raw vegetables so that you can eat these when you are hungry.
* Increase the amount of exercise you take each day.

When you are dieting it is important to remember that all foods are potentially fattening. There are very few that can be eaten in large quantities without causing you to put on weight. Some of the foods that can cause problems include:

Crispbreads Some people still think that they can eat as many crispbreads as they like because they are low in calories. Although they *are* lower in calories, only two or three can replace a slice of bread.

Unsweetened fruit juice Because it says unsweetened one automatically assumes that large quantities can be drunk on a diet. However the calorie content of a small glass (per 100ml) of fruit juice is approximately 50 kilocalories, therefore just over 2 pints (approximately 1 litre) of fresh fruit juice would contain approximately 500 kilocalories – which is half a day's calorie allowance for some slimmers.

Butter and margarine Both these spreads have the same number of calories unless they are called low fat spreads, when they have half the number of calories. Low fat spreads are basically water and fat, hence the lower number of calories. Take care not to spread twice as much.

Salad dressing and sauces These can be included on a diet but with caution. If it is obviously a fatty-type sauce such as a cream- or oil-based sauce, the amounts consumed should be extremely small. There are low calorie dressings available, or you can make your own version based on low fat natural yoghurt or lemon juice.

Cheese Although cheese can be included in a diet, you should limit the quantity of high fat cheese to no more than 8oz (230g) a week. There are now low fat, hard cheeses available, and these should be substituted for high fat cheeses.

Pies and pastries As these are high in calories they really should be excluded from a diet. Instead of using a pie topping, use mashed potato. This will have many fewer calories than a pastry topping as only a small amount of fat, if any, need be added to the potato.

Alcohol Ideally alcohol should not be included in a diet because it provides "empty" calories – i.e. calories that provide no nutritional benefits. However, if you have been used to consuming large quantities of alcohol before dieting, you could allow yourself a couple of drinks at the weekend. Further tips on cutting down on drinking are given on pages 270-1. You should not, of course, drink if you have been advised against it for medical reasons.

CHILDREN AND SLIMMING

Dieting can be hard for everyone, but it can be particularly difficult for the overweight child. Those who are most successful have the help and co-operation of their parents, not only in terms of general support, but in providing the meals and snacks that are suitable for the child and making the rest of the family eat similar food. In addition to dieting, it is also important to encourage children to exercise. Many overweight children do not like school sports, so it is important that you help them find some form of exercise that they enjoy. If necessary join them yourself. It will do you good as well!

As children are growing rapidly, weight-reducing diets should not be too restrictive. The aim is to achieve weight maintenance rather than weight loss so that as they grow they will lose weight indirectly. Too restrictive a diet can result in a child feeling isolated not only from his friends but also within his own family.

Relatives and friends can be a problem if a child is trying to diet. Instead of letting them give sweets to the child, suggest that they bring comics, crayons or something that is needed for the latest hobby.

Reducing a child's normal food intake by approximately 500 calories a day should result in a weight loss of between ½-1lb (0.23-0.45kg) a week. Reducing the diet by this amount should not result in any "real" hunger, and the child will be more likely to find the diet acceptable.

Many of the pointers about dieting that have already been discussed also apply to children. First, they need to learn what healthy eating is all about. For example, to help them reduce their calorie intake they should cut out all sugary foods and drinks and substitute sugar-free drinks. They should cut down on the amount of fat consumed by changing their milk to skimmed or semi-skimmed milk, using less butter or margarine on bread and less oil in cooking, and grilling foods instead of frying them. Try to encourage the use of wholemeal bread and breakfast cereals. If necessary, alternate white bread with wholemeal at first.

Children like fast food, so it is important to explain how they can include these in their diet. This will help them feel less isolated from their friends. However, it can be helpful if they avoid these foods for the first couple of months while they re-educate their eating habits. Hamburgers, fishfingers, fish cakes, bread rolls from cafés, some Chinese and Indian food can all be included on a diet but try to choose small portions. For advice look at the section on eating out (pages 202-4).

Relatives and friends can be a problem if a child is trying to diet. Instead of letting them give sweets to the child, suggest that they bring comics, crayons or something that is needed for the latest hobby. Pocket money can be saved for a special purchase rather than frittering it away on sweets. And instead of buying sweets, they could buy a diet drink or a piece of fruit or start a collection of stickers.

Once the child has lost some weight he or she can be allowed a treat food once a week or once a day so that they don't feel totally deprived of all sweets, cakes or biscuits. If a treat food is included, the calorie intake should be reduced accordingly. You may well find they choose the same treat food all the time.

Treat foods:
1 mini chocolate bar
1 packet of crisps
1 3½oz (100g) small portion large oven chips
1 large scoop ice cream
1 small piece of cake
1 crunchy bar
1 small chocolate wafer biscuit

If you feel that you need extra help contact your local doctor or dietitian.

THE OVERWEIGHT INFANT
Many parents worry that their chubby baby will become an overweight child/adult. However, most babies grow out of the "Winston Churchill" stage of their own accord, either when they start to crawl or as a result of a natural reduction in their

appetite in the second year. If you have an overweight infant (over 6 months old) there are a few points to check:

1. Avoid giving sugary foods such as rusks, even the low sugar versions.
2. Offer water instead of sweetened drinks. You can give diluted unsweetened fruit juice once a day.
3. Avoid fatty foods; give lean meat, fish and plenty of fruit and vegetables.
4. Check that you are not making any bottlefeeds too concentrated.
5. Once a baby is eating solids three times a day, make sure you are not giving more than 1 pint (0.6 litre) of milk. Milk must be the full-fat variety at this age.
6. If in doubt, seek the advice of your doctor or dietitian.

WEIGHT-REDUCING PLAN FOR CHILDREN

There should be a daily allowance of 1 pint (0.6 litre) skimmed or semi-skimmed milk for use in tea and coffee, and three pieces of fruit a day plus one glass fresh fruit juice. In this menu one piece of fruit can be eaten in addition to the other two pieces of fruit on the menu. In addition, offer plenty of vegetables (except avocado or potato). The 1,200-kilocalorie diet includes five exchanges and the 1,500-kilo-calorie diet includes seven exchanges (see page 262). The exchange list allows the diet to be more flexible. Instead of all the exchanges being eaten as, say, bread, the system allows the child to include rice, pasta, potato or breakfast cereals. Rather than eating all the exchanges at one meal try to split them up throughout the day as suggested below. Many children can lose weight on the 1,500-calorie diet as their energy output is far greater than this. Occasionally, however, a lower intake will have to be advised. Instead of using the chicken and tuna as suggested in the sample menu, use a portion of other lean meat, fish, eggs, low fat cheese, beans or other vegetarian dish.

1,200 kilocalories	*1,600 kilocalories*
Breakfast:	
1 glass orange juice	1 glass orange juice
1 slice wholemeal bread	2 slices wholemeal bread
(1 exchange)	(2 exchanges)
⅓oz (10g) peanut butter	¾oz (20g) peanut butter
Lunch:	
2 slices wholemeal bread	2 slices wholemeal bread
(2 exchanges)	(2 exchanges)
2¾oz (75g) tuna, drained of brine	2¾oz (75g) tuna, drained of brine
Cucumber and grated carrot	Cucumber and grated carrot
Less than ¼oz (5g) polyunsaturate margarine	Less than ¼oz (5g) polyunsaturate margarine
1 banana	1 banana
Evening:	
3½oz (100g) chicken breast*	3½oz (100g) chicken breast*
3½oz (100g) cooked brown rice	5¼oz (150g) cooked brown rice
(2 exchanges)	(3 exchanges)

Salad of beansprouts, carrot, raisin and tomatoes or cooked vegetables
1 pear

Salad of beansprouts, carrot, raisin and tomatoes or cooked vegetables
1 pear

*Marinaded in 1tsp (5ml) soy sauce, 1tsp (5ml) oil, 1tsp (5ml) cumin, 2tsp (10ml) lemon juice and some crushed garlic. Leave for at least 1 hour then grill.

Exchanges:
1 slice wholemeal or white bread
½ bread roll – wholemeal or white
1¾oz (50g) cooked rice – brown or white
1 digestive biscuit
3½oz (100g) cooked beans
3 crispbreads
2¾oz (75g) boiled/jacket potato
3tbsp (55ml) breakfast cereal – high fibre
1 Weetabix or Shredded Wheat
1¾oz (50g) cooked pasta – wholemeal or white or spinach
1 small bowl porridge.

Foods allowed freely:
All vegetables – e.g., cauliflower, carrots, green beans, tomato, mushrooms, peas, turnips, swedes, lettuce, broccoli, onion, aubergine, peppers, parsnip and beetroot.
    Water, tea, coffee, diet drinks, tomato juice, clear soups, beef and yeast extract drinks.
    All herbs and spices.
    Low calorie salad dressings in moderation.

Foods to avoid:
Sweets, sugar, honey, syrup, jams, marmalade, ice cream, jelly, cakes, chocolate, sweet biscuits, pastries, puddings.
Squashes and fizzy drinks that contain sugar. Sweetened malt or chocolate drinks. Milkshake syrups.
Butter, margarine, oil except from the daily allowance. Salad creams or mayonnaise except low calorie ones in moderation. Fatty meats such as salami, pâté and liver sausage. Visible fat on meat. All cream.
Tinned, packet or cream soups. Thick sauces or gravy. Pickles and chutneys.
Products intended for diabetics.

CHAPTER 13

DRINKS

D rinks are not only a necessary part of the diet (as outlined on page 50), but they also have an important place in our social life. Drinks are usually offered and consumed much more frequently than food during the day. Therefore what we choose to drink should be considered with as much care as what we choose to eat.

—*WATER*—

In many parts of the world the water supplies are a major carrier of diseases like cholera and dysentery, but in countries like the UK we take clean water for granted. The fact that we are able to have clean water is due to the efforts of a huge water industry, which keeps water clean and constantly checks for accidental contamination that may occur from industrial effluents, from heavily fertilized agricultural land or from piping materials.

Some chemicals like chlorine, lime and ferric sulphate are deliberately added to water supplies as part of the general purification and treatment processes, and levels of these are closely controlled. There are three items in water that are of most public concern and have been researched extensively. These are lead, nitrate and fluoride.

LEAD

Lead gets into our water either from the pipes that transport water from the street to the house or from household lead plumbing. The levels of lead are usually highest in water that is soft and acidic. A government report on lead in water indicated that 9 per cent of all households in the UK have tap water containing more than 0.1mg lead in their first draw of water, whereas only 4 per cent of all households will have this level during daytime samples. In Scotland, where water is primarily soft, the figures were 28 per cent and 21 per cent respectively. Although this survey indicates how much lead is in water, it doesn't state how much this contributes to our total intake of lead. Soft water may also dissolve other materials, including copper and cadmium, but whether in suf-

6
There are three items in water that are of most public concern and have been researched extensively. These are lead, nitrate and fluoride.
9

263

ficient amounts to damage human health is not known.

FLUORIDE

It is widely held by the medical authorities that a level of 1ppm (part per million) fluoride in drinking water is beneficial to teeth. This is equivalent to a daily intake of about 3mg fluoride for an adult drinking water containing this concentration of fluoride. In most parts of the UK the water supplies naturally contain between one-tenth and one-fifth of this amount. However in parts of Bedfordshire, Buckinghamshire, Cleveland, Derbyshire, Dorset and Essex the natural ground water contains more than 1ppm of fluoride. About thirty water authorities fluoridate their water supplies in order to bring the natural amounts up to the recommended level.

The only other useful source of fluoride in the diet is from tea. A tea infusion contains about 1ppm (or 2ppm if made with fluoridated water) leading to an average daily intake of 1mg from tea alone. Although tea consumption may be useful in areas where the water supply is low in fluoride, it is unlikely to benefit young children who need it most. For this reason dentists advise that babies and young children, living in an area with a low level of fluoride in the water, should be given fluoride tablets or drops.

NITRATES

Nitrates occur naturally in drinking water and are thought to be harmless in low concentrations. However, since 1945 there have been dramatic increases in the amount of nitrates present in some parts of the country. These high levels are probably due to the greatly increased use of fertilizers, usually nitrate-based, on agricultural land, but the problem may be more complex as it can take up to thirty years for the effects of nitrates to be shown in the water supply. The EEC has suggested that levels for nitrates in water should be 25mg/litre, but the WHO set the higher maximum level of 50mg/litre. The limit was set because high levels of nitrate have been associated with infantile methaemoglobinemia, a rare form of anaemia found in bottlefed babies under 6 months of age. If it is recognized early this condition is reversible, but it can lead to death if unchecked. The incidence of this disease in the UK is low, although in areas where cases have been cited, such as parts of East Anglia, bottled water is sometimes used for feeds as a precaution.

The concern about nitrates is based on the fact that nitrates can be converted to nitrites in the body, and these in turn can combine with amines to form nitrosamines, which are believed to be a cause of stomach cancer. About three-quarters of the nitrate present in our diet comes from food, either because the nitrates are naturally present but usually because they have been added as preservatives. Nitrates and nitrites are used in meat products because they act as a deterrent against botulism.

For all these reasons the levels of nitrates and nitrites in the water supply and foods are carefully monitored. Despite the increased use of nitrates in the soil, the incidence of stomach cancer in industrialized countries has been going down over the last twenty years. Nevertheless, the nitrate contribution made by drinking water is relatively small, approximately 30 per cent of that from food. Therefore it may be more relevant to pay greater attention to the amount of nitrates added to food than to water.

OTHER CONTAMINANTS

Tap water varies in composition, reflecting the geological background of its source as well as the processing it has received (chlorination, fluoridation, etc.). Two common mineral salts in tap water are calcium and magnesium, and the levels of these mineral salts determine whether the water is classified as hard or soft – the higher the concentration, the harder the water. Hard water deposits scale on metal surfaces and in pipes, and will affect cooking utensils such as kettles and coffee makers. It can also affect the texture and appearance of some cooked vegetables.

BOTTLED WATER

There are many different kinds of bottled water: some from wells, some from natural springs and some from ordinary tap water that has been reprocessed. Some of the most famous brands are Ashbourne, Highland Spring, Evian, Vichy, Perrier and Malvern.

Bottled waters may be still, naturally carbonated (in which case they are labelled "naturally carbonated natural mineral waters"), or artificially carbonated (and so are labelled "carbonated natural mineral water"). Some contain considerable amounts of dissolved minerals, which may be either naturally present or have been artificially added, while others may have a low mineral content. Most of the waters are mildly alkaline, and the greater the mineral content and the more alkaline the water, the stronger will be its taste. Tap water often has a mineral content similar to bottled waters, although the nitrate level may be higher.

Some of the bottled waters contain high amounts of sodium, which may need to be considered by those who are trying to lower their salt intake.

SODIUM CONTENT OF MINERAL WATERS

	mg/100ml
Perrier	1.4mg
Vichy Saint Yorre	113.8mg
Badoit	13.8mg
Volvic	0.8mg
Evian	0.5mg
Contrexeville	1.0mg
Buxton	2.4mg
Highland Spring	5.5mg
Ashbourne	2.4mg
Malvern	1.5mg
Soda water	25-30mg
Tap water	0-6mg
	(average 2-3mg)

All bottled waters are controlled by different laws. Natural mineral water is controlled by an EEC directive, under which manufacturers are not allowed to make any therapeutic claims about bottled water. Other types of water are controlled by local rules on public water supply. Recent studies have discovered that water kept in plastic bottles may have a higher bacterial colony count. This seems to be due to the plastic rather than the water itself. Therefore to ensure that your water is not contaminated it is advisable to buy it in a glass bottle.

There has been much interest recently in filtering tap water at home to remove any chemicals such as chlorine, copper and lead. The main component of a water filter is charcoal (or its equivalent) or activated carbon. Some also incorporate silver, which acts as a disinfectant against bacteria. The charcoal or carbon works like blotting-paper and absorbs or soaks up the various unwanted elements. Although this may be beneficial, filtering also removes valuable minerals such as calcium and magnesium. Although some manufacturers dispute this claim it is hard to see how the filtering processes can differentiate among all the elements present in water.

——TEA AND COFFEE——

In Britain we are still a nation of tea drinkers, consuming on average four cups of tea every day compared with two cups of coffee. Tea contains caffeine, usually less than coffee although this depends on the strength of the tea or coffee. The average cup of tea contains 50-80mg of caffeine, and an average consumption of tea represents a daily intake of 200-300mg of caffeine. Because as a nation we tend to drink tea rather than coffee, it is likely that tea provides more of our daily caffeine intake than coffee does.

Tannin is another constituent of tea. Again, the precise amount depends on the strength of the cup of tea, but it has been measured at 40-140mg/100ml. Tannin does not appear to have any side-effects, although some people find that it causes indigestion. Drinking tea with milk helps to neutralize the effect of tannin. But tannin and caffeine are not the only constituents of tea and coffee.

Although caffeine is the strongest stimulant in tea and coffee, these drinks also contain other "xanthine" compounds such as theobromine and theophylline, which have a stimulating effect.

Although tea is still more popular, coffee drinking has risen since World War II. In 1982 coffee was consumed by 70 per cent of the population while tea was consumed by 86 per cent. Recent figures show that consumption of both tea and coffee is declining.

Cola drinks contain extracts from the kola nut. They originated in the United States in 1886 and are now manufactured throughout the world. The precise formulations for different brands of cola drinks are closely guarded secrets, but they usually contain approximately 55mg caffeine per 330ml drink. In the US caffeine-free soft drinks have been introduced for children, who are thought to be particularly sensitive to the stimulating effects of caffeine, which they absorb readily into their smaller bodies.

Cocoa also contains caffeine, although less than tea or coffee. It is not drunk with such regularity by adults, but it is popular with children and should be taken into account as a source of caffeine. Cocoa contains other substances such as theobromine, tyramine and phenylethylamine, which may also cause headaches.

Although caffeine is found in these drinks, some of it is combined with other chemicals and so not all of it is absorbed by the body. Caffeine has been shown to have a stimulating effect on the brain. It affects the cerebral cortex, which is concerned with thought, and the medulla, which regulates heart rate, respiration and

THE CAFFEINE CONTENT OF EVERYDAY DRINKS

Drink	Caffeine per cup
Brewed ground coffee	125-150mg
Tea (strong)	80-125mg
Tea (average strength)	50-80mg
Tea (weak)	20-50mg
Instant coffee	35-75mg
Decaffeinated coffee	3mg
Cola drinks	55mg per 330ml
Most herbal teas	0
Coffee-grain blends such as Barley Cup	14-37mg

muscular co-ordination. Too much caffeine can cause palpitations, indigestion, irritability and insomnia, so drinking too much coffee can result in a person feeling on edge, anxious, jittery and wide awake. Caffeine can also raise the basal metabolic rate and thus increase the number of calories the body burns. This may be a slight aid in weight control, but approximately three cups of strong black coffee have been shown to trigger the release of insulin, which causes blood sugar to drop, thus producing feelings of hunger!

Caffeine also stimulates the heart muscles and can cause the heart to beat more quickly. Although one study indicated that those who drank large amounts of coffee were more prone to heart disease, other studies have not confirmed this. As coffee can make the heart beat abnormally fast, it has been suggested that caffeine can also increase blood pressure. However, despite much research there is little evidence that moderate coffee consumption increases the risk of heart disease. Caffeine also relaxes the muscles of the respiratory system and the digestive tract. It also has a diuretic effect thus causing the kidneys to increase the output of urine.

Those of us who imagine we don't function so well without caffeine may well be correct, as small amounts of caffeine can stimulate, especially when feeling fatigued. Those who consume caffeine regularly can become mildly addicted. At present no one knows precisely how much caffeine is required to become psychologically and physically dependent, but there are people who have reported withdrawal symptoms, such as feeling drowsy, after they have stopped drinking only 3 or 4 cups of coffee a day.

Caffeine is a pharmacological agent and like any drug it can have drawbacks. However, it has probably received more bad press than it deserves. It has been suggested that caffeine is connected with heart disease, cancer and digestive disorders. In a study in America a link was found between the consumption of freshly ground coffee and cancer of the pancreas. However there appeared to be no connection between instant coffee or tea and the incidence of the cancer.

Some people, especially those who suffer from heartburn, may find that coffee irritates the stomach. This is probably the result of the acids present in coffee rather than the amount of caffeine. Decaffeinated coffee does not help as acids, which include tannic, nicotinic, formic and citric acid, are still present. However, these irritants can be reduced by the addition of milk in tea and coffee.

Decaffeinated coffee has become readily available over the last five years.

Although some experts think that decaffeinated fresh ground coffee has a superior taste to the instant decaffeinated coffee, the percentage of people who drink it in the UK is relatively small, possibly because the British drink more instant coffee than fresh-ground coffee. Most decaffeination processes involve the use of a chemical solvent, which is mixed with steamed coffee beans before being removed by further heating. The high temperature destroys some of the delicate flavours, so manufacturers are now switching to other processes in an attempt to reduce this loss of flavour.

GRAIN-BASED AND PLANT DRINKS

These are usually made from a mixture of grains such as barley, rye and wheat, which means that no caffeine is present in the final drink. These grain-based drinks, such as Barley Cup, are usually available only from health food shops.

Carob powder, which is made from the pulp of the carob or locust bean, is now being used by some health food manufacturers to replace cocoa, not only in drinks but also in cooking. Carob powder contains no caffeine or theobromine.

Dandelion and chicory coffee were used during the war when coffee was in short supply. Some people use them today as they find they help digestion.

TYPICAL ANALYSIS OF CAROB AND COCOA POWDER

| | Content per 100g | | Kcals per 8g (2tsps) | |
	Carob	Cocoa	Carob	Cocoa
Calories	177	295	14	24
Crude fat	0.7	23.7	0.06	1.9
Carbohydrates (Natural sugar)	46.0	5.5	3.7	0.4
Crude fibre	7.0	4.3	0.6	0.3
Other CHO	35.4	38.5	2.8	3.1
Iron (mg)	50.0	10.0	4.0	0.8
Caffeine	nil	0.16	nil	0.01
Theobromine	nil	1.1	nil	0.09

HERBAL TEAS

These have been gaining in popularity recently, although "tisanes", another name for herbal teas, have been around for centuries. Herbal teas are infusions of fresh or dried leaves, flowers or roots such as mint leaves, raspberry leaves and orange petals. Herbs do contain small amounts of drugs and as such they should be used with caution; brew a fresh cup of tea each time to avoid strong concentrations of any chemicals. It is safer to buy herbal teas from a shop than to make your own infusions with leaves etc. from the garden. Most herbal teas are caffeine-free, while their tannin content, although variable, is generally much less than that of ordinary tea. Some, like matté tea, contain no tannin at all. Others, like rosehip tea, also provide vitamin C. The flavour of herb teas deteriorates with long storage and, like ordinary tea, they should always be stored in an airtight tin.

LEVEL OF TANNIN IN DIFFERENT TEAS

Beverage	Per cent tannin mg
Black tea	7.3-15.1
Matté	5.86
Peppermint	4.0
Mixed fruit	3.0
Rosehip (some brands)	2.27
Coffee	2.0
Fennel	1.85
Camomile	1.69

(Research conducted by Leatherhead Food Research Association.)

—SOFT DRINKS—

Sales of soft drinks increased dramatically in the 1960s and 1970s, and although sales are still increasing overall, it is now mainly the diet drinks and fruit juices that are gaining ground. Soft drinks can be divided into three categories: squashes, fresh fruit juices and fizzy drinks.

SQUASHES

These remain popular because they are cheap, but recent concern about dental health, particularly over the "health drinks", has led more parents to switch to fresh fruit juices or low calorie drinks. Highly sweetened drinks are not necessarily the best way to quench the thirst as the sugar actually increases the body's need for water. Water and diluted fresh fruit juice are a better alternative. One glass of fruit squash or 1 glass of diluted fruit juice (half water and half fruit juice) provide approximately 2tsp (10ml) of sugar. From the point of view of teeth both drinks are undesirable between meals, although fruit juice does have the advantage of being a good source of vitamin C.

There are many varieties of fruit squash, including the recent addition of high juice fruit squash. All squashes have by law to contain a certain minimum proportion of fruit juice.

Fruit squashes These must by law contain 25 per cent of fruit juice for undiluted citrus squash; and 10 per cent of fruit juice for non-citrus fruit squashes.

Cordials These are filtered fruit squash and contain the same amount of fruit juice as fruit squashes. Curiously, labelling regulations in the UK stipulate that lime cordial cannot be labelled lime squash, but other citrus cordials can be called either squash or cordial.

Barley water This must contain at least 15 per cent of fruit juice when undiluted. It also contains citrus juice, sugar and barley flour.

Fruit drinks These may be sold ready diluted or as concentrates. Concentrates have to contain at least 7 per cent whole fruit and 10-15 per cent sugar, plus some preservative so they remain safe during storage. Ready diluted fruit drinks that are often sold in cartons have no restriction on fruit or sugar content.

High juice fruit squashes These usually contain 35-50 per cent fruit juice, but there is no legal minimum as to the amounts that should be added.

FRUIT JUICES

Since the introduction of Ultra Heat Treated fruit juice in Tetra packs in the 1980s consumption has increased dramatically. Not only does the fruit juice taste better than canned fruit juice, but the cartons – unlike cans – can be put into the refrigerator once they are open. The availability of smaller cartons has also made them popular with children. However, it is also possible to buy fruit drinks in the same type of cartons that contain added sugar. Check the list of ingredients carefully.

Fruit juices are not lower in calories but they do contain essential vitamins and minerals. One glass of orange or grapefruit juice, for example, contains the daily requirement of vitamin C. For the young and old, who may not eat much fresh fruit, this is a useful way of ensuring that they obtain their daily requirement.

If your children drink large quantities of fresh fruit juice, try to persuade them to have other drinks occasionally. Low calorie-saccharin- or aspartame-sweetened drinks may be acceptable alternatives, for a child who likes sweet-tasting drinks. Diluting fruit juice will help reduce the acidity as well as the sugar content. Concentrated fruit juices may contain small amounts of preservatives but no artificial sweeteners, or other additives.

Recently there has been the introduction of fizzy fresh fruit juices, particularly apple and grape. These are basically carbonated fruit juices. They are naturally high in sugar and contain little vitamin C.

FIZZY DRINKS

Although sugary fizzy drinks account for the majority of the sales, there has been a recent trend towards consuming sugar-free drinks. These were initially sold as low calorie drinks for those on a diet but with the public's recent interest in "sugar-free" foods and drinks there has been an increase in sales. A 12fl oz (330ml) can or almost 2 glasses of fizzy drink (not sugar-free) such as cola contains the equivalent of 7tsp (42ml) of sugar.

—ALCOHOL—

In the past twenty years, alcohol consumption has doubled in the UK, and intake has increased most among adolescents and women. Alcohol is not commonly regarded as a food, but it is a source of energy and can account for anything up to 9 per cent of an average adult's energy intake. A recent report (1986) suggested that the average alcohol consumption should be reduced by one-third.

Once alcohol is consumed, it is rapidly absorbed into the bloodstream from where it is carried to the liver. Here it is metabolized and detoxified at a fixed rate. Some alcoholic drinks supply small amounts of vitamins and minerals, although the quantities are trivial. (For further information on alcohol see pages 19-22.)

TIPS TO CUT DOWN DRINKING

Take non-alcoholic drinks like alcohol-free lagers and wines, mineral waters and fruit juices. Sometimes the action of pouring a drink, for example on getting home from work, is more important than the actual drink itself, so a soft drink may do just as well. If tomato or orange juice draw unwanted attention to yourself, then drinking mixers like tonic or mineral water will be less obvious. (See pages 188-9 for a list of non-alcoholic drinks.)

Occupy yourself with other enjoyable activities while drinking to distract attention from the glass.

Drink for taste if it is the flavour you particularly want to enjoy. Drink more slowly, putting down the glass between sips. Count the number of sips and increase the number next time.

Change the drink. Changing the type of drink can help break old habits and reduce the amount drunk. (Beer drinkers seem to underestimate the amount they consume far more than spirit or wine drinkers.)

Imitate the slow drinker. Copy someone who drinks slowly, only picking up the glass when they do.

Slow down on the "rounds". Either buy your own drinks (like smokers smoke their own cigarettes these days rather than offering the packet round), or when it is your turn for a round, don't buy yourself a drink.

Take days off. If you usually drink every day, take one day off from alcohol, then two and three. On the other hand don't give up alcohol on four or five days and then "make up" for it with binges at weekends.

Learn to refuse drinks. Say you are cutting down or that you don't want to get sleepy, or that you want to keep a clear head.

Make non-alcoholic drinks available to other people. Always have a jug or bottle of water on the table at mealtimes; display non-alcoholic drinks so that people can see they have the choice; don't make people feel guilty or a killjoy if they don't ask for an alcoholic drink and if they ask for a small measure, don't give them a large one.

CHAPTER 14

BUYING, STORING AND COOKING FOOD

*F*or most people eating more healthily not only means eating less of some foods but, perhaps more importantly, eating more of other foods such as cereals, fruit, vegetables, pulses and fish. But this is not always as simple as it sounds. You may be willing to try out new dishes, but you first have to buy the basic ingredients and, having bought them, you need to know what to do with them. And it is here that difficulties may arise. For example, many people find displays of fish attractive, but when it comes to making a purchase they find it difficult to know what to choose. Most of us have got so used to the ubiquitous fillets of cod and fish-fingers that the art of cooking fish is forgotten.

FRUIT AND VEGETABLES
Fruit has the advantage of being sweet but at the same time fairly low in calories, and a good source of vitamins and minerals. Even if you don't eat much in the way of puddings, different combinations of fruits can add interest and variety to salads and grain dishes. Fruit juices can also be used in marinades, salad dressings and sauces. Fruit is also good combined with yoghurt and low fat cheese, and makes a starter to a meal.

Always try to buy soft fruit the day you want to eat it. Fruits such as strawberries, blackcurrants and raspberries should be firm yet soft, and you should never buy soft fruit that looks wet or mouldy as it is likely to be a few days old or it may even have been picked when wet. Stone fruit such as peaches, mangoes, apricots, plums and cherries should be firm to touch and not bruised. Avoid any fruit with split or discoloured skins or soft spots. Stone fruits too are best eaten on the day of purchase, but they may be kept for another day, especially if they are bought a little under-ripe. Apples and pears should also be firm to touch. Avoid any that have brownish bruises. It's not worth trying to store damaged fruit or windfalls; instead cook them and use to make purées or crumbles.

Adding vegetables to stews and casseroles is a traditional way of adding flavour and making the dish go further. They can also be used to lighten and add interest to rice or pasta, and vegetable purées make good sauces. You can also make excellent pâtés, dips, fillings for pancakes and alternative layers for pasta dishes like lasagne. Side salads make a refreshing first or final course to a meal.

When you buy vegetables, avoid those that are dull, wilted, limp, damaged or discoloured. Freshness is again the key, so choose those that are bright and plump-looking. Remember to take account of the recent weather. After a heavy frost, vegetables such as Brussels sprouts could look all right but still be badly frost-damaged inside and unpleasant to eat. Similarly, wet lettuces may be fine on the outside but rotten in the middle. Smell the vegetables to check that they are really fresh. Some vegetables, especially potatoes, can be bought in bulk, and this can represent a substantial saving if they are stored correctly.

Even after picking and cropping, fruit and vegetables are still living organisms that "breathe", taking in oxygen and giving off carbon dioxide. The key to prolonging the storage life of fruits and vegetables is therefore to slow down this rate of respiration by keeping the produce in a controlled atmosphere. This means keeping most, but not all, crops at a cool or cold temperature and, more difficult, at the correct humidity. To store fruit and vegetables in the home at a higher humidity than is normally found in the fridge, keep them in polythene bags (aerated with a few holes). In much the same way commercially stored produce can be kept for several weeks and sometimes months.

Unfortunately the actual process of buying fruit and vegetables can shorten their storage life, as they get squeezed and thrown into shopping trolleys, boxes and finally into the vegetable basket or fridge at home. Damaged and roughly handled produce withers and decays more quickly, both because a damaged or broken skin allows disease organisms to enter and because rough handling and inappropriate storage conditions increase the "breathing" rate of the crop, so making it decay more rapidly.

In order to prolong the storage life of fruits and vegetables they should be stored as follows:

In the fridge in a polythene bag or cellophane wrapping Apples, apricots, berries, cherries, figs, grapes, nectarines, peaches, pears, persimmons, plums, pomegranates, rhubarb. Asparagus, broccoli, Brussels sprouts, cabbage, cauliflower, carrots, celeriac, celery, endive, globe artichokes, kohlrabi, leeks, lettuce, mushrooms, parsley, parsnips, peas, radishes, salsify, sweetcorn, turnips, watercress.
In a cold larder or the salad compartment of the fridge without covering Aubergines, courgettes, cranberries, cucumbers, grapefruit, lemons, limes, lychees, melons, okra, oranges and tangerines, peppers, tomatoes.
In a cool place Aubergines, avocados (or in the airing cupboard for ripening), bananas, grapefruit, guavas, ginger, mangoes, melons, papayas, pineapples, potatoes, sweet potatoes, tomatoes.
At room temperature or in a cool place Garlic, onions.

FISH

Fish is an excellent source of protein and minerals. The white varieties are low in calories – provided they are not accompanied by rich sauces – and oily fish contains the special long chain polyunsaturates that are currently the subject of much research (see page 18).

Fresh fish, whether oily or white, can be recognized by firm flesh, clear and full shiny eyes, bright red gills and a clean smell. Steaks and fillets should be firm with

'
All fish is best used within 12 hours of purchase.
'

closely packed flakes. A watery appearance is an indication that the fish is stale. If the skin has a blue or green tinge, the fish is definitely not fresh. Trout with a blackish or very reddish appearance are in breeding condition and will not be as good as bright silvery specimens. Fresh shellfish should look crisp and dry. Prawns, scampi and shrimps should be firm to the touch and not flaccid. Any broken mussels, scallops or oysters or those that do not close when tapped should be discarded. All fish is best used within 12 hours of purchase.

Fishmongers are much less common today than they used to be. However, more and more large supermarkets are opening up fish counters. Take the fishmonger's advice on what is best for the time of year. Most white fish are at their best in the winter before they start to breed. Fish that are about to breed or that have just bred are usually unpleasant to eat.

Cook fish as follows:

Flat fish suitable for steaming, grilling, baking, frying and casseroling Brill, dab, flounders, halibut (needs careful cooking otherwise it loses its flavour), John Dory, plaice, skate (any smell of ammonia disappears on cooking and the bones come away easily), sole and turbot (similar to sole in flavour). Those who find fish like these somewhat insipid may like the added bite that can be given by cooking with lemons, limes, kumquats or anchovy essence.

White fish, which may be easily flaked and is suitable for fish pies or fish cakes Cod, coley, haddock, hake (the flesh comes easily away from bones) and whiting.

Round, firm-fleshed fish for poaching, baking, steaming, casseroling and grilling White fish, such as cod, haddock, hake and monkfish (which has a good flavour and the bones are easily identified); oily fish, such as bass, salmon, sea bream and trout.

Oily fish for grilling, baking, barbecuing, frying or casseroling Herring, mackerel (which should be eaten as fresh as possible as it stales quickly), red mullet, sardines, sprats, trout and tuna.

Shellfish for garnishes, soups, casseroles, starters and shellfish dishes Clams, crayfish, mussels, oysters, prawns, scallops, shrimps and whelks.

MEAT

Lean meat is an excellent source of iron and other minerals in addition to protein. Lamb and pork tend to be fattier than beef (depending on the cut), although pork and lamb are now, because of modern farming practices, much less fatty than they used to be. It is fairly easy to see how much fat there is on a joint, but it is much more difficult to tell how much fat there is when meat is sold as mince. On average mince contains 16 per cent fat, although the proportions will vary widely, and many supermarkets are now declaring the fat content of mince on the labels so it is possible to choose those that have a lower fat content.

When you buy meat remember that the colour is only an indication, not a guarantee, of quality. Meat is often displayed under slightly warm lighting, which makes it look redder and juicier than it actually is. Beef should be a plum red, pork should be a pale pink, and lamb should be pink with a touch of red. The fat should be creamy to white, depending on the meat, and not yellow. Although much emphasis is placed on reducing the fat in the diet, it is commonly thought that a certain amount of fat is necessary for meat to be juicy and flavoursome. A covering of fat traditionally helped to keep in the juices of a roasting joint, but nowadays foil, roasting bags and the practice of "sealing in the juices" at a high temperature for the first 10 minutes of cooking time can achieve the same end.

From the point of view of flavour, probably the most important factor is the way meat is treated at the time of slaughter. In the past, the meat was usually hung for at least five days, preferably fifteen, to allow the flavours to develop. Now, new methods being evolved in meat science can cut down the time to a matter of hours. Enzymes that are naturally present in the animal cause the tenderizing of the meat, and their activity can be markedly speeded up by using the fast chilling method.

Meat will keep for about three days in the refrigerator. Never let raw meat come in contact with cooked meat – for example, by using the same knife to cut both without cleaning it in between or by letting raw meat accidentally drip on to cooked meat in the fridge. Bacteria in the raw meat will contaminate the cooked.

Poultry Chicken and particularly turkey are low fat meats, and it is possible to reduce the fat content of chicken further by removing the skin and any lumps of fat, especially from the body cavity, before cooking.

Today poultry is available fresh, chilled and frozen. Generally, the larger the bird, the better value it will be because the proportion of meat to bone is higher. Poultry should always look firm and shiny. Check to see if there is any bruising on the leg and breast, and avoid bruised birds. Today the giblets are often not included with the bird, and if you enjoy chicken liver or want to make a stock, make sure you know what you are buying. Poultry should be eaten within three days of purchase. Frozen chicken should be thoroughly defrosted before cooking, as bacteria within the body cavity of the bird are a frequent source of food poisoning if partially defrosted meat is cooked inadequately.

Game Game birds and animals are wild, so their flesh tends to be leaner, coarser and tougher than intensively reared birds and animals. Hanging softens the flesh as well as bringing out the flavours.

It can be difficult to distinguish between "good" and "bad" game, but look for clean and soft-spurred feet and pliable breastbones. The flesh should also look soft and shiny. Buying and storing game is a specialized business, so it is a good idea always to buy from a good game dealers or supermarket. Make sure that game birds have not been too damaged by shot, and when you eat them be careful not to break a tooth on a stray bit of lead!

Offal Liver has always been much favoured by nutritionists because it is not only an excellent source of iron and vitamins but is also one of the cheapest cuts of meat. Liver and other forms of offal are usually very lean meats. In general, offal should look bright and shiny, and it should be clean-smelling. Offal does not store well. Either use it on the day of purchase, keeping it in the refrigerator before use, or buy it frozen and keep it in the freezer for up to one month. Some people do not like the strong flavour of offal, but a little chopped liver or kidney added to a vegetable-based stew can add much flavour to the dish.

Sausages The nutritional value of sausages has recently come under scrutiny as interest in eating foods that are lower in fat has developed. By law, pork sausages must contain 65 per cent meat, but only half of that meat must be lean. Beef

Meat is often displayed under slightly warm lighting, which makes it look redder and juicier than it actually is.

sausages must contain 50 per cent meat (again with only half that amount needing to be lean). The meat content can come from any part of the animal, including the udder, rind and the fat.

Sausage manufacturers sometimes add breadcrumbs or rusk to sausages. Although they help to bind the sausages, bread crumbs also help to keep in the unwanted fat. Sausages are pink because of the addition of red colouring.

NUTRITIONAL COMPOSITION OF SAUSAGES (per 100g)

	kcals	Protein	CHO	Fat
		g	g	g
Pork sausages, grilled	318	13.3	11.5	24.6
Beef sausages, grilled	265	13.0	15.2	17.3
Low fat sausages, grilled	210	15.8	12.2	11.9
Frankfurters	274	9.5	3.0	25.0
Salami	491	19.3	1.9	45.2

DAIRY PRODUCTS

The standard dairy products – milk, cheese and eggs – are well known to all, but there are now some interesting alternatives available. Many of the low fat dairy foods, like skimmed and semi-skimmed milk and the lower fat cheeses, are now widely accepted as everyday items of our diet. People who try these products for the first time often find that some of the flavour is lost, particularly in skimmed milk. However, this reaction is usually only temporary – rather like stopping having sugar in tea and coffee, you at first wonder how on earth you will be able to drink one cup let alone get used to the change permanently! Yet eventually you wonder how you ever managed to drink tea and coffee with sugar in the first place. Semi-skimmed milk tastes like ordinary silver-top without the cream on top. Although the fat and energy content of skimmed and semi-skimmed milk is reduced, most of the important nutrients, for example calcium and protein, are unaffected. These products can be used in our diet without affecting our overall nutrition.

However, there are one or two new products that are low or lower in fat than more conventional items.

Smetana is a Russian product. It can be used to replace soured cream but has the advantage of being lower in fat.

Fromage frais is rather like a low fat yoghurt. As its name suggests, this is a French product with a thick, creamy taste that is suitable for eating with baked potatoes, in dips and in desserts. Mixed with fruit purée it also makes a good cake filling. Because it is less acid than yoghurt, many people find it more acceptable. Look for the lower fat varieties of 1 or even 0 per cent, but if you can't find *fromage frais*, you can make your own by liquidizing curd cheese with skimmed milk.

Quark is another low fat soft cheese. It closely resembles *fromage frais* but is slightly coarser and more acid. There are varieties with added garlic and onion, which can be used instead of the cream cheese versions of these products. There are three types of quark: with 10 per cent fat, 4.5 per cent fat and practically no fat at all. Quark is also available mixed with fruit, but unfortunately these varieties also contain added sugar. As with yoghurt, it is possible to make fruit quark at home using fresh fruit, frozen or dried fruit, or tinned fruit in natural juices.

Greek yoghurt is available both strained and unstrained and made from either cow's or sheep's milk. The strained version is thicker as more of the whey has been removed. Greek yoghurt is particularly high in fat and therefore contains more calories than other yoghurts, but its thickness and sweetness make it a good substitute for cream.

CALORIE AND FAT CONTENT OF DIFFERENT YOGHURTS COMPARED WITH CREAM AND LOW FAT SOFT CHEESE

	Fat per 100g	kcals per 100g
Most yoghurts	1.0	70-100
Light/diet yoghurts	0.1	40-50
Thick yoghurts	3.0	90-110
Greek cow's yoghurt	10.0	135
Half cream	12.0	135
Single/sour cream	18.0	190
Sterilized cream	23.0	230
Whipping cream	35.0	335
Double cream	48.0	450
Clotted cream	55.0	500
Quark	0.3	77
Fromage frais	0.4	50
Smetana	10.0	130
Buttermilk	0.1	40

Cheese Many of the traditionally made speciality cheeses are high in fat, and it is difficult to see how this can change to any great extent. Low fat cheeses are available, but they are probably most useful for cooking and in the preparation of other dishes. If you are a hard- or cream-cheese lover you should perhaps consider having bread and cheese as a meal in its own right, rather than having cheese and biscuits at the end of a meal. A cheese course after a meat-based first course could result in an extremely fatty meal.

Specialist cheese shops in the UK may provide over 150 different types of cheese. In general, however, the cheese should look fresh and bright, and it should not be dry when it is bought. Soft cheeses, such as Brie and Camembert, do not keep well. They should only be bought in small quantities and used as soon after purchase as possible. Ideally, cheese should be stored in a cool room or cellar, but a refrigerator will suffice. Wrap cheese in aluminium foil or waxed paper and cover it with a plastic bag. Take cheese out of the refrigerator and unwrap it one hour before it is to be eaten so that the flavour is improved.

All cheese manufacturers within the EEC will soon have to comply with regulations requiring them to use the same system to express the fat content of their cheeses. At the moment there is much confusion because different manufacturers use different systems. Some express fat as a percentage of dry matter, i.e. excluding water; others express fat as an overall percentage. The latter system is to be used.

Low fat hard cheeses are usually lower fat versions of ordinary hard cheese but made with semi-skimmed milk instead of full fat milk. Although there are no legal requirements governing the fat content of low fat hard cheese, most contain approximately 15g of fat and 260 kilocalories per 100g. They also contain slightly lower proportions of calcium than hard fat cheeses – 300mg per 100g instead of 800mg. However, both these amounts make a valuable contribution to the diet.

Other low fat cheeses include ricotta and curd cheese. Ricotta is made from whey rather than curd, and its nutritional value is therefore different from most other cheeses: it has a lower calcium and protein content. Ricotta can be used either on its own or in cooking. It is particularly well suited to Italian cookery, and can be used to fill pancakes, lasagnes and ravioli. It can also be used like many other low fat cheeses to make dips and desserts.

Curd cheese is probably the most widely available of these low fat products. Its fat content will depend on the type of milk from which it is made. Look out for the one made from skimmed milk. Curd cheese can be used to replace cottage cheese in many dishes.

TABLE SHOWING THE FAT CONTENT OF MANY DIFFERENT CHEESES

High Fat 30-50% fat
Cheddar, Stilton, Danish Blue, Lymeswold, Parmesan, cream cheese, Cheshire, Lancashire, Leicester, Roquefort, Dolcelatte, Bel Paese, Cambozola, Gouda.

Medium Fat 15-30% fat
Brie, Edam, Camembert, mozzarella, low fat Cheddar, curd cheese, St Paulin, feta, Baby Bel, Gervais Petit Suisse, provolone, Emmenthal, Gruyère.

Low Fat 0-15% fat
Cottage cheese, low fat soft cheese, curd cheese, ricotta cheese.

Eggs As a nation we are eating fewer eggs than in the past, and this is probably the result of the waning interest in cooked breakfasts. Eggs are particularly useful for setting fruit and vegetable purées and for vegetable-based flans. Whether you buy white or brown, free-range or battery eggs, they are nutritionally much the same. Eggs will keep for two to three weeks in the refrigerator or a cool place. Because eggshells are porous they should be kept away from strong-smelling foods.

FATS AND OILS

There is now a wide variety of fats available: low fat spreads, margarines high in polyunsaturates, spreads that are made of a mixture of butter and vegetable oils, and ordinary margarines and butter. There is also a plethora of different oils. Some oils, like olive oil, may be refined to different levels. This affects their flavour but has little effect on the level of fatty acids.

The following list will help you to choose fats and oils low in saturated fat:

Fat and oils high in polyunsaturates Sunflower oil, safflower oil, soya oil, walnut oil, corn oil and margarine high in polyunsaturates.
Fats and oils high in monounsaturates Olive oil, peanut oil and low fat spread.

Fats and oils high in saturates Palm oil, coconut oil, butter, lard, dripping, hard margarine and suet.

BREAD

Bread is something we should all be eating more of, and the simplest way to do this is to provide bread with every meal. Bread comes in many shapes and sizes and the choice depends on personal taste. Some people like crusty bread; others prefer their bread slightly less done. If slightly stale, some breads, like pitta and crusty bread, can be refreshed by sprinkling them with water and placing them in a hot oven or under the grill. Bread should be stored in a polythene bag in a cool place, but if you buy hot bread this should be left to cool first.

Bread made with preservatives and kept sealed in a polythene bag can be kept for a week or more before it goes stale, but traditionally baked breads will start to stale after only one or two days. Preservatives are added to bread to inhibit the growth of mould, but there is little benefit from preservatives if you shop frequently.

Flour, bread, rice and pasta are not the only grain and cereal foods available, of course. Health food shops and supermarkets now display a wide range of other wholegrain cereals to choose from.

Barley In the past barley was eaten regularly, usually in stews and milk puddings. It has a lower gluten content than wheat and is not suitable for making bread, but it still contains high levels of protein, fibre, calcium, iron and the B vitamins. It does not require any soaking before cooking, and can be cooked by simmering for 50-60 minutes. Pot or Scotch Barley is whole barley with the outer husks removed: only about 7 per cent of the B vitamins are retained after processing. Pearl barley is even more refined, a larger amount of the skin having been removed, and it is highly polished like white rice. Flaked barley, which is now widely available, is quicker to cook than the other types.

Buckwheat Although not technically a grain but the seed of a herbaceous plant, buckwheat can be used in a similar manner to most grains. It has a distinctive flavour and texture. It can be bought both raw and roasted, although it must always be roasted before using. Buckwheat flour and noodles are also available, and these are perhaps the most usual ways of cooking buckwheat, although it can also be used to make buckwheat pancakes or in soups.

Bulgar and cracked wheat These are often used as substitutes for rice in Middle Eastern cooking, bulgar and cracked wheat are produced by soaking wholewheat grains and then roasting them to a very high temperature until they crack. Because the grains have been pre-cooked, they take only 15-20 minutes to complete the cooking process. Their nutritional content is similar to wheat. It can be used to make a satisfyingly substantial base for a salad.

Corn, maize or polenta Although corn is used in many countries as a staple part of the diet, in the UK it is used mainly for cornflakes, cornflour, as an occasional vegetable and to make oil. As corn does not contain any gluten it cannot be used to make leavened bread. It is high in protein but deficient in nicotinic acid. The calorie count varies depending on the product, but the vegetable corn is about 25 calories per ounce (approximately 28g), whereas products like cornflour are about 90 calories per ounce.

Couscous This is made from the inner part of the wheat grain – the semolina part

– couscous is now available in wholewheat versions. A staple food in North African cuisine, it is nutritionally similar to wheat. It is best steamed for about 20 minutes before being used in dishes like pilaus.

Millet Millet is used mainly in the East and in Africa where it can easily be harvested in the arid conditions. The nutritional content of millet is like the rest of the cereal group, and, like corn, it lacks gluten and so cannot be used for making bread. Roasting millet before cooking gives it more flavour. Millet is then boiled for 30-40 minutes.

Oats A valuable source of protein, the B vitamins and fibre, oats have been shown to be particularly beneficial to health as the fibre may help to lower blood cholesterol. There are three main types of oats: whole oat grain (not commonly found), which can be used as an alternative to rice; oatmeal, which comes in varying degrees of coarseness and can be used to make porridge; and rolled oats, some types of which have been pre-treated and so take less time to cook.

Rice One of the staple grains of many countries in Asia, America and Europe, rice comes in numerous forms depending on the variety grown and the degree of treatment. It can be used with savoury dishes and in sweet dishes. It can be firm and nutty, like brown rice, or sweet and sticky, like glutinous rice. From the nutritional point of view, brown rice is the best, for not only is it higher in fibre but also in the B vitamins and protein than de-husked and polished white rice. Although brown rice takes longer to cook, there is less chance of the final product sticking together. The more refined the product the fewer the vitamins and minerals and the more calories per ounce. For example, rice flour contains about 90 calories per ounce and fewer vitamins and minerals than white rice.

Wild rice Wild rice is not strictly a rice at all but the seed of a wild grass. It is extremely expensive, and so it is best to cook it with brown rice. But as it takes slightly longer to cook than brown rice, it should be cooked on its own first for between 10 and 15 minutes.

Whole rye Although whole rye is difficult to find, its flour is available from most specialist shops. Rye has a distinctive flavour and is not suitable for many dishes. Rye flour is low in gluten, and therefore bread made with it will rise less and be flatter than high-gluten cereals such as wheat. Rye bread is usually a mixture of wheat and rye and is eaten quite widely in Eastern Europe and the Soviet Union.

Wheat The majority of wheat, the main staple of the West, is converted into flour to make bread, breakfast cereals, pasta and pastry. Wholewheat grains can also be cooked but need to be soaked overnight and then cooked for an hour. In the average British diet wheat provides one-quarter of our protein; whereas in the past wheat probably provided about one-half to three-quarters of the protein intake. Unrefined wheat also provides dietary fibre, the vitamin B group, calcium and iron.

Sorghum A major cereal throughout Asia and Africa, sorghum is a very hardy, drought-resistant type of millet. There are several types of sorghum grains, but the differences are of size. Sorghum may also be referred to as kaffir, durra, milo, fetentas and shallu. Its nutritional composition is similar to that of millet.

Mixed rice and grains One manufacturer has recently come out with a product that consists of brown rice, whole oats, barley, wheat, rye, buckwheat and sesame seeds. By mixing combinations of rice, grains and seeds the protein and calcium content is substantially increased over other cereals. If you prefer, you could make your own combination of cereals but it is practical to choose those that have similar cooking times.

NUTS

Many people regard nuts as a snack food, not as part of a main meal. Nuts are high in fibre and most are also high in fat, mainly monounsaturates and polyunsaturates. Some people may find this a disadvantage, but others who cannot consume the bulk of bread or potatoes find nuts a useful filler. Some varieties, such as macadamia and pine nuts, are very expensive; to lower the proportion of fat and nuts consumed, they can be eaten with dried fruit.

Because most nuts are high in protein they are extremely useful in vegetarian or vegan diets. They are also quick to cook compared with pulses, which need lengthy cooking. Even in a non-vegetarian diet they are a useful contribution to dishes as not only do they add another taste and texture but they can also be used so that less meat needs to be included. For example, nuts can be used in dishes such as stir-fried chicken, or with brown rice and beef risotto. They can also be included very easily with pulses and lentils to make nut roasts and rissoles.

Nuts do not vary widely in their nutritional value. Most contain around 170 kilocalories per ounce (28g), a relatively high amount of fat, fibre, protein, potassium, phosphorus, iron and calcium and vitamins B and E. Nuts were, in fact, used in Europe until the 18th century as an alternative form of milk, when ground and mixed with water. Chestnuts are a notable exception being considerably lower in calories and containing more carbohydrate than other nuts.

Do not buy more than one month's supply of unshelled nuts at a time as the fat tends to go rancid and the flavour deteriorates. Whenever possible store nuts in air-tight jars. Buying nuts in vacuum packs helps, as the removal of oxygen helps them to keep better. Unshelled nuts will keep for up to six months as they are protected by the kernel.

SEEDS

Seeds were regarded throughout the East as a symbol of immortality, and although in the West we may not view them with the same esteem, they are certainly beginning to gain acceptance in our diet, especially among vegetarians and vegans. In countries such as Greece and Turkey, seeds have been used for centuries as a dietary supplement. Today we are probably most familiar with the ready-hulled varieties of poppy, sesame, sunflower and pumpkin seeds. The most common use for seeds in the UK is as decoration in cereal dishes, on salads, in cakes and with vegetbles. Larger quantities of seeds are used in some spreads and nut dishes. Sesame seed paste – or tahini – is reasonably well known, and sunflower seeds often form part of nut stews and loaves.

Nutritionally seeds are similar to nuts. They contain high levels of protein, fibre and fat, little carbohydrate and approximately the same amount of calories.

> *Seeds were regarded throughout the East as a symbol of immortality, and although in the West we may not view them with the same esteem, they are certainly beginning to gain acceptance in our diet, especially among vegetarians and vegans.*

281

They also contain the same vitamins and minerals. Because of their high fat content, seeds should be stored in the same way as nuts to ensure that they maintain their freshness.

SEA VEGETABLES

There are many varieties of sea vegetables such as nori, dulse, kombu, wakame, arame, agar and carrageen. All are high in calcium, iron, iodine, traces of vitamin B_{12}. Their main culinary use is as setting agents or as seasoning. Sea vegetables are usually bought dried and need to be soaked for at least 5 minutes before they are cooked. Dried dulse needs to be rinsed and soaked again for 10 minutes before it can be used. The sea vegetables most often used in Japanese cookery are arame, nori and dulse.

PULSES

Pulses – peas, beans and lentils – are an excellent source of protein, minerals and some vitamins. Most are also low in fat and high in fibre, although a few, notably soya beans, are rich in fat, particularly of the polyunsaturated type.

Pulses have a firm place in many cuisines – including the British diet – even though they may go unnoticed. Pulses are not always dried, and they are more versatile than is often imagined. Peas, runner beans, French beans and broad beans are usually eaten fresh. Cooked, dried beans are often an important vegetable – like baked beans and the dhal that accompany curries or the pease pudding that was traditionally eaten with gammon in this country. Certain traditional dishes could not be made without them. Chilli con carne, for example, contains red kidney

Common name	Other names	Varieties	Availability
Aduki bean	Adzuki bean		Dried or as a flour
Bean		Black beans; haricot beans; kidney beans; pinto beans; canellini beans; borlotto beans; Boston beans	Dried or canned
Black-eyed bean	Cow pea		Dried or canned
Broad bean	Faba bean; Windsor bean; horse bean		Fresh, dried, frozen, canned
Butter bean		Lima beans	Dried or canned
Chick pea	Bengal gram; garbanzos		Canned, dried or as flour
French bean	Haricot verts		Fresh, frozen or canned
Ful medames			Dried or canned
Lentil	Split pea; lentil; dhal	Red, brown, green, yellow	Canned, dried, split or whole
Mung bean	Green gram	Urd bean	Dried, whole or split, sprouted
Pea		Petit pois	Fresh, canned, frozen, dried or processed
Soya bean	Soy beans	Chinese black bean	Curd fresh, flour, oil, dried, fermented, margarine, texturized vegetable protein (TVP)

beans and hummus is impossible without chick peas.

Dried pulses tend to take a long time to prepare. Most have to be soaked over-night and then cooked for one to two hours. All beans must be boiled for the first 10 minutes of cooking. Soya beans sometimes need up to four hours cooking, but not all need such a lengthy preparation time: lentils and mung beans do not need soak-ing and will cook in 15-20 minutes.

Rather than preparing beans each time you want to use them, prepare them in bulk and freeze them in small quantities. They can also be bought ready cooked in cans, although this is an expensive way of buying them. It is possible to speed up the process of soaking by bringing the beans to the boil, boiling for 2-3 minutes and then leaving them to soak for 1 hour.

SPROUTED BEANS OR GRAINS
Bean sprouts are familiar to many households who have eaten Chinese cooking. Bean sprouts are usually grown from mung beans, but there are many other vari-eties that can be grown at home, including those from wheat, alfalfa, lentil and aduki beans.

Beans that are sprouted change their nutritional value and become higher in vitamin C and in protein. Sometimes the vitamin B content is also increased. They are useful in cooking, in salads and in sandwiches. All you need to do sprout beans is to add a couple of tablespoons to a jam jar, cover the beans with water and leave in a warm place. The beans need to be rinsed with fresh water and drained twice a day. (This is a good activity to do with young children.)

SOYA PRODUCTS
The protein-rich soya bean has been exploited by food manufacturers and made into many valuable products. Perhaps the most versatile of all the pulses, soya beans are one of the commonest sources of vegetable oil, flour and "milk" which can be made from them; when fermented they are a major ingredient in Chinese cookery; and they may be found both fresh and dried. Food technologists have been able to make imitation meat and fruit products from soya beans, although these have never become particularly popular. The main disadvantage of the soya bean is that it takes a long time to cook, but it is now possible to buy soya splits or soya grits, which are similar to split peas but made from soya beans. They take less time to cook and therefore may be a useful alternative.

Tofu has been made from the yellow soya bean for over a thousand years. ("Tofu" is the Japanese name; "doufu" is the Chinese equivalent.) Tofu is soya bean curd and there are two varieties: firm, and the silken junket-like variety. The firm tofu is sold in small white blocks in specialist shops. Tofu is most commonly used in Oriental dishes for stir-frying or steaming. Store it in fresh water in a covered container for up to 5 days.

The silken tofu is more widely available, but it is really only suitable for making dips, salad dressings or ice creams. It is often sold in cartons. All tofu is high in pro-tein but low in fat, and because of its bland flavour it can be readily combined with other ingredients.

Tamari sauce is more commonly known as soya sauce. Unlike some soya sauces, that have caramel and wheat added during their manufacture, this is made by the

> *There is no substantial nutritional difference between white or brown sugar, syrup, treacle or honey. All are equally undesirable from the point of view of dental health and all provide similar amounts of calories.*

traditional method of fermenting water and soya beans for 1 to 3 years. Tamari is a fairly thick, rich, dark brown sauce. It is available from most specialist shops and will keep for 18 months once opened.

Tamari sauce is used mainly to flavour soups, vegetables, stir-fried dishes, cereals and rice dishes. However tamari sauce (and soya sauce) is very high in salt and should be used sparingly.

Miso, which is fermented in a similar way to soya sauce, is a thick paste. It can be added to meatless dishes to give extra flavour and can be used in soups instead of stock. There are three main varieties of miso available: mugi miso (fermented soya with barley and sea salt); genmai miso (fermented soya with brown rice and sea salt); and hatcho miso (fermented soya and sea salt). The main difference between the three varieties is that of taste. Miso is readily available in most specialist shops and will keep for 18 months in the refrigerator once opened.

SUGARS AND PRESERVES

There is no substantial nutritional difference between white or brown sugar, syrup, treacle or honey. All are equally undesirable from the point of view of dental health and all provide similar amounts of calories. Although these are the best known forms of sugar, many other varieties appear on food labels but may not be immediately recognizable as forms of sugar – glucose, dextrose, fructose or fruit sugar, malt, lactose, invert syrup, glucose syrup and high fructose syrup. When the word "sugar" appears on a label it usually refers to sucrose, the white, packet sugar; so if the label says the product is low in sugar it may only be low in sucrose. Any claim that a product has reduced sugar needs to be checked with the list of ingredients. The product may indeed be low in sucrose, but it may contain other sugars in the form of glucose syrups or fruit concentrates. The only small advantage that natural fruit sugars or fruit juices have over sucrose or syrups is that they tend to be used in smaller quantities so that the products are less sweet.

There are now many products on the market that are low in sugar – sugar-reduced jams, for example – where a large part, if not all, of the added sugar is substituted with alternative sweeteners such as isomalt, xylitol, sorbitol, hydrogenated glucose syrup, aspartame, acesulfame K, thaumatin and, of course, saccharin. These alternative sweeteners are not harmful to teeth and are very low in calories.

Reduced-sugar products may be particularly useful if they help you get accustomed to less sweet foods. Not all foods can be made with less sugar, but those that can include soft drinks, biscuits, some cakes, desserts and canned fruit. Pie fillings, jams, pickles and sauces can also be made with less sugar, but these products either need a preservative to replace the sugar or they should be stored in a refrigerator.

——STORING FOODS——

Houses are no longer built with a cellar, which was the traditional place for keeping many foods. Today we rely on kitchen cupboards, the refrigerator and the deep freeze to keep our foodstuffs as fresh as possible.

The ideal temperature for the storage of perishable items is just above freezing point, because this temperature will not alter the structure of food. Refrigerators operate at temperatures between 1 and 7°C (34-45°F). In addition most refrigerators also have a deep freeze compartment. These vary from one star to four stars:

One Star Temperature at approximately –6°C (21°F). Already-frozen food can be kept for up to one week.

Two Star Temperature at approximately –12°C (10°F). Already-frozen food can be kept for up to four weeks.

Three Star Temperature at approximately –18°C (0°F). Already-frozen food can be kept up to three months.

Four Star Freezer compartments can be used to freeze unfrozen food, which can then be kept for up to three months.

The top of the refrigerator, just beneath the freezer compartment, is the coldest part and is where perishable foods such as meat should be kept. The door area is the warmest part of the refrigerator. Never put warm or hot food in the fridge – leave it to cool to room temperature first. Like the freezer, a refrigerator should be defrosted regularly.

STORING FOODS IN THE REFRIGERATOR

Food	Storage time	Comments
Bacon, smoked	7 to 10 days	Keep wrapped
Bacon, green	Slightly shorter than smoked bacon	Keep wrapped
Butter and fats	2 to 3 weeks	Keep wrapped or covered
Cheese, soft (except Brie, Camembert)	4 to 5 days	Keep in covered carton Remove 1 hour before serving
Cheese, hard	8 to 9 days	Keep covered with foil
Fish	1 to 2 days	Keep tightly covered or wrapped in foil
Fruit, soft and green vegetables	1 to 5 days	Keep covered but allow some air to reach the fruit
Leftovers (containing meat, sauces or potatoes)	1 day	Keep meat tightly covered
Meat and poultry	1 to 3 days	Store in the chiller tray, or immediately below it; keep meat and poultry loosely wrapped in foil. Remove poultry giblets
Meat joints, large	4 days	Drain off meat juices; cover loosely
Milk and cream	3 to 5 days	Keep covered
Eggs	2 to 3 weeks	

THE GOLDEN RULES

1. Defrost food thoroughly, so that when it is cooked it will reach a high temperature right through, not just the outer layers.

2. Heat food thoroughly to kill off bacteria.

3. Eat food within one hour of cooking.

4. If food is to be stored, it should be cooled in about an hour or less and then refrigerated, or frozen. If food has been cooked in bulk, such as rice or casseroles, it will need to be divided up into small portions to ensure it cools rapidly.

5. Make sure your fridge is working properly and keeping the temperature below

4°C (0°F). Follow the manufacturer's instructions concerning freezer use and temperatures.
6. Raw and cooked food, and the utensils used with them, must be kept entirely separate, otherwise live bacteria in the raw food will contaminate the cooked.
7. When food is being reheated it must reach a boiling temperature throughout. Food in tins is sterilized during the canning process and does not have to be boiled in the same way as other previously cooked dishes.

The following produce may be kept for the time indicated. Check stored food from time to time to ensure that it is still in good condition.

Nuts Shelled nuts should be used within a month; unshelled nuts will keep for about 6 months.
Savoury biscuits are best used within 2 months.
Flour is best used within 3-6 months.
Sea vegetables such as arame or wakame will keep for about 4 months once the packets are opened.
Oils are best used within 6 months.
Dried fruit will keep for a year in airtight containers, although it is best used within 6 months.
Dried beans are best used within 6 months. They will keep for up to a year but will take longer to cook.
Breakfast cereals are best used within 6 months, although some can be used up to a year after purchase.
Pasta is best eaten within a year.
Rice is best eaten within a year.
Whole grains will keep about a year in a cool dark place.
Dried herbs and spices are best used within a year.

——*KITCHEN EQUIPMENT*——

Healthy eating depends on the ingredients, but it can also be influenced by the cooking equipment available. Eating healthily is all very well in theory, but good intentions tend to fall by the wayside if trying new recipes takes up too much time or is generally inconvenient. The right tools are helpful if healthy eating is to become a part of daily life. For example, a good-quality non-stick frying pan can do much to help cut down the fat in cooking, and if baked potatoes are popular a microwave will cut down the cooking time from hours to minutes.

MICROWAVE OVENS AND COMBINATION MICROWAVE COOKERS
It took several years for microwave ovens to become popular in Britain. Initially there was some concern that food didn't brown and was unevenly cooked – and because it was thought they might constitute a health risk (see page 145). Since the early models, developments in microwave technology now ensure that the air circulates throughout the oven so that the food is cooked evenly. Some recent models also incorporate a conventional oven to help brown the food so that it looks more like food cooked in an ordinary oven.

As we have seen (pages 144-5) microwave ovens cook by making the moisture in food vibrate at such a high speed that sufficient heat is generated to cook it. A vent at the sides, top or back of the oven allows the excess steam to escape. The heat inside the oven is moist which prevents the food from shrinking or drying out but also prevents the food from browning.

Microwaves are ideal for heating individual portions of food and can be particularly valuable if members of a household want to eat at different times or to have different foods. Microwave cooking also means much less in the way of cooking smells – a great advantage when it comes to cooking fish. Fish is, in fact, often better cooked by the moist heat of a microwave rather than the dry heat of a conventional cooker, and fruit and vegetables keep their colour and shape better when cooked in a microwave. Food can also be reheated with little deterioration to either the taste, texture or nutritional value. However, as in conventional cooking, smaller portions will cook more quickly than larger ones. If several items are to be cooked at the same time, they should be reasonably equal in size, weight and shape, so that they will cook in the same time.

As the volume of food being cooked is increased, so must be the cooking time. This is because the amount of energy the oven gives out remains constant but has to be shared out among a larger amount of food. For example, one jacket potato would take about 4 minutes to cook in a microwave oven; four jacket potatoes would take about 14 minutes to cook.

Although most foods can be cooked in a microwave – two exceptions are boiled eggs and deep-fried foods – some foods, such as roast meat, bread, pastry and cakes, are better suited to conventional cooking methods. Although these dishes can be browned under a hot grill or in a special browning dish after being cooked in a microwave, the final product is often unsatisfactory. The solution to this problem has been the development of the combination microwave cooker.

The combination microwave cooker includes both a conventional oven or a convection oven, which uses a fan to circulate the heat more evenly, with a microwave oven. The more sophisticated models also include a grill. The added advantage of these is that they allow food to be cooked quickly while at the same time ensuring that it browns.

Microwaves or combination cookers allow busy people to prepare food in a hurry. For example, you may have in the freezer a pre-prepared frozen dish that can be prepared in half the time in a microwave oven.

Like microwave ovens, the combination cooker should not use metal bakeware or foil when the microwave part of the cooker is in use. The metal causes "arcing" – i.e. the energy rebounds off the metal surface so that the food does not cook properly and with large quantities of metal the oven may be damaged. Yoghurt cartons and ordinary plastic bags are also unsuitable as they melt with the heat from the hot food and, unless the label says it is safe for use in cooking, cling-film should not be used as components in the plastic can be transferred into the food during the heating process. One of the advantages of microwave cooking is that the oven and dishes usually remain cool. With combination cookers the dishes will be become hot whenever the conventional heat source is used. All microwave ovens and combination cookers sold in this country incorporate stringent safety measures. As we saw in Chapter 7, much of the anxiety about microwave cookers stems from fear of the unknown.

FOOD PROCESSORS

Food processors can perform a whole range of tasks from mixing dough, pastry and cake mixtures to grating and chopping vegetables, mincing meat and liquidizing. Some models also have special attachments for beating egg whites and for making fruit juice. A food processor performs a wide range of tasks adequately but perhaps not as well as more specialized pieces of individual equipment. Liquidizers make smoother soups, juices and purées and mix better cakes. So if you do a lot of baking and soup making, a mixer with a liquidizer attachment is probably a better buy.

However, if you seem to be forever grating and chopping fruit, vegetables and nuts, a food processor is useful. Don't used the processor to chop everything or you will find all your ingredients will be of a uniform size and shape. Some food processors are particularly good at mincing meat, which is useful for those who want to ensure that lean meat is used to make mince, and they can also be used to purée quantities of food that would be too large for a liquidizer to manage properly – for example, cooked chick peas.

Both food processors and food mixers are fairly bulky and take up a good deal of space on the work surface. You must be able to justify this loss of space (and the cost of the machine) by regular use. Keeping the food processor in the cupboard is no solution for it must be easily available to allow maximum use.

COFFEE GRINDER

Herbs, spices, lemon juice and chopped onion not only make interesting alternatives to salt but they have been used in many cuisines to add zest and bite to staple foods like rice and other grains. If you use a lot of spices in your cooking, you will find that freshly ground ones are much the best from the point of view of both flavour and convenience. A coffee grinder can be indispensable for grinding these small quantities evenly – but use a separate grinder for the spices and the coffee beans because the flavour of the spices will almost certainly taint the coffee, however well the grinder is cleaned. If you don't have a food processor, a coffee grinder will also grind nuts and make small quantities of breadcrumbs.

FREEZER

Whether you decide to purchase a refrigerator with a small freezing compartment or to buy a large chest or upright freezer, the freezer can act as a useful storage unit. Someone living alone could buy a cheap family pack of chicken and freeze the items individually or use the freezer to store double portions of cooked food. It is also possible to keep meat or fish to save on shopping, to keep leftovers or to store ready-prepared dishes for use when someone has turned up unexpectedly. The freezer can store foods that are either not easy to obtain, such as fresh yeast, fresh herbs or soft fruits that are available fresh for only a limited period.

Keeping foods in a freezer maintains their condition as near to their original quality in terms of colour, flavour and nutritional value as possible. Texture, however, sometimes suffers. Older methods of preserving food, such as canning, salting and drying, do tend to alter the food, particularly the flavour. The nutritional value of frozen food can often be better than fresh food, because it is frozen soon after harvesting and so retains more of the goodness. If frozen foods don't seem to be as good as their fresh equivalent it may be because poor quality materials were used. You may, for example, find you achieve better quality by freezing fresh meat from the butcher rather than buying frozen meat. However, it is crucial that you ensure that the "fresh" meat has not been frozen before.

Herbs can be stored in a freezer bag so that you break off what you require each time, or they can be chopped, placed in an ice cube tray and frozen with water to form herb "ice cubes", which are excellent in soups, casseroles and stews. A freezer is extremely useful if you are organized enough to make double the quantity of casseroles, nut and bean loaves, or anything else that freezes well. This allows you to have another meal later on without too much effort.

With all the interest in healthy eating most of us should be eating more fish. Frozen fish can help us to do this. Not only does fish freeze well but it also defrosts quickly or can sometimes be cooked from frozen which is useful for the unexpected meal. (For suggestions for other suitable standby foods see page 179.)

CHECKLIST FOR FREEZING FOOD

1. Blanch all vegetables (except herbs) before freezing so that they maintain their colour, flavour and nutritive value.

2. Open-freeze vegetables or fruits on a tray and pack into bags once frozen to avoid having a solid block of fruit or vegetables.

3. Freeze food as quickly as possible so that fewer ice crystals form, thus destroying the texture of the food. For this reason fruit and vegetables should initially be frozen spread out on trays.

4. Pack food in the portion sizes that you and your family are most likely to use.

5. Where possible, keep pre-cooked dishes in oven-to-tableware dishes to save on both containers and washing up.

6. Make sure packets of food are as airtight as possible, otherwise the food will deteriorate more rapidly.

7. Use proper packaging such as freezer bags or plastic containers so that moisture from the interior of the freezer does not migrate into the food and damage it.

8. Label the food with a date by which it should be eaten so that you don't end up with poor quality food because it has been in the freezer too long.

9. Never put anything hot or warm into the freezer as it is important to maintain a steady storage temperature of −18°C (0°F).

10. Defrost the freezer at least once a year, preferably when stocks are low.

Frozen food should never be refrozen. However if food thaws partially – provided that there are still ice crystals – it can be frozen again, although the quality may be poorer. Cakes and fruit can be refrozen because the sugar and acid in them acts as a preservative. Frozen food keeps for different lengths of time:

Bread: 1 month
Shellfish: 1 month
Bacon and gammon: 1-2 months
Cooked meat or fish casseroles: 2 months
Fish: 3 months
Cakes and pastries: 3 months
Raw meat, nuts, pulses, herbs, fruit and vegetables: 4 months
Soft fruit: 12 months

Foods that are unsuitable for freezing include:

Cooked eggs and raw eggs (unless the yolk is separated from the white)
Cooked sliced potatoes, which can go leathery
Mashed potato that has had milk added before freezing, which will go slushy after
    defrosting
Salad items, such as lettuce, watercress, celery, which go limp and mushy
Custard
Mayonnaise
Garlic is best added to dishes when they have been thawed
Dishes with a high proportion of gelatine
Milk, unless it states otherwise on the container

PRESSURE COOKER

Although considered by some to be an outmoded form of cookery, many people find pressure cookers extremely useful. All pressure cookers have safety valves, and it is important to ensure these are working correctly. Automatic timers have made pressure cookers more reliable.

Pressure cookers are ideal for cooking such items as beans and pulses and brown rice risottos as it can cook them faster than a microwave. Pressure cookers can also be used for pot roasts, soups, bottling and cooking vegetables. The nutritive value remains much the same as in conventional methods, and it may occasionally be better as more water soluble nutrients are retained. When choosing a pressure cooker, select a large stainless-steel one, which can be used for cooking large quantities of, for instance, pasta.

STEAMER

A steamer is invaluable for cooking vegetables especially if you don't have a microwave. Steaming retains more of the vitamins and minerals, and steamed vegetables are less likely to be overcooked than boiled vegetables. Fish, too, is excellent steamed and should be tried.

There are three types of steamer: the Chinese bamboo type, the metal non-collapsible version and the metal collapsible version. The collapsible metal variety is probably the most versatile as it will fit any sized saucepan and can be used to steam something that is flat or in a bowl. The best but most expensive are the stainless steel steamers that fit one on top of each other so that you can steam more than one vegetable at a time. Bamboo steamers are adequate but they tend to go out of shape after a while.

WOK

If you like Oriental cookery such as Chinese food, you will find that a wok will be essential. Chinese food has long been popular, both as takeaway food and in restaurants, but it wasn't until the mid-1970s that people started to cook it for themselves. Stir-frying was perhaps one of the first Chinese cooking styles to be tried at home, and with stir-frying came the wok. This pan quickly gained popularity as people found that it was easier to use than a large frying pan and enabled less fat to be used. Cooking with a wok is quicker than many other forms of cooking because of the high temperatures of the pan surface and the use of bite-sized pieces, traditional in Eastern cuisine.

Although flat-bottomed woks can be used on electric stoves, they are not as successful as the round-bottomed woks used on gas. Choose a wok about 14in (35cm) in diameter to give you enough space to stir and turn food, and choose one made of carbon steel, which allows the rapid transfer of heat thus ensuring that the high temperatures needed are achieved. The best woks are those that have a wooden handle to allow them to be manoeuvered while the food is cooking. This type of pan is known as a pau wok.

Although stir-frying does use some oil, the amount used is small if the pan has been prepared properly; in fact if the pan has been carefully prepared it can be used almost like a non-stick pan. Seasoning a wok makes the difference between easy cooking and cleaning and very hard work! When you buy a wok you may find it has been covered with a layer of oil to protect it while it is in the shop. First remove this oil by washing the wok with hot soapy water. Sometimes a cream cleanser may be required, but the instructions usually indicate if this is necessary. Dry the wok and put it over a low heat. Add about 2fl oz (55ml) oil and rub this round the inside of the wok. Slowly increase the heat and cook for 8-10 minutes. Wipe away the excess oil with kitchen paper and repeat this process until no more black appears on the kitchen paper. Your wok is now ready to use. Never use washing-up liquid on a wok unless it is absolutely necessary; if you do, you will have to reproof it. Used carefully, woks get better and better with use.

NON-STICK PANS

A non-stick frying pan with a lid to keep the moisture in is invaluable for cooking many different foods with the minimal amount of fat. It can also be used for porridge or scrambled egg and will save washing-up time. The new non-stick finishes are far superior to the earlier versions, as they will heat to much higher temperatures without flaking.

It is possible to "dry fry" many foods in a good quality non-stick pan. "Dry frying" is usually done with either no oil or a tiny amount – no more than a teaspoon – into which you put the food that you are frying once the pan is hot. Thereafter, the food is cooked slowly over a low heat so that it doesn't burn in the pan.

SKEWERS

These are, of course, useful for cooking kebabs, but if you thread jacket potatoes on a skewer before putting them in the oven you will find that they cook in one-third less time than potatoes that are just placed in the oven. Buy skewers made of fairly thick aluminium so that they don't buckle.

BARBECUE

Barbecuing food has become popular over the last five years, and barbecues not only add some fun to the family meal but also a different flavour. Don't choose too large a barbecue or you will use a lot of charcoal. Even a fairly small one will serve four or five people. If you feel you need bigger ones for parties, it might be worth buying two small ones rather than being stuck with a large one that you rarely use. A smaller barbecue is also more portable, and you could take it with you on picnics or camping. Always buy a barbecue that has some air vents underneath; they are essential on days when there is no wind.

Whether you use briquettes or lumpwood, the barbecue should be lit at least half an hour before cooking. Never start cooking until the coals are red or white as the temperature will not be hot enough to cook the food safely.

Food can be given a different flavour by marinades or by herbs such as rosemary, which should be placed under the food. Other spices, the dried stems of fennel and so on, can be spread on the coals. Chicken breasts, fish and vegetables may need to be basted in a small amount of oil to stop them drying out, but most other foods can be barbecued without extra fat. It is also possible to cook foods such as potatoes (which need to be partially boiled), mushrooms and courgettes wrapped in foil over the barbecue, and to use the barbecue to cook vegetarian rissoles, although these may need to be put in a gridiron to stop them breaking up.

Recent years have seen some concern about the carcinogenic effect of barbecued food. Although more potential carcinogens are produced by barbecued or smoked food, these were found when food was overcooked rather than to the levels that we would expect in the home. It was noted that meats with the highest fat content, such as sausages, acquired the highest levels of carcinogens – yet another reason for cutting down on fatty types of meat in the diet.

BEAN SPROUTER

If you're a bean enthusiast, buy a sprouter with separate tiers, which will make life easier than using the old-fashioned jam jar method – although this is quite simple (see page 283). Sprouts seem to come into their own in the winter when there are fewer winter salad vegetables. Sprouted wheat will take two or three days while mung beans are ready after four or five days, when they taste like fresh peas. Sprouted beans contain small amounts of protein and vitamins B and C. Most beans and grains will sprout unless they are the split variety.

KNIVES

A good knife is probably the most valuable piece of kitchen equipment, yet one that is neglected by many cooks. Chopping, crushing and peeling all become much easier and faster with good knives. The best are made from either carbon steel or from stainless steel. It is important that the metal tang of the blade goes all the way through the handle to ensure that the knife will not break for many, many years. Keep all your knives sharp and out of the reach of children.

——COOKING FOOD——

Although cooking results in a loss of vitamins and minerals, the nutritional value of the overall diet should not be affected if it consists of a variety of foods. The nutrients most commonly destroyed by cooking (and storage) are vitamin C and folic acid, and so it is important that some fruit and vegetables are eaten raw.

NUTRIENT LOSSES DURING DIFFERENT METHODS OF COOKING

Cooking or processing method	Nutrients lost
Boiling	40-70% vitamin C and some B and potassium.
Steaming and pressure cooking	Some vitamin C and B but less than boiling.
Toasting	10-30% loss of thiamin.
Dehydration	50% of vitamin C and some A.
Baking	Some vitamin B, particularly thiamin, and C.
Chilling	A little vitamin C and B.
Freezing	Most losses are the result of blanching of vegetables before freezing: 30% loss of vitamin C; some iron and B vitamins may be lost from the "drip" in meat and fish during defrosting.
Microwaving	Vitamin C but less than conventional cooking; vitamin B losses similar to conventional cooking.
Canning	30% vitamin C and some B during processing.

FOOD COMPOSITION TABLES

This table will give you an approximate guide to the major nutrients in foods, bearing in mind that portion sizes and differences in recipes between brands can vary considerably. The figures can be used for comparing the proportions of nutrients in foods but they may not be suitable reference for anyone who is receiving medical advice (such as someone who has been instructed to go on a very low protein or low sodium diet as part of medical treatment).

| Food | Energy value | | Water | Protein | Total |
100g/Portion g	kcals	kJ	g	g	Fats g
BREAD					
Wholemeal 100g	216	918	39.7	8.8	2.7
med. slice 30g	65	254	11.9	2.6	0.8
Brown 100g	223	948	39.0	8.9	2.2
med. slice 30g	67	280	11.7	2.7	0.7
White 100g	233	991	39.0	7.8	1.7
med. slice	70	297	11.7	2.3	0.5
Bread roll (white) 100g	290	1231	28.8	11.6	3.2
1 55g	160	677	15.8	6.4	1.8
Bread roll (brown) 100g	282	1194	31.0	11.7	6.4
1 55g	155	648	17.0	6.4	3.5
Pitta bread 100g	265	1127	32.7	9.2	1.2
1 60g	219	915	19.6	5.5	0.7
Chapati 100g	328	1383	28.5	8.1	1.0*
CEREALS					
Flour, white 100g	350	1493	13.0	9.8	1.2
Flour, self raising 100g	339	1443	13.0	9.3	1.2
Flour, wholemeal 100g	318	1351	14.0	13.2	2.0
Oats 100g	401	1698	8.9	12.4	8.7
Barley, pearl 100g	360	1535	10.6	7.9	1.7
Millet flour 100g	354	1481	13.3	5.8	1.7
Couscous 100g	227	950	40.0	5.7	1.0
Rye flour 100g	335	1428	15.0	8.2	2.0
Pasta, uncooked 100g	370	1574	10.4	13.7	2.0
Pasta, cooked 100g	117	499	71.5	4.3	0.6
2 hpd tbsp 60g	70	293	42.9	2.6	0.4
Rice, uncooked 100g	361	1536	11.7	6.5	1.0
Rice, cooked 100g	123	522	69.9	2.2	0.3
2 hpd tbsp 60g	74	313	41.9	1.3	(Tr)
Rice, brown					
uncooked 100g	357	1518	13.9	6.7	2.8
cooked 100g	119	506	4.6	2.3	0.9
2 hpd tbsp 60g	71	298	2.8	1.4	0.5

n.a. = not available
Tr = Trace
100g = 3½oz
28g = 1oz

(Satu-rates) g	Total Carbo-hydrate g	(Sugars) g	Fibre g	Sodium mg	(Salt equivalent) g	Comment
(0.7)	41.8	(2.1)	8.5	540	(1.4)	
(0.2)	12.5	(0.6)	2.6	162	(0.4)	
(0.6)	44.7	(1.8)	5.1	550	(1.4)	
(0.2)	14.9	(0.6)	1.7	183	(0.5)	
(0.5)	49.7	(1.8)	2.7	540	(1.4)	
(0.2)	14.9	(0.5)	0.8	162	(0.4)	
(1.0)	57.2	(2.1)	3.1	630	(1.6)	
(0.5)	31.5	(1.2)	1.7	347	(0.9)	
(1.8)	47.9	(1.9)	5.4	620	(1.6)	
(1.0)	26.3	(1.0)	3.0	341	(0.9)	
(n.a)	57.9	(2.1)	4.3	520	(1.4)	
(n.a)	34.7	(1.3)	2.6	312	(0.8)	
(n.a)	50.2	(1.8)	3.7	130	(0.3)	*If made with fat 12.6g/100g
(0.2)	80.1	(1.7)	3.4	2	(0)	
(0.2)	77.5	(1.4)	3.7	350	(0.9)	
(0.5)	65.8	(2.3)	9.6	3	(0)	
(0.6)	72.8	(Tr)	7.0	33	(0)	
(0.4)	83.6	(Tr)	6.5	3	(0)	
(n.a)	75.4	(n.a)	(n.a)	21	(Tr)	
(n.a)	51.3	(n.a)	(n.a)	(n.a)	(n.a)	
(0.4)	75.9	(Tr)	(n.a)	1	(0)	
(0.4)	79.2	(Tr)	(n.a)*	26	(Tr)	*Wholewheat pasta has 10g/100g fibre
(0)	25.2	(Tr)	(n.a)	8	(0)	
(0)	15.1	(Tr)	(n.a)	4	(0)	
(0.3)	86.8	(Tr)	2.4	6	(0)	
(0)	29.6	(Tr)	0.8	2	(0)	
(0)	17.8	(Tr)	0.5	1.2	(0)	No salt added during cooking
(n.a)	81.3	(Tr)	4.2	1	(0)	
(n.a)	27.1	(Tr)	1.6	0	(0)	
(n.a)	16.3	(Tr)	1.0	0	(0)	

Food 100g/Portion g	Energy value kcals	kJ	Water g	Protein g	Total Fats g
Spaghetti in tomato sauce 100g	59	250	83.1	1.7	0.7
1 small tin 200g	118	500	166.2	3.4	1.4
Pastry, white, shortcrust					
raw 100g	455	1900	19.5	5.9	27.8
cooked 100g	527	2202	6.9	6.9	32.2
Pastry, white, flaky					
raw 100g	427	1780	29.6	4.4	30.6
cooked 100g	565	2356	7.3	5.8	40.5
BREAKFAST CEREALS					
All Bran 100g	273	1156	2.3	15.1a	5.7
1 bowl 28g	76	319	0.6	4.2	1.6
Bran wheat flakes 100g	330	1390	2.5	9.9	1.8
1 bowl 28g	92	386	0.7	2.7	0.5
Muesli 100g	368	1556	5.8	12.9	7.5
2 tbsp 30g	110	461	1.7	3.9	2.2
Cornflakes 100g	368	1567	3.0	8.6	1.6
1 bowl 25g	92	385	0.8	2.2	0.4
Rice Crispies 100g	372	1584	3.8	5.9	2.0
1 bowl 28g	104	444	1.1	1.7	0.6
Frosted cornflakes 100g	397	1704	3.0	6.1	0.2
1 bowl 25g	99	415	0.8	1.5	0
Puffed Wheat 100g	325	1386	2.5	14.2	1.3
1 bowl 16g	52	218	0.4	2.1	0.2
Weetabix 100g	340	1444	3.8	11.4	3.4
2 biscuits 40g	136	578	1.5	4.6	1.4
Shredded Wheat 100g	324	1378	7.6	10.6	3.0
2 biscuits 44g	143	606	3.3	4.7	1.3
Porridge 100g	44	188	89.1	1.4	0.9
1 bowl 113g	50	212	100.7	1.6	1.0
BISCUITS AND CRISPBREADS					
Crispbread, rye 100g	321	1367	6.4	9.4	2.1
1 18g	58	246	1.2	1.7	0.4
Cream cracker 100g	440	1857	4.3	9.5	16.3
1 10g	44	186	0.4	1.0	1.6
Digestive, plain 100g	471	1981	4.5	9.8	20.5
1 14g	66	277	0.6	1.4	2.9
Digestive, chocolate 100g	493	2071	2.5	6.8	24.1
1 17g	84	350	0.4	1.2	4.1
Biscuit, semi-sweet 100g	457	1925	2.5	6.7	16.6
1 10g	46	193	0.3	0.7	1.7
Muesli bar 100g	400	1672	n.a	10.0	20.0
1 33g	135	564	n.a	3.3	6.6

(Saturates) g	Total Carbohydrate g	(Sugars) g	Fibre g	Sodium mg	(Salt equivalent) g	Comment
(n.a)	12.2	(3.4)	n.a	500	(1.3)	
(n.a)	24.4	(6.8)	n.a	1000	(2.5)	
(n.a*)	48.2	(1.0)	2.0	410	(1.0)	*The saturates content will depend on the type of fat used during cooking: lard being 43% saturates whereas a poly-unsaturate margarine is 25%
(n.a)	55.8	(1.2)	2.4*	480	(1.2)	*Wholemeal pastry has 6.7g fibre/100g
(n.a)	35.8	(0.8)	1.5	350	(0.9)	
(n.a)	47.4	(1.1)	2.0	470	(1.2)	
(1.1)	43.0	(15.4)	26.7	1670	(4.2)	
(0.3)	12.0	(4.3)	7.5	468	(1.8)	
(0.4)	71.9	(16.7)	15.4	760	(1.9)	
(0.1)	20.1	(4.7)	4.3	213	(0.5)	
(1.5)	66.2	(26.2)	7.4	180	(0.5)	
(0.4)	19.9	(7.9)	2.2	54	(Tr)	
(n.a)	85.1	(7.4)	11.0	1160	(2.9)	
(n.a)	23.7	(1.9)	2.8	290	(0.7)	
(0.6)	88.1	(9.0)	4.5	1110	(2.8)	
(0.2)	24.7	(2.5)	1.3	311	(0.8)	
(0)	88.9	(30.8)	0.4	n.a	(n.a)	
(0)	22.2	(7.7)	0.1	n.a	(n.a)	
(0.3)	68.5	(1.5)	15.4	4	(0)	
(Tr)	!1.0	().2	2.5	0.6	(0)	
(0.3)	70.3	(6.1)	12.7	360	(0.9)	
(Tr)	28.1	(2.4)	5.1	144	(0.4)	
(0.6)	67.9	(0.4)	12.3	8	(0)	
(0.3)	29.9	(0.2)	5.4	4	(0)	
(0.2)	8.2	(Tr)	0.8	580	(1.5)	
(0.2)	9.3	(Tr)	0.9	655	(1.6)	
(0.4)	70.6	(3.2)	11.7	220	(0.6)	
(Tr)	12.7	(0.6)	2.1	40	(Tr)	
(6.0)	68.3	(Tr)	3.0	610	(1.5)	
(0.6)	6.8	(0)	0.3	61	(Tr)	
(10.3)	66.0	(16.4)	5.5	440	(1.1)	
(1.5)	9.2	(2.3)	0.8	62	(Tr)	
(12.8)	66.5	(28.5)	3.5	450	(1.1)	
(2.8)	11.3	(4.8)	0.6	77	(Tr)	
(8.3)	74.8	(22.3)	2.3	410	(1.0)	
(0.9)	7.5	(2.2)	0.6	41	(Tr)	
(n.a)	45.0	(23.4)	14.0	n.a	(Tr)	
(n.a)	15.0	(7.8)	4.6	n.a	(Tr)	

Food 100g/Portion g	Energy value kcals	kJ	Water g	Protein g	Total Fats g
CAKES AND PASTRIES					
Jam tart 100g	384	1616	19.2	3.5	14.9
1 40g	154	646	7.7	1.4	6.0
Chocolate eclair 100g	376	1569	34.8	4.1	24.0
1 medium 50g	188	785	17.4	2.0	12.0
Current bun 100g	302	1279	28.6	7.4	7.6
1 35g	106	448	10.0	2.6	2.7
Doughnut 100g	349	1467	26.4	6.0	15.8
1 32g	112	469	8.5	1.9	5.1
Fruit pie, pastry top 100g	369	1554	22.9	4.3	15.5
1 slice 160g	590	2486	36.6	6.9	24.8
Sponge cake 100g	464	1941	14.9	6.4	26.5
1 slice 50g	232	971	7.5	3.2	13.3
Iced cake 100g	407	1717	12.7	3.8	14.9
1 slice 85g	346	1459	10.8	3.2	12.7
Rich fruit cake 100g	332	1403	46.7	3.7	11.0
1 slice 85g	282	1193	39.7	3.1	9.4
MILK AND MILK PRODUCTS					
Milk – whole 100g	65	272	87.6	3.3	3.8
1 pint 556g	361	1512	487.0	18.3	21.1
1 glass 170g	111	462	148.9	5.6	6.5
in hot drink 28g	18	76	24.5	0.9	1.0
Milk, semi-skimmed 100g	47	196	89.0	3.5	1.6
1 pint 556g	261	1092	495.0	19.5	8.9
1 glass 170g	80	334	151.0	6.0	15.1
in hot drink 28g	13	55	30.0	1.0	0.4
Milk, skimmed 100g	33	142	90.9	3.4	0.1
1 pint 556g	183	767	505.4	18.9	0.6
1 glass 170g	56	241	154.5	5.8	0.2
in hot drink 28g	9.2	39	25.4	1.0	Tr
Dried skimmed milk 100g	355	1512	4.1	36.4	1.3
1 tsp 5g	18	75	0.2	1.8	Tr
Yogurt, low fat 100g	52	216	85.7	5.0	1.0
1 carton, plain 150g	78	324	128.5	7.5	1.5
Fruit yogurt 100g	95	405	74.9	4.8	1.0
1 carton 150g	147	615	112.3	6.8	1.4
Flavoured yogurt 100g	81	342	79.0	5.0	0.9
1 carton 150g	122	143	118.5	7.5	1.4
Cheese, hard type 100g	406	1682	37.0	26.0	33.5
cube 30g	122	505	11.1	7.8	10.0
as a meal 60g	244	1009	22.2	15.6	20.1
Stilton 100g	462	1915	28.2	25.6	40.0
cube 30g	139	579	8.4	7.7	12.0
Brie/Camembert 100g	300	1246	47.5	22.8	23.2
cube 30g	90	376	14.2	6.8	7.0
Cream cheese 100g	439	1807	45.5	3.1	47.4
cube 30g	132	551	13.7	0.9	14.2

(Satu-rates) g	Total Carbo-hydrate g	(Sugars) g	Fibre g	Sodium mg	(Salt equivalent) g	Comment
(7.7)	62.8	(37.5)	1.7	230	(0.6)	
(3.1)	25.1	(15.0)	0.9	92	(Tr)	
(n.a)	38.2	(26.3)	n.a	160	(0.4)	
(n.a)	19.1	(13.2)	n.a	80	(Tr)	
(n.a)	54.5	(14.0)	n.a	100	(0.3)	
(n.a)	19.1	(4.9)	n.a	35	(Tr)	
(n.a)	48.8	(15.0)	n.a	60	(Tr)	
(n.a)	15.6	(4.8)	n.a	19	(Tr)	
(n.a)	56.7	(30.9)	2.6	210	(0.5)	
(n.a)	90.7	(49.4)	4.2	336	(0.8)	
(10.6)	53.2	(30.5)	1.0	350	(0.8)	
(5.3)	26.6	(15.3)	0.5	175	(0.4)	
(9.7)	68.8	(54.0)	2.4	250	(0.6)	
(8.3)	58.5	(27.0)	2.0	213	(0.5)	
(5.2)	58.3	(20.6)	3.5	170	(0.4)	
(4.4)	49.5	(17.5)	3.0	145	(0.4)	
(2.2)	4.7	(4.7)*	0	50	(Tr)	*All the sugar is the milk sugar lactose
(12.0)	26.1	(26.1)	0	278	(0.7)	
(37.1)	8.0	(8.0)	0	85	(Tr)	
(0.6)	1.3	(1.3)	0	14	(Tr)	
(0.9)	4.95	(4.95)*	0	51	(Tr)	
(5.0)	27.5	(27.5)	0	284	(0.7)	
(8.6)	8.4	(8.4)	0	87	(Tr)	
(0.20)	1.4	(1.4)	0	14	(Tr)	
(Tr)	5.0	(5.0)	0	52	(Tr)	
(0.3)	27.8	(27.8)	0	289	(0.7)	
(0.1)	8.5	(8.5)	0	88	(Tr)	
(Tr)	1.4	(1.4)	0	10	(Tr)	
(0.7)	52.8	(52.8)	0	550	(1.4)	
(Tr)	2.6	(2.6)	0	27	(Tr)	
(0.6)	6.2	(6.2)	0	76	(Tr)	
(0.9)	9.3	(9.3)	0	114	(0.3)	
(0.6)	17.9	(17.9)	0	64	(Tr)	
(0.8)	27.0	(27.0)	0	96	(0.3)	
(0.6)	14.0	(14.0)	0	64	(Tr)	
(0.8)	21.0	(21.0)	0	96	(0.3)	
(19.0)	Tr	(0)	0	610	(1.5)	*Includes Cheddar, Gruyère, Cheshire, Emmental
(5.7)	Tr	(0)	0	183	(0.5)	
(11.4)	Tr	(0)	0	366	(1.0)	
(22.8)	Tr	(0)	0	1150	(2.9)	
(6.8)	Tr	(0)	0	345	(0.9)	
(13.2)	Tr	(0)	0	1410	(3.5)	
(4.0)	Tr	(0)	0	423	(1.0)	
(27.0)	Tr	(0)	0	300	(0.8)	
(8.1)	Tr	(0)	0	90	(0.2)	

Food 100g/Portion g	Energy value		Water g	Protein g	Total Fats g
	kcals	kJ			
Feta 100g	245	1017	55.8	16.5	19.9
cube 30g	74	307	16.7	5.0	6.0
Parmesan 100g	408	1696	28.0	35.1	29.7
1tblsp 30g	122	512	8.4	10.5	8.9
Edam type 100g	304	1262	43.7	24.4	22.9
cube 30g	91	381	13.1	7.3	6.9
Cottage cheese 100g	92	402	78.8	13.6	4.0
1 tblsp 30g	28	121	23.6	4.1	1.2
Cream, single 100g	212	876	71.9	2.4	21.2
1 tblsp 15g	32	131	10.8	0.4	3.2
Cream, double 100g	447	1841	48.6	1.5	48.2
1 tblsp 15g	67	280	7.3	0.2	7.2
Whipping cream 100g	332	1367	61.5	1.9	35.0
on fruit/pie 30g	100	410	18.5	0.6	10.5
EGGS					
Egg 100g	147	612	74.8	12.3	10.9
1 size 3 egg 55g (no shell)	81	337	41.1	6.8	6.0
Egg yolk 100g	339	1402	51.0	16.1	30.5
1 17g	58	238	8.7	2.7	5.2
Egg white 100g	36	153	88.3	9.0	(Tr)
1 31g	11	47	27.4	2.8	(Tr)
Fried egg 100g	232	961	63.3	14.1	19.5
1 50g	116	481	31.7	7.0	9.8
Poached egg 100g	155	644	74.7	12.4	11.7
1 48g	74	309	35.9	6.0	5.6
Scrambled 100g	246	1018	62.2	10.5	22.7
2 eggs 130g	320	1337	80.9	13.7	29.5
Omelette 100g	190	787	68.8	10.6	16.4
2 eggs 130g	247	1032	89.4	13.8	21.3
FATS AND OILS					
Butter 100g	740	3041	15.4	0.4	82.0
individual pat 10g	74	304	1.5	(Tr)	8.2
Margarine, hard 100g	730	3000	16.0	0.1	81.0
individual pat 10g	73	300	1.6	(Tr)	8.1
Margarine, soft 100g	730	3000	16.0	0.1	81.0

(Satu-rates) g	Total Carbo-hydrate g	(Sugars) g	Fibre g	Sodium mg	(Salt equivalent) g	Comment
(11.3)	Tr	(0)	0	1260	(3.1)	
(3.4)	Tr	(0)	0	378	(0.9)	
(16.9)	Tr	(0)	0	760	(1.9)	
(5.1)	Tr	(0)	0	228	(0.6)	
(13.1)	Tr	(0)	0	980	(2.5)	*Includes Gouda and St Paulin
(3.9)	Tr	(0)	0	294	(0.7)	
(2.3)	1.4	(1.4)	0	450	(1.1)	
(6.8)	0.4	(0.4)	0	135	(0.3)	
(12.0)	3.2	(3.2)	0	42	(Tr)	
(1.8)	0.5	(0.5)	0	6	(0)	
(27.5)	2.0	(2.0)	0	27	(Tr)	
(4.1)		( )	0	4	(Tr)	
(20.0)	2.5	(2.5)	0	34	(Tr)	
(6.0)	0.6	(0.6)	0	10	(0)	
(3.9)	Tr	(0)	0	140	(0.4)	
(2.1)	Tr	(0)	0	77	(Tr)	
(11.0)	Tr	(0)	0	50	(Tr)	An egg yolk provides 1mg iron, but in a poorly absorbed form, and 1 microg of vitamin D
(1.9)	Tr	(0)	0	9	(0)	
(0)	Tr	(0)	0	190	(0.5)	
(0)	Tr	(0)	0	59	(Tr)	
(n.a)	Tr	(0)	0	220	(0.6)	
(n.a)	Tr	(0)	0	110	(0.3)	
(3.2)	Tr	(0)	0	110	(0.3)	
(1.6)	Tr	(0)	0	53	(Tr)	
(n.a)	Tr	(0)	0	1050	(2.6)	
(n.a)	Tr	(0)	0	1365	(3.4)	
(n.a)	Tr	(0)	0	1030	(2.6)	
(n.a)	Tr	(0)	0	1339	(3.3)	
(46.7)	Tr	(0)	0	870	(2.2)	Good source of vitamin A 750 microg/ 100g
(4.7)	Tr	(0)	0	87	(Tr)	
(30.8)	0.1	(0.1)	0	800	(2.0)	
(3.1)	0	(0)	0	80	(0.2)	
(25.1)	0.1	(0.1)	-	800	(2.0)	All margarines and similar spreads are fortified with vitamin A: 900 microg/100g and vitamin D: 8 microg/100g

Food 100g/Portion g	Energy value kcals	kJ	Water g	Protein g	Total Fats g
individual pat 10g	73	300	1.6	(Tr)	8.1
Margarine, polyunsaturate 100g	730	3000	16.0	0.1	81.0
individual pat 10g	73	300	1.6	(Tr)	8.1
Low fat spread 100g	366	1506	57.1	0	40.7
individual pat 10g	37	151	5.7	0	4.1
Oil, vegetable 100g	899	3696	(Tr)	(Tr)	99.9
1 tblsp 20g	180	739	(Tr)	(Tr)	20.0
Lard 100g	891	3663	1.0	(Tr)	99.0

MEAT, POULTRY AND MEAT PRODUCTS

Food	kcals	kJ	Water	Protein	Fats
Beef, roast, lean and fat 100g	284	1182	54.3	23.6	21.1
Steak, grilled 100g	218	912	59.3	27.3	12.1
1 medium 170g	371	1549	100.1	46.4	20.6
Mince, raw 100g	221	919	64.5	18.8	16.2*
cooked with salt 100g	229	955	59.1	23.1	15.2
Lamb, roast leg 100g	266	1106	55.3	26.1	17.9
shoulder 100g	316	1311	53.6	19.9	26.3
breast 100g	410	1697	43.6	19.1	37.1
Lamb chop, lean 100g	222	928	58.9	27.8	12.3
1 large or 2 small 140g	311	1299	82.5	38.9	17.2
Pork, roast 100g	286	1190	51.9	26.9	19.8
lean only 100g	185	777	61.6	30.7	6.9
1 chop, large, lean 140g	316	1323	78.5	45.2	15.0
Gammon joint, boiled, lean 100g	167	703	62.7	29.4	5.5
Chicken, roast & skin 100g	216	902	61.9	22.6	14.0
dark meat 100g	155	648	68.2	23.1	6.9
white meat 100g	142	599	68.5	26.5	4.0
lean only 100g	148	621	68.4	24.8	5.4
Turkey, roast & skin 100g	171	717	65.0	28.0	6.5
dark meat 100g	148	624	67.7	27.8	4.1
white meat 100g	132	558	68.4	29.8	1.4
Duck, roast 100g	339	1406	49.6	19.6	29.0
lean only 100g	189	789	64.2	25.3	9.7
Pheasant, roast 100g	213	892	56.9	32.2	9.3
Hare, stewed 100g	192	804	60.7	29.9	8.0
Venison 100g	198	832	56.8	35.0	6.4
Liver, calf's, fried 100g	254	1063	52.6	26.9	13.2

(Saturates) g	Total Carbohydrate g	(Sugars) g	Fibre g	Sodium mg	(Salt equivalent) g	Comment
(2.5)	0	0	0	80	(0.2)	
(20.2)	0.1	(0.1)	0	800	(2.0)	
(2.0)	0	0	0	80	(0.2)	
(11.0)	0	(0)	0	690	(1.7)	
(1.1)	0	(0)	0	69	(Tr)	
(14–75)*	0	(0)	0	Tr	(0)	*Negligible vitamins and minerals present
(3–15)	0	(0)	0	Tr	(0)	
(43.6)	0	(0)	0	2	(0)	
(10.1)	0	(0)	0	54	(Tr)	Also 1.9mg iron/ 100g. Iron from all meats is well-absorbed
(5.8)	0	(0)	0	50	(Tr)	
(9.9)	0	(0)	0	85	(Tr)	
(7.8)	0	(0)	0	86	(Tr)	*Lean varieties can contain up to 50% less fat
(7.3)	0	(0)	0	320	(0.8)	
(9.3)	0	(0)	0	65	(Tr)	
(13.7)	0	(0)	0	73	(Tr)	
(19.3)	0	(0)	0	61	(Tr)	
(6.4)	0	(0)	0	75	(Tr)	
(8.9)	0	(0)	0	105	(0.3)	
(8.3)	0	(0)	0	79	(Tr)	
(2.9)	0	(0)	0	79	(Tr)	
(6.3)	0	(0)	0	118	(0.3)	
(2.3)	0	(0)	0	1110	(2.8)	
(4.8)*	0	(0)	0	72	(Tr)	*The skin accounts for up to two-thirds of the fat
(2.3)	0	(0)	0	91	(Tr)	
(1.4)	0	(0)	0	71	(Tr)	
(1.8)	0	(0)	0	81	(Tr)	
(2.4)	0	(0)	0	52	(Tr)	
(1.5)	0	(0)	0	71	(Tr)	
(0.5)	0	(0)	0	45	(Tr)	
(8.4)	0	(0)	0	76	(Tr)	
(2.8)	0	(0)	0	96	(0.3)	
(3.3)	0	(0)	0	100	(0.3)	
(n.a)	0	(0)	0	40	(Tr)	
(n.a)	0	(0)	0	86	(Tr)	
(5.4)	7.3	(Tr)	Tr	170	(0.4)	Rich in vitamin A; 17,400 microg/100g and folic acid 320 microg/ 100g

Food 100g/Portion g	Energy value kcals	kJ	Water g	Protein g	Total Fats g
ox, stewed & seasoning 100g	198	831	62.6	24.8	9.5
Kidney, lamb's 100g	155	651	66.5	24.6	6.3
2 fried 56g	87	365	39.9	13.8	3.5
Bacon, grilled, lean 100g	292	1218	46.0	30.5	18.9
1 back rasher 30g	122	504	10.8	7.6	10.1
2 streaky rashers 30g	127	529	10.3	7.3	10.8
Sausage, pork, grilled/fried 100g	318	1320	45.1	13.3	24.6
2 large/4 small 80g	254	1056	36.1	10.6	19.7
Sausage, beef, grilled/fried 100g	265	1104	47.9	13.0	17.3
2 large/4 small 80g	212	886	38.3	10.4	13.8
Haggis 100g	310	1292	46.2	10.7	21.7
Black pudding, fried 100g	305	1270	44.0	12.9	21.9
Frankfurter 100g	274	1135	59.5	9.5	25.0
Salami 100g	491	2031	28.0	19.3	45.2
in a sandwich 28g	137	569	7.8	5.4	12.7
Liver sausage 100g	310	1283	51.8	12.9	26.9
in a sandwich 28g	87	359	14.5	3.6	7.5
Ox tongue 100g	293	1216	48.6	19.5	23.9
1 slice 28g	82	340	13.6	5.5	6.7
Ham 100g	120	502	72.5	18.4	5.1
1 slice 28g	34	140	20.3	5.2	1.4
Corned beef 100g	217	905	58.5	26.9	12.1
1 slice 28g	61	254	16.4	7.5	3.4
Steak and kidney pie 100g	323	1349	42.6	9.1	21.2
individual 142g	459	1916	60.5	7.7	30.1
Pork pie 100g	376	1564	36.8	9.8	27.0
individual 142g	534	2221	52.3	13.9	38.3
Sausage roll 100g	479	1991	23.0	7.2	36.2
1 56g	268	1115	12.9	4.0	20.3
Cornish pasty 100g	332	1388	39.2	8.0	20.4
1 190g	631	2637	74.5	15.2	38.8
Beefburger, fried 100g	264	1099	53.0	20.4	17.3
1 38g	102	426	20.1	7.7	6.6

FISH AND FISH PRODUCTS
Cod/Haddock, grilled/baked/poached

Food 100g/Portion g	Energy value kcals	kJ	Water g	Protein g	Total Fats g
100g	95	402	78.0	20.8	1.3
portion 120g	114	482	93.6	25.0	1.6
Cod/haddock, battered 100g	199	834	60.9	19.6	10.3
portion 170g	338	1418	103.5	33.3	17.5
Cod/haddock, smoked 100g	101	429	71.6	23.3	0.9
portion 120g	120	515	86.0	28.0	1.1
Crab, fresh, boiled 100g	127	534	72.5	20.1	5.2
Crab, tinned 100g	81	341	79.2	18.1	0.9
portion (tinned) 42g	34	143	33.3	7.6	0.4
Halibut, steamed 100g	99	417	53.8	18.0	3.0
portion 120g	119	500	64.6	21.6	3.6
Herring, fried in oatmeal 100g	234	975	58.7	23.1	15.1
edible portion 90g	211	878	52.8	20.8	13.6

(Saturates) g	Total Carbohydrate g	(Sugars) g	Fibre g	Sodium mg	(Salt equivalent) g	Comment
(4.7)		(0)	0	110	(0.3)	
(3.5)	0	(0)	0	270	(0.7)	Source of iron
(1.9)	0	(0)	0	151	(0.4)	
(7.9)	0	(0)	0	2240	(5.6)	
(4.2)	0	(0)	0	606	(1.5)	
(4.5)	0	(0)	0	597	(1.5)	
(10.3)*	11.5	(n.a)	0.5	1000	(3.0)	*Sausages lose fat during frying as well as grilling
(8.3)	9.2	(n.a)	0.4	800	(2.0)	
(7.6)	15.2	(n.a)	0.6	1100	(2.8)	
(6.0)	12.2	(n.a)	0.5	880	(2.2)	
(n.a)	19.2	(n.a)	1.8	770	(1.9)	
(n.a)	15.0	(n.a)	0.6	1210	(3.0)	
(10.5)	3.0	(0)	0.1	980	(2.5)	
(19.0)	1.9	(0)	0.1	1850	(4.6)	
(5.3)	0.5	(0)	0	518	(1.3)	
(10.5)	4.3	(0)	0.2	860	(2.2)	
(2.9)	1.2	(0)	0	240	(6.0)	
(11.5)	0	(0)	0	1000	(2.5)	
(3.2)	0	(0)	0	280	(0.6)	
(2.1)	0	(0)	0	1250	(3.1)	
(0.6)	0	(0)	0	350	(0.9)	
(5.8)	0	(0)	0	950	(2.4)	
(1.6)	0	(0)	0	266	(0.7)	
(9.1)	25.6	(n.a)	1.1	510	(1.3)	
(12.9)	36.4	(n.a)	1.5	724	(1.8)	
(11.6)	24.9	(n.a)	1.0	720	(1.8)	
(16.5)	35.4	(n.a)	1.4	1022	(2.5)	
(15.6)	33.1	(n.a)	1.3	590	(1.5)	
(8.7)	18.5	(n.a)	0.6	330	(0.8)	
(8.7)	31.1	(n.a)	1.3	590	(1.5)	
(16.7)	59.1	(n.a)	2.5	1121	(2.8)	
(8.3)	7.0	(n.a)	0.3	880	(2.2)	
(3.2)	2.7	(n.a)	0.1	334	(0.8)	
(0.3)	0	0	0	91	(Tr)	
(0.4)	0	0	0	109	(0.3)	
(n.a)	7.5	(n.a)	0.3	100	(0.3)	
(n.a)	12.6	(n.a)	0.5	170	(0.4)	
(0.2)	0	(0)	0	1220	(3.0)	
(0.2)	0	(0)	0	1464	(3.7)	
(0.8)	0	(0)	0	370	(0.9)	
(0.1)	0	(0)	0	550	(1.4)	
(Tr)	0	(0)	0	231	(0.6)	
(0.7)	0	(0)	0	84	(Tr)	
(0.8)	0	(0)	0	101	(0.3)	
(n.a)	1.5	(0)	0	100	(0.3)	
(n.a)	1.4	(0)	0	90	(Tr)	

Food 100g/Portion g	Energy value kcals	kJ	Water g	Protein g	Total Fats g
Kipper/Smoked Mackerel 100g	205	855	58.7	25.5	11.4
1 fish 168g	344	1436	98.6	42.8	19.2
Mussels (shelled) 100g	87	366	79.0	17.2	2.0
portion 56g	49	205	44.2	9.6	1.1
Prawns (shelled) 100g	107	451	70.0	22.6	1.8
portion 56g	60	253	39.2	12.7	1.0
Salmon, fresh, steamed 100g	160	666	53.0	16.3	10.5
portion 120g	192	803	63.6	19.6	12.6
Salmon/Tuna, tinned 100g	155	649	70.4	20.3	8.2
portion in brine (drained) 70g	109	454	49.3	14.2	5.7
smoked 100g	142	598	64.9	25.4	4.5
portion 28g	40	167	18.2	7.1	1.3
Sardines, canned 100g	217	906	58.4	23.7	13.6
4 small, drained 56g	122	507	32.7	13.3	7.6
Scallops, steamed 100g	105	446	73.1	23.2	1.4
Scampi, fried 100g	316	1321	39.4	12.2	17.6
portion 85g	269	1123	33.5	10.4	15.0
Sole/Plaice, fried 100g	216	904	60.4	16.1	13.0
portion 170g	367	1535	103	27.4	22.1
steamed 100g	91	384	77.2	20.6	0.9
portion 120g	109	456	92.6	24.7	1.0
Taramasalata 100g	446	1837	35.9	3.2	46.4
Trout, steamed 100g	135	566	70.6	23.5	4.5
1 170g	230	962	120.0	40.0	7.7
Fish fingers 100g	196	819	55.6	13.2	8.9
1 grilled 28g	55	230	15.6	3.7	2.5
Fish cakes, fried 100g	188	785	63.3	9.1	10.5
2 bought 120g	226	942	76.0	10.9	12.6
VEGETABLES (all cooked [with no added salt], unless otherwise stated)					
Artichokes, globe 100g (as served)	7	28	36.3	0.5	Tr
Asparagus 100g (1 serving)	18	75	46.2	3.4	Tr
Aubergine, raw 100g	14	62	93.4	0.7	(Tr)
1 average 198g	28	123	185.0	1.4	(Tr)
Beans, French 100g (1 serving)	7	31	95.5	0.8	Tr
Beans, Runner 100g (1 serving)	19	83	90.7	1.9	0.2
Beans, Broad 100g (1 serving)	48	206	83.7	4.1	0.6
Beansprouts, canned 100g	9	40	95.4	1.6	Tr
Beetroot 100g	44	189	82.4	1.8	Tr
1 medium 120g	52	227	98.9	1.0	Tr

(Satu-rates) g	Total Carbo-hydrate g	(Sugars) g	Fibre g	Sodium mg	(Salt equivalent) g	Comment
(2.6)	0	(0)	0	990	(2.5)	
(4.4)	0	(0)	0	1663	(4.2)	
(n.a)	0	(0)	0	210	(0.5)	
(n.a)	0	(0)	0	118	(0.3)	
(0.4)	0	(0)	0	1590	(4.0)	
(0.2)	0	(0)	0	890	(2.2)	
(2.4)	0	(0)	0	87	(Tr)	(Salmon/Tuna tinned) vitamin D: 12 microg/100g for salmon and 6 microg/100g for tuna
(2.9)	0	(0)	0	104	(0.3)	
(1.9)	0	(0)	0	570	(1.4)	
(1.3)	0	(0)	0	396	(1.0)	
(1.0)	0	(0)	0	1880	(4.7)	
(0.3)	0	(0)	0	526	(1.3)	
(2.9)	0	(0)	0	650	(1.6)	Vitamin D 7.5 microg/100g
(1.6)	0	(0)	0	364	(0.9)	
(0.4)	0	(0)	0	270	(0.7)	
(n.a)	28.9	(n.a)	1.2	380	(1.0)	
(n.a)	24.6	(n.a)	1.0	323	(0.8)	
(n.a)	9.3	(n.a)	0.4	140	(0.4)	
(n.a)	15.8	(n.a)	0.7	238	(0.6)	
(0.2)	0	(0)	0	120	(0.3)	
(0.2)	0	(0)	0	144	(0.4)	
(n.a)	0	(0)	0	650	(1.6)	
(1.0)	0	(0)	0	88	(Tr)	
(1.8)	0	(0)	0	150	(0.4)	
(n.a)	17.2	(n.a)	0.7	350	(0.9)	
(n.a)	4.3	(n.a)	0.2	88	(Tr)	
(n.a)	15.1	(n.a)	0.7	500	(1.3)	
(n.a)	18.1	(n.a)	0.8	600	(1.5)	
(0)	1.2	(0)	n.a	6	(0)	
(0)	0.6	(0.6)	0.8	1	(0)	Vitamin C 20mg/100g
(0)	3.1	(2.9)	2.5	3	(0)	
(0)	6.1	(2.8)	5.0	6	(0)	
(0)	1.1	(0.8)	3.2	3	(0)	
(Tr)	2.7	(1.3)	3.4	1	(0)	
(0.2)	7.1	(0.6)	4.2	20	(Tr)	Vitamin C 15mg/100g
(0)	0.8	(0.4)	3.0	80	(Tr)	
(0)	9.9	(9.9)	2.5	64	(Tr)	
(0)	11.9	(11.9)	3.0	77	(Tr)	

Food 100g/Portion g	Energy value kcals	kJ	Water g	Protein g	Total Fats g
Broccoli 100g	18	78	89.0	3.1	Tr
(1 serving) Cabbage, white, raw 100g	22	93	90.3	1.9	Tr
cooked 100g	15	66	93.0	1.7	Tr
(1 serving) Cabbage, green, cooked 100g	9	40	95.7	1.3	Tr
(1 serving) Carrots 100g	19	79	91.5	0.6	Tr
(1 serving) Cauliflower 100g	9	40	92.7	1.6	Tr
(1 serving) Celery, raw 100g	8	36	93.5	0.9	Tr
1 large stick 56g	5	20	52.4	0.5	Tr
Chicory, raw 100g	9	38	96.2	0.8	Tr
1 serving 28g	3	11	26.9	0.2	Tr
Courgettes, raw 100g	25	105	92.2	1.6	0.4
Cucumber, raw 100g	10	43	96.4	0.6	0.1
in salad 56g	6	24	54.0	0.3	Tr
Leeks 100g (1 serving)	31	128	90.8	1.9	Tr
Lettuce, raw 100g	12	51	95.9	1.0	0.4
in salad 30g	4	15	29.0	0.3	0.1
Marrow 100g (1 serving)	7	29	97.8	0.4	Tr
Mushrooms, raw 100g	13	53	91.5	1.8	0.6
fried 100g	210	863	64.2	2.2	22.3
Onion, raw 100g	23	99	92.8	0.9	Tr
fried 100g	345	1424	42.0	1.8	33.3
Parsley, raw 100g	21	88	78.7	5.2	Tr

(Satu-rates) g	Total Carbo-hydrate g	(Sugars) g	Fibre g	Sodium mg	(Salt equivalent) g	Comment
(0)	1.6	(1.5)	4.1	6	(0)	Vitamin A 416 microg/100g; vitamin C 34mg/100g; iron 1mg/100g
(0)	3.8	(3.7)	2.7	7	(0)	Vitamin C 15-25mg/100g cooked; raw has 40mg/100g vitamin C but 8mg are lost with shredding. Vitamin A: 2500mg/100g in dark outer leaves but only 50 microg/100g in the heart
(0)	2.3	(2.2)	2.8	4	(0)	
(0)	1.1	(1.1)	2.5	8	(0)	
(0)	4.3	(4.2)	3.1	50	(Tr)	Vitamin A 2000 microg/100g
(0)	0.8	(0.8)	1.8	4	(0)	Vitamin C 20mg/100g
(0)	1.3	(1.2)	1.8	140	(0.4)	
(0)	0.7	(0.7)	1.0	78	(Tr)	
(0)	1.5	(n.a)	n.a	7	(0)	
(0)	0.4	(n.a)	n.a	2	(0)	
(n.a)	4.5	(n.a)	n.a	1	(0)	Vitamin C 16mg/100g
(0)	1.8	(1.8)	0.4	13	(0)	
(0)	1.0	(1.0)	0.2	7	(0)	
(0)	4.6	(4.6)	3.9	6	(0)	Vitamin C 15mg/100g; iron 2mg/100g
(Tr)	1.2	(1.2)	1.5	9	(0)	
(0)	0.4	(0.4)	0.2	3	(0)	
(0)	1.4	(1.3)	0.6	1	(0)	
(0.2)	0	(0)	2.5	9	(0)	
(n.a)	0	(0)	4.0	11	(Tr)	
(0)	5.2	(5.2)	1.3	10	(Tr)	
(n.a)	2.7	(2.7)	1.3	7	(0)	
(0)	Tr	(0)	—	33	(Tr)	Vitamin A 1166 microg/100g and vitamin C 150mg/100g

Food 100g/Portion g	Energy value kcals	kJ	Water g	Protein g	Total Fats g
garnish 5g	1	4	3.7	0.3	Tr
Parsnip, boiled 100g (1 serving)	56	238	83.2	1.3	Tr*
Peas, fresh 100g	52	223	80.0	5.0	0.4
Peas, frozen 100g (1 serving)	41	175	80.7	5.4	0.4
tinned (1 serving)	47	201	81.6	4.6	0.3
Pepper, raw 100g	15	65	93.5	0.9	0.4
in salad 28g	4	52	26.2	0.3	0.1
cooked 100g	14	59	93.7	0.9	0.4
medium 150g	21	89	140.5	1.4	0.6
Potatoes, old, boiled 100g	80	343	80.5	1.4	0.1
2 medium 120g	96	412	96.6	1.7	0.1
mashed (in margarine and milk) 100g	119	499	76.9	1.5	5.0
2 scoops 120g	143	597	92.4	1.8	6.0
roast 100g	157	662	64.3	2.8	4.8
2 medium 110g	173	722	70.7	3.0	5.3
baked & skin 100g	105	448	71.0	2.6	0.1
1 large 200g	210	896	142.0	5.2	0.2
chipped 100g	253	1065	47.0	3.8	7-15g (av. 11g)
1 serving 113g	286	1203	53.1	4.3	12.3
Oven chips 100g	188	786	47.0	3.8	6.2
1 serving 113g	212	888	53.1	4.3	7.0
Crisps 100g	533	2224	2.7	6.3	35.9
1 packet 28g	141	586	0.8	1.9	10.0
Crisps, lower fat 100g	485	2029	2.7	6.0	26.0
1 packet 28g	121	507	0.7	1.5	6.5
Potatoes, new, boiled 100g	76	324	78.8	1.6	0.1
1 serving 113g	86	359	89.0	1.8	0.1

(Satu-rates) g	Total Carbo-hydrate g	(Sugars) g	Fibre g	Sodium mg	(Salt equivalent) g	Comment
(0)	Tr	(0)	—	2	(0)	
(0)	13.5	(2.7)	2.5	4	(0)	*If roasted 6.5g fat
(0.2)	7.7	(1.8)	5.2	Tr	(0)	Vitamin C 13-15mg/100g; tinned 8mg/100g and processed none. Iron 1.4mg/100g
(0.2)	4.3	(1.0)	12.0	2	(0)	
(0.1)	7.0	(3.6)	6.3	230	(0.6)	
(0.1)	2.2	(2.2)	0.9	2	(0)	Vitamin C 100mg/100g raw and 60mg/100g cooked
(0)	0.6	(0.6)	0.3	1	(0)	
(0.1)	1.8	(0.1)	0.9	2	(0)	
(0.1)	2.7	(0.1)	1.3	4	(0)	
(0)	19.7	(0.4)	1.0	3	(0)	Because of the large quanities eaten, potatoes are reasonable sources of protein, iron (0.8mg/100g) and vitamin C (8-30mg/100g – depending on the length of storage time)
(0)	23.6	(0.5)	1.2	4	(0)	
(n.a)	18.0	(0.6)	0.9	24	(Tr)	
(n.a)	23.6	(0.6)	1.2	29	(Tr)	
(n.a)	27.3	(n.a)	n.a	9	(0)	
(n.a)	27.6	(n.a)	n.a	10	(Tr)	
(0)	25.0	(0.6)	2.5 + 1.9	8	(0)	
(0)	50.0	(1.2)	5.0 + 3.8	16	(Tr)	
(n.a)	37.5	(1.1)	2.0	12	(Tr)	
(n.a)	42.4	(1.1)	2.3	14	(Tr)	
(n.a)	31.8	(0.7)	2.0	12	(Tr)	
(n.a)	35.9	(0.4)	2.3	14	(Tr)	
(17.0)	49.3	(0.7)	11.9	550	(1.4)	
(4.3)	11.6	(0.2)	3.1	150	(0.4)	
(10.5)	60.4	(0.9)	13.5	300	(0.9)	
(2.6)	12.1	(0.2)	3.4	75	(0.2)	
(0)	18.3	(0.7)	2.0	41	(Tr)	
(0)	20.7	(0.8)	2.3	46	(Tr)	

Food 100g/Portion g	Energy value		Water g	Protein g	Total Fats g
	kcals	kJ			
Spinach 100g	30	128	85.1	5.1	0.5
Spring onion, raw 100g	35	151	86.8	0.9	Tr
in salad 14g	5	21	12.2	0.1	Tr
Sprout 100g	18	75	91.5	2.8	Tr
(1 serving)					
Sweetcorn 100g	123	520	65.2	4.1	2.3
(1 serving)					
canned 100g	76	325	73.4	2.9	0.5
(1 serving)					
Sweet potato 100g	85	363	72.0	1.1	0.6
(1 serving)					
Turnip 100g	14	60	94.5	0.7	0.3
Tomato, raw 100g	14	60	93.4	0.9	Tr
1 medium 56g	8	34	52.3	0.5	Tr
Watercress, raw 100g	14	61	91.1	2.9	Tr
in salad 14g	2	8	12.7	0.4	Tr
PULSES (dried) 100g	304	1293	12.2	23.8	1.0
Lentils (cooked) 100g	99	420	72.1	7.6	0.5
Baked beans 100g	64	270	73.6	5.1	0.5
1 serving 113g	72	305	83.2	5.8	0.6
Beans, Red Kidney, dried 100g	272	1159	11.0	22.1	1.7
Black-eyed, dried 100g	340	1423	11.5	22.7	1.6
Haricot, cooked 100g	93	396	69.6	6.6	0.5
Butter beans, cooked 100g	95	405	70.5	7.1	0.3

(Satu-rates) g	Total Carbo-hydrate g	(Sugars) g	Fibre g	Sodium mg	(Salt equivalent) g	Comment
(Tr)	1.4	(1.2)	6.3	120	(0.3)	Vitamin A 1000 microg/100g; vitamin C 25mg/100g; iron 4mg/100g. The huge loss of water accounts for the high concentration of nutrients in the cooked form.
(0)	8.5	(8.5)	3.1	13	(0)	
(0)	1.2	(1.2)	0.4	2	(0)	
(0)	1.7	(1.6)	2.9	2	(0)	Vitamin C 40mg/100g
(n.a)	22.8	(1.7)	4.7	1	(0)	
(n.a)	16.1	(8.9)	5.7	310	(0.8)	
(0.3)	20.1	(9.1)	2.3	18	(Tr)	Vitamin A – dark yellow varieties 200 microg/100g but white varieties only trace amounts; vitamin C 15mg/100g
(0)	2.3	(2.3)	2.2	28	(Tr)	Vitamin C 17mg/100g (same for swede)
(0)	2.8	(2.8)	1.5	3	(0)	Vitamin C 20mg/100g
(0)	1.6	(1.6)	0.8	2	(0)	
(0)	0.7	(0.6)	3.3	60	(Tr)	Vitamin A 1500 microg/100g and vitamin C 60mg/100g (210 microg and 8mg per serving)
(0)	Tr	(Tr)	0.5	8	(0)	
(n.a)	53.2	(2.4)	11.7	36	(Tr)	
(n.a)	17.0	(0.8)	3.7	12	(Tr)	
(0.1)	10.3	(5.2)	7.3	480	(1.2)	Pulses, on average, contain 1.5-2.5mg iron/100g
(0.1)	11.6	(5.9)	8.6	542	(1.4)	
(n.a)	45.0	(3.0)	25.0	40	(Tr)	
(n.a)	56.8	(n.a)	n.a	6	(0)	
(n.a)	16.6	(0.8)	7.4	15	(Tr)	
(n.a)	17.1	(1.5)	5.1	16	(Tr)	

Food 100g/Portion g	Energy value kcals	kJ	Water g	Protein g	Total Fats g
Chickpeas, cooked as dahl 100g	144	610	65.8	8.0	3.3
Hummus 100g	185	773	61.4	7.6	12.6
Mung beans, cooked as dalh 100g	106	447	72.5	6.4	4.2
Soyabeans, raw 100g	403	1686	10.0	34.1	17.7
Tofu, steamed 100g	70	291	85.0	7.4	4.2
fried 100g	302	1264	47.4	21.6	25.1
NUTS (shelled)					
Almonds 100g	565	2336	4.7	16.9	53.5
Brazil 100g	619	2545	8.5	12.0	61.5
Chestnuts 100g	170	720	51.7	2.0	2.7
Coconut, fresh 100g	351	1446	42.0	3.2	36.0
Hazelnuts 100g	380	1570	41.1	7.6	36.0
Peanuts, plain 100g	570	2364	4.5	24.3	49.0
handful 28g	160	667	1.3	6.8	13.7
roasted 100g	570	2364	4.5	24.3	49.0
& salted 28g	160	667	1.3	6.8	13.7
Walnuts 100g	525	2166	23.5	10.6	51.5
FRUIT					
Apple, eating 100g	46	196	84.3	0.3	Tr
1 average 135g	62	265	113.8	0.4	Tr
Apple, cooker 100g	39	165	85.6	0.3	Tr
stewed, no sugar 170g	66	280	144.5	0.5	Tr
Apricot 100g	28	117	79.6	0.6	Tr
1 average 60g	17	70	47.8	0.4	Tr
Avocado (½ average) 100g	223	922	68.7	4.2	22.2
Banana 100g	79	337	70.7	1.1	0.3
1 average, peeled 150g	120	674	105.1	1.6	0.5
Blackberries, fresh 100g	29	125	82.0	1.3	Tr

(Satu-rates) g	Total Carbo-hydrate g	(Sugars) g	Fibre g	Sodium mg	(Salt equivalent) g	Comment
(n.a)	22.0	(5.2)	6.0	850	(2.1)	
(n.a)	11.1	(n.a)	n.a	665	(1.7)	
(n.a)	11.4	(0.8)	6.4	820	(2.0)	
(n.a)	28.6	(n.a)	n.a	5	(0)	
(n.a)	0.6	(n.a)	0.3	4	(0)	
(n.a)	3.9	(n.a)	n.a	8	(0)	
(4.3)	4.3	(4.3)	14.3	6	(0)	
(16.0)	4.1	(1.7)	9.0	2	(0)	
(0.5)	36.6	(7.0)	6.8	11	(Tr)	
(30.0)	3.7	(3.7)	13.6	1	(0)	
(2.5)	6.8	(4.7)	6.1	1	(0)	
(7.4)	8.6	(3.1)	8.1	6	(0)	
(2.1)	2.4	(0.9)	2.3	2	(0)	
(7.4)	8.6	(3.1)	8.1	440	(1.1)	
(2.1)	2.4	(0.9)	2.3	123	(0.3)	
(6.2)	5.0	(3.2)	5.2	3	(0)	
(0)	11.9	(11.8)	2.0	2	(0)	The commonest apples are low in vitamin C (3mg/100g). Some varieties have 10 times this amount. Most vitamin C is in the peel. Bramley Seedlings (cookers) have 15mg vitamin C peeled (20mg/100g unpeeled)
(0)	16.1	(15.9)	2.7	3	(0)	
(0)	10.0	(9.6)	2.5	2	(0)	
(0)	17.0	(16.3)	4.3	1	(0)	
(0)	6.2	(6.2)	1.9	Tr	(0)	Vitamin A 250 microg/100g
(0)	3.7	(3.7)	1.1	Tr	(0)	
(12.3)	1.8	(1.8)	2.0	2	(0)	The fattiest fruit, so high in calories. Vitamin C 15mg/100g and folic acid 66 microg/100g
(0.1)	19.2	(16.2)	3.4	1	(0)	Rich in carbohydrate and calories
(0.3)	38.4	(32.4)	6.8	2	(0)	
(0)	6.4	(6.4)	7.3	4	(0)	A high fibre fruit. Vitamin C 20mg/100g

Food 100g/Portion g	Energy value		Water g	Protein g	Total Fats g
	kcals	kJ			
1 serving, stewed, no sugar 113g	68	283	95.6	1.1	Tr
Cherries (20) 100g	41	175	71.0	0.5	Tr
Currants, Black/Red, fresh 100g	28	121	77.4	0.9	Tr
1 serving, stewed, no sugar 113g	27	113	91.2	0.9	Tr
Gooseberries, fresh 100g	17	73	89.9	1.1	Tr
Grapes (20) 100g	63	268	79.3	0.6	Tr
Grapefruit (½) 100g	11	45	43.5	0.3	Tr
Lemon, whole 100g	15	65	85.2	0.8	Tr
Melon (Canteloupe & Honeydew) 100g	24	102	93.6	1.0	Tr
1 wedge 227g	55	232	212.5	2.3	Tr
Nectarine (1 small) 100g	50	214	85.0	0.9	Tr
1 large 142g	71	304	121.0	1.3	Tr
Orange 100g	35	150	86.1	0.8	Tr
1 large, peeled 120g	42	180	103.3	0.9	Tr
squeezed juice 100g	38	161	87.7	0.6	Tr
1 glass 170g	65	270	149.0	1.0	Tr
Peach 100g	32	137	75.1	0.6	Tr
1 large 170g	51	213	127.7	1.0	Tr
Pear 100g	41	175	83.2	0.3	Tr
1 medium 150g	62	263	124.8	0.5	Tr
Pineapple 100g	46	194	84.3	0.5	Tr
1 slice 150g	69	288	126.5	0.8	Tr
Plums/Damsons, fresh 100g	36	153	79.1	0.5	Tr
stewed, no sugar 170g	34	142	136.5	0.7	Tr

(Satu-rates) g	Total Carbo-hydrate g	(Sugars) g	Fibre g	Sodium mg	(Salt equivalent) g	Comment
(0)	6.2	(6.2)	7.1	3	(0)	
(0)	10.4	(10.4)	1.5	2	(0)	
(0)	6.6	(6.6)	8.7	3	(0)	High fibre. Iron 1.3mg/100g. Blackcurrants are very rich in vitamin C 200mg/100g, redcurrants 40mg/100g
(0)	6.3	(6.3)	8.4	3	(0)	
(0)	3.4	(3.4)	3.2	2	(0)	Vitamin C 40mg/100g
(0)	16.1	(16.2)	0.9	2	(0)	Only 3mg/100g of vitamin C – little to recommend them for the sick!
(0)	5.3	(5.3)	0.6	1	(0)	Vitamin C 40mg/100g
(0)	3.2	(3.2)	5.2	6	(0)	Calcium 110mg/100g. With the skin vitamin C 80mg/100g, juice 50mg/100g
(0)	5.3	(5.3)	1.0	14	(Tr)	Vitamin C 25mg/100g, folic acid 30 microg/100g. Vitamin A in Canteloupes 330 microg/100g
(0)	12.0	(12.0)	2.3	32	(Tr)	
(0)	12.4	(8.1)	1.7	9	(0)	
(0)	17.6	(11.5)	2.4	13	(Tr)	
(0)	8.5	(8.5)	2.0	3	(0)	Vitamin C 50mg/100g; folic acid 37 microg/100g
(0)	10.2	(10.2)	2.4	4	(0)	
(0)	(9.4)	(9.4)	0	2	(0)	
(0)	16.0	(16.0)	0	3	(0)	
(0)	7.9	(7.9)	1.2	2	(0)	
(0)	13.4	(13.4)	2.0	3	(0)	
(0)	10.6	(10.6)	2.3	2	(0)	
(0)	15.9	(15.9)	3.5	3	(0)	
(0)	11.6	(11.6)	1.2	2	(0)	Vitamin C 25mg/100g
(0)	17.4	(17.4)	1.8	3	(0)	
(0)	9.0	(9.0)	2.0	2	(0)	
(0)	8.2	(8.2)	3.4	3	(0)	

Food 100g/Portion g	Energy value		Water g	Protein g	Total Fats g
	kcals	kJ			
Raspberries 100g	25	105	83.2	0.9	Tr
1 serving 113g	28	118	94.0	1.0	Tr
Rhubarb, stewed 100g	6	25	94.6	0.6	Tr
1 serving no sugar 170g	10	42	160.8	1.0	Tr
Strawberries 100g	26	109	88.9	0.6	Tr
1 serving 125g	33	136	111.1	0.8	Tr
Tangerine 100g	34	143	86.7	0.9	Tr
1 peeled 60g	60	86	52.0	0.5	Tr
DRIED FRUIT					
Apricots 100g	182	776	14.7	4.8	Tr
stewed 170g	112	469	116.2	3.0	Tr
Currants 100g	243	1039	22.0	1.7	Tr
Dates 100g	213	909	12.6	1.7	Tr
Figs 100g	213	908	16.8	3.6	Tr
Prunes 100g	134	570	23.3	2.0	Tr
stewed, no sugar 170g	126	526	93.7	1.9	Tr
Raisins 100g	246	1049	21.5	1.1	Tr
Sultanas 100g	250	1066	18.3	1.8	Tr
SUGARS AND PRESERVES					
Sugar, white/brown 100g	394	1681	Tr	0.5	0
1 level tsp 5g	20	84	Tr	Tr	0
Golden syrup 100g	298	1269	79.0	0.3	0
1 portion 10g	30	127	7.9	Tr	0
Jam/Marmalade/Jelly 100g	261	1114	29.8	0.6	0
1 portion 10g	26	111	3.0	Tr	0

(Saturates) g	Total Carbohydrate g	(Sugars) g	Fibre g	Sodium mg	(Salt equivalent) g	Comment
(0)	5.6	(5.6)	7.4	3	(0)	Rich in fibre.
(0)	6.3	(6.3)	8.4	3	(0)	Iron 1.2mg/100mg, vitamin C 25mg/100g
(0)	0.9	(0.9)	2.4	2	(0)	
(0)	1.5	(1.5)	4.0	3	(0)	
(0)	6.2	(6.2)	2.2	2	(0)	Vitamin C 60mg/100g
(0)	7.8	(7.8)	2.8	3	(0)	
(0)	8.0	(8.0)	1.9	2	(0)	Vitamin C 30mg/100g
(0)	4.8	(4.8)	1.1	1	(0)	
(0)	43.4	(43.4)	24.0	56	(Tr)	Iron 2.5mg/100g in a stewed portion
(0)	33.8	(33.8)	15.1	36	(Tr)	
(0)	63.1	(63.1)	6.5	20	(Tr)	Iron 1.8mg/100g
(0)	54.9	(54.9)	7.5	4	(0)	Iron 1.4mg/100g
(0)	52.9	(52.9)	18.5	87	(Tr)	Iron 4.2mg/100g
(0)	40.3	(40.3)	16.1	12	(Tr)	Laxative action due to presence of derivatives of hydroxyphenylisatin. Iron 1.4mg/100g
(0)	31.6	(31.6)	12.6	10	(Tr)	
(0)	64.4	(64.4)	6.8	52	(Tr)	Iron 1.6mg/100g
(0)	64.7	(64.7)	7.0	53	(Tr)	Iron 1.8mg/100g
(0)	99.9	(99.9)	0	Tr	(Tr)	
(0)	5.0	(5.0)	0	Tr	(Tr)	
(0)	79.0	(79.0)	0	270	(0.7)	Iron 1.5mg/100g (Black Treacle 9.2mg/100g)
(0)	7.9	(7.9)	0	27	(Tr)	
(0)	69.0	(69.0)	1.1	16	(Tr)	Jams made with stone fruit have no vitamin C, jams from seed fruit contain 10mg/100g and blackcurrant has 24mg/100g
(0)	6.9	(6.9)	0.1	2	(0)	

Food 100g/Portion g	Energy value kcals	kJ	Water g	Protein g	Total Fats g
Honey 100g	288	1229	76.4	0.4	Tr
1 portion 10g	29	123	7.6	Tr	Tr
Peanut butter 100g	623	2581	1.1	22.6	53.7
1 portion 10g	62	258	0.1	2.3	5.4
DESSERTS					
Ice cream, dairy 100g	167	704	64.4	3.7	6.6
1 portion 50g	84	35	32.2	1.9	3.3
Custard, packet 100g	118	496	74.7	3.8	4.4
2 tblsp (made with whole milk) 40g	47	198	29.9	1.5	1.8
Egg 100g	118	497	76.8	5.8	6.0
2 tblsp (made with whole milk) 40g	47	197	30.7	2.3	2.4
Gelatin 100g	338	1435	Tr	84.4*	0
Jelly cubes 100g	259	1104	29.9	6.1*	0
portion made up with water 113g	67	284	94.9	1.6*	0
Fruit salad, tinned 100g	95	405	71.1	0.3	Tr
1 small tin 220g	209	891	156.4	0.7	Tr
CONFECTIONARY					
Boiled sweets 100g	327	1397	Tr	Tr	Tr
1 small packet 113g	370	1579	Tr	Tr	Tr
Liquorice allsorts 100g	313	1333	6.6	3.9	2.2
1 small bag 113g	354	1478	7.5	4.4	2.4
Milk chocolate 100g	529	2214	2.2	8.4	30.3
1 small bar 50g	265	1107	1.1	4.2	15.2
Peppermints 100g	392	1670	0.2	0.5	0.7
1 small bag 113g	443	1887	0.2	0.6	0.8
BEVERAGES					
Coffee powder 100g	100	424	3.4	14.6	0
1 tsp 3g	3	13	0.1	0.4	0
Drinking chocolate 100g	366	1554	2.1	5.5	6.0
2 heaped tsp 12g	44	186	0.3	0.7	0.7
Soft drink (cola) 100g	39	168	89.8	Tr	0
1 can 330g	129	538	296.3	Tr	0
Squash/Fruit drink, undiluted 100g	107	456	71.2	Tr	0
1 glass, diluted 170g 1:5 (28g)	30	125	162.0	Tr	0

(Satu-rates) g	Total Carbo-hydrate g	(Sugars) g	Fibre g	Sodium mg	(Salt equivalent) g	Comment
(0)	76.4	(76.4)	n.a	11	(Tr)	Trace amounts of minerals but even less than in Golden syrup
(0)	7.6	(7.6)	n.a	1	(0)	
(9.7)	13.1	(6.7)	7.6	350	(0.9)	
(1.0)	1.3	(0.7)	0.8	35	(Tr)	
(3.5)	24.8	(22.6)	0	80	(Tr)	
(1.7)	12.4	(11.3)	0	40	(Tr)	
(2.7)	16.8	(11.6)	0	76	(Tr)	
(1.1)	6.7	(4.6)	0	30	(Tr)	
(n.a)	11.0	(11.0)	0	78	(Tr)	
(n.a)	4.4	(4.4)	0	31	(Tr)	
(0)	0	(0)	0	27	(Tr)	*An essential amino acid is missing, so it is useless as a source of protein
(0)	62.5	(62.5)	0	25	(Tr)	
(0)	16.0	(16.0)	0	7	(0)	
(0)	25.0	(25.0)	1.1	2	(0)	Vitamin C 3mg/100g
(0)	55.0	(55.0)	2.4	4	(0)	
(0)	87.3	(86.9)	0	25	(Tr)	
(0)	98.6	(98.2)	0	28	(Tr)	
(n.a)	74.1	(67.2)	0	75	(Tr)	Iron 8.1mg/100g
(n.a)	83.7	(75.9)	0	85	(Tr)	
(18.5)	59.4	(56.5)	0	120	(0.3)	Iron 1.6mg/100g
(9.3)	29.7	(28.2)	0	60	(Tr)	
(n.a)	102.2	(102.2)	0	9	(0)	
(n.a)	115.4	(115.4)	0	10	(Tr)	
(0)	11.0	(6.5)	0	41	(Tr)	
(0)	0.3	(0.2)	0	1	(0)	
(3.7)	77.4	(73.8)	0	250	(0.6)	
(0.4)	9.3	(8.9)	0	30	(Tr)	
(0)	10.5	(10.5)	0	8	(0)	Sugars content equivalent to 7tsp/can
(0)	34.7	(34.7)	0	26	(Tr)	
(0)	28.5	(28.5)	0	21	(Tr)	Sugars content equivalent to 1½tsp/glass
(0)	8.0	(8.0)	0	6	(0)	

| Food | Energy value | | Water | Protein | Total |
100g/Portion g	kcals	kJ	g	g	Fats g
Blackcurrant cordial undiluted 100g	229	956	39.8	0.1	0
1 glass, diluted 1:5 (28g) 170g	64	268	170	Tr	0
Apple juice, unsweetened 100g	45	188	85	Tr	0
1 glass 170g	77	320	144.5	Tr	0
Orange juice, unsweetened 100g	33	143	88.7	0.4	Tr
1 glass 170g	56	234	150.7	0.7	Tr
Tomato juice 100g	16	66	93.3	0.7	Tr
1 glass 170g	27	114	158.6	1.2	Tr
Lucozade/Glucose drink 100g	68	288	81.7	Tr	0
1 glass 170g	116	483	138.9	Tr	0
PICKLES AND MISCELLANEOUS					
Beef extract 100g	174	737	38.7	38.0	0.7
1 tsp 5g	9	36	1.9	1.9	Tr
Yeast extract 100g	179	759	25.4	39.7	0.7

(Saturates) g	Total Carbohydrate g	(Sugars) g	Fibre g	Sodium mg	(Salt equivalent) g	Comment
(0)	60.9	(60.9)	0	20	(Tr)	Sugars content equivalent to 3½tsp/glass. Vitamin C 210mg/100g but soon lost once bottle is opened and stored in the light. Economy sized bottles therefore do not make sense if the drink is bought for its vitamin C content
(0)	17.1	(17.1)	0	6	(0)	
(0)	11.8	(11.8)	0	8	(0)	Sugars content equivalent to 4tsp/glass. Vitamin C 5mg/100g
(0)	20.1	(20.1)	0	14	(Tr)	
(0)	8.5	(8.5)	0	4	(0)	Sugars content equivalent to 3tsp/glass. Vitamin C 35mg/100g
(0)	14.5	(14.5)	0	7	(0)	
(0)	3.4	(3.2)	0	230	(0.6)	Sugars content equivalent to 1tsp/glass. Vitamin C 20mg/100g
(0)	5.8	(5.8)	0	391	(1.0)	
(0)	18.0	(9.0)*	0	29	(Tr)	If intermediate sugars are added they account for the whole carbohydrate content and are equivalent to 6tsp/glass
(0)	30.6	(15.3)*	0	49	(Tr)	
(0.3)	2.9	(0)	0	4800	(12.0)	Good for B vitamins including folic acid
(0)	0.1	(0)	0	240	(0.6)	
(0)	1.8	(0)	0	4500	(11.2)	Good for B vitamins including folic acid

Food 100g/Portion g	Energy value kcals	kJ	Water g	Protein g	Total Fats g
1 tsp 5g	5	16	1.3	2	Tr
Stock cubes 100g	229	969	9.1	38.3	3.4
1 cube 10g	23	97	0.9	3.8	0.3
French dressing/Vinaigrette 100g	658	2706	23.5	0.1	73.0
1 tblsp 15g	99	413	3.5	Tr	10.9
Mayonnaise 100g	718	2952	28.0	1.8	78.9
1 tblsp 15g	108	450	4.2	0.3	11.8
Oil-reduced 100g	346	1430	55	1.5	35.0
1 tblsp 15g	52	216	8.5	0.2	5.3
Salad cream 100g	311	1288	52.7	1.9	27.4
1 tblsp 15g	47	195	7.9	0.3	4.1
Soy sauce, light 100g	64	268	70.6	5.2	0.5
1 tblsp 15g	10	40	11.0	0.8	Tr
Chutney, mango 100g	285	1202	34.8	0.4	10.9
1 dstsp 20g	57	240	7.0	0.1	2.2
Sweet pickle 100g	134	572	58.9	0.6	0.3
1 dstsp 20g	27	116	11.6	0.1	Tr
Tomato purée 100g	67	286	65.7	6.1	Tr
1 small tin 70g	27	200	46.0	4.3	Tr
Tomato ketchup 100g	98	420	64.8	2.1	Tr
1 tblsp 17g	17	71	11.0	0.4	Tr
Vinegar 100g	4	16	—	0.4	0
Salt – 1 tsp 5g	0	0	0	0	0
Mustard powder 100g	452	1884	0	28.9	28.7
1 tsp 5g	23	95	0	1.4	1.4
Baking powder 100g	163	693	6.3	5.2	Tr
1 tsp 5g	8	34	0.3	0.3	0
ALCOHOL					
Beer (bitter/lager) 100g	32	132	3.1	0.3	Tr
½ pint 285g	91	376	8.8	0.9	Tr
Strong ale 100g	72	301	6.6	0.7	Tr
½ pint 285g	205	858	18.8	2.0	Tr
Cider, dry, sweet 100g	36	152	3.8	Tr	0
½ pint 285g	103	429	10.8	Tr	0
vintage 100g	101	421	10.5	Tr	0
½ pint 285g	288	1203	29.9	Tr	0
Sherry/Vermouth, dry, medium 100g	116	481	15.0	0.2	0
1 measure 60g	70	291	9.0	Tr	0
Sweet 100g	151	631	14.0	Tr	0
60g	91	379	8.4	Tr	0
Spirits 100g	222	919	31.7	Tr	0
1 measure 28g	62	257	8.9	Tr	0
Wine, red 100g	68	284	9.5	0.2	0
1 glass 110g	75	312	10.5	0.2	0
Wine, white-dry 100g	66	275	9.1	0.1	0
1 glass 110g	73	303	10.0	0.1	0
sweet 100g	94	394	10.2	0.2	0
1 glass 110g	103	432	11.2	0.2	0

(Satu-rates) g	Total Carbo-hydrate g	(Sugars) g	Fibre g	Sodium mg	(Salt equivalent) g	Comment
(0)	Tr	(0)	0	225	(0.6)	
(n.a)	12.0	(n.a)	0	10300	(25.8	
(n.a)	1.2	(n.a)	0	1030	(2.6)	
(10.9)*	0.2	(0.2)	0	960	(2.4)	*If made with olive oil
(1.6)*	0	(0)	0	144	(0.4)	
(n.a)	0.1	(0.1)	0	360	(0.9)	
(n.a)	0	(0)	0	54	(Tr)	
(n.a)	6.7	(n.a)	0	745*	(1.9)	*American figures
(n.a)	1.0	(n.a)	0	112	(2.8)	
(n.a)	15.1	(13.4)	n.a	840	(2.1)	
(n.a)	2.3	(2.0)	n.a	126	(0.3)	
(Tr)	8.3	(n.a)	n.a	5720	(14.3)	
(0)	1.2	(n.a)	n.a	858	(2.1)	
(n.a)	49.5	(n.a)	1.6	1090	(2.7)	
(n.a)	9.9	(n.a)	0.3	218	(0.5)	
(Tr)	34.4	(32.6)	1.7	1700	(4.2)	
(0)	7.0	(6.5)	0.3	340	(0.9)	
(0)	11.4	(11.4)	0	20	(Tr)	
(0)	8.0	(8.0)	0	14	(Tr)	
(0)	24.0	(22.9)	0	1120	(2.8)	
(0)	4.1	(3.9)	0	190	(0.5)	
(0)	0.6	(0.6)	0	20	(Tr)	
(0)	0	(0)	0	1943	(4.9)	
(n.a)	20.7	(n.a)	n.a	5	(0)	
(n.a)	1.0	(n.a)	n.a	0.5	(0)	
(0)	37.8	(Tr)	n.a	11800	(29.5)	
(0)	1.9	(0)	n.a	590	(1.5)	
(0)	2.3	(2.3)	0	12	(Tr)	
(0)	6.6	(6.6)	0	34	(Tr)	
(0)	6.1	(6.1)	0	15	(Tr)	
(0)	17.4	(17.4)	0	43	(Tr)	
(0)	3-4	(3-4)	7	(0)		
(0)	8-12	(8-12)	0	20	(Tr)	
(0)	7.3	(7.3)	0	2	(0)	
(0)	20.8	(20.8)	0	6	(0)	
(0)	1.4	(1.4)	0	10	(Tr)	
(0)	0.8	(0.8)	0	6	(0)	
(0)	6.9	(6.9)	0	13	(Tr)	
(0)	4.1	(4.1)	0	8	(0)	
(0)	Tr	(0)	0	Tr	(0)	
(0)	Tr	(0)	0	Tr	(0)	
(0)	0.3	(0.3)	0	10	(Tr)	
(0)	0.3	(0.3)	0	10	(Tr)	
(0)	0.6	(0.6)	0	4	(0)	
(0)	0.7	(0.7)	0	4	(0)	
(0)	5.9	(5.9)	0	13	(Tr)	
(0)	6.5	(6.5)	0	14	(Tr)	

—USEFUL ADDRESSES—

British Diabetic Association
10 Queen Anne Street
London
W1M 0BD

The British Dietetic Association
Daimler House
Paradise Circus Broadway
Birmingham
B1 2BJ

Coeliac Society of the United Kingdom
PO Box No 181
London
NW2 2QY

The Consumers' Association
14 Buckingham Street
London
WC2N 6DS

The Coronary Prevention Group
60 Great Ormond Street
London
WC1N 3HR

Disabled Living Foundation
380/384 Harrow Road
London
W9 2HU

The Health Education Authority
78 New Oxford Street
London
W1A 1AH

Hyperactive Children's Support Group
59 Meadowside
Angmering
Nr. Littlehampton
West Sussex
BN16 4BW

Migraine Trust
45 Great Ormond Street
London
WC1N 3HD

National Childbirth Trust
9 Queensborough Terrace
London
W2 3TB

National Eczema Society
Tavistock House North
Tavistock Square
London
WC1H 9SR

The Scottish Health Education Group
Woodburn House
Canaan Lane
Edinburgh
EH10 4SG

The Vegan Society
47 Highlands Road
Leatherhead
Surrey

The Vegetarian Society
53 Marloes Road
London
W8 6LA

National Centre for Anorexic Family Aid
Sackville Place
44/8 Magdalen Street
Norwich
NR3 1JP

Weight Watchers
11 Fairacres
Dedworth Road,
Berks.
SL4 4UY

La Lèche League
BM Box 3424
London
WC1N 3XX

British Naturopathic/Osteopathic Assoc.
6 Netherhall Gardens,
London NW3 5RR